Drugs and the Athlete

CONTEMPORARY EXERCISE AND SPORTS MEDICINE SERIES
ALLAN J. RYAN, M.D., Editor-in-Chief

Drugs and the Athlete

**GARY I. WADLER, M.D., F.A.C.P.,
F.A.C.S.M., F.A.C.P.M., F.C.P.**
Clinical Associate Professor of Medicine
Cornell University Medical College
Attending, Department of Medicine
North Shore University Hospital
Manhasset, New York
Tournament Physician
U.S. Open Tennis Championships

BRIAN HAINLINE, M.D.
Assistant Professor of Neurology
Cornell University Medical College
Assistant Attending, Department of Neurology
North Shore University Hospital
Manhasset, New York

CONTEMPORARY EXERCISE AND SPORTS MEDICINE SERIES
ALLAN J. RYAN, M.D., Editor-in-Chief

F. A. DAVIS COMPANY • Philadelphia

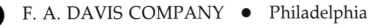

Printed in the United States of America

Last digit indicates print number: 10 9 8 7 6 5 4 3   Hardbound Edition
Last digit indicates print number: 10 9 8 7 6 5 4 3 2   Paperback Edition

NOTE: As new scientific information becomes available through basic and clinical research, recommended treatments and drug therapies undergo changes. The author(s) and publisher have done everything possible to make this book accurate, up-to-date, and in accord with accepted standards at the
time of publication. However, the reader is advised always to check product information (package
inserts) for changes and new information regarding dose and contraindications before administering
any drug. Caution is especially urged when using new or infrequently ordered drugs.

Library of Congress Cataloging-in-Publication Data

Wadler, Gary I., 1939–
    Drugs and the athlete.
    Includes bibliographies and index.
    1. Doping in sports.   I. Hainline, Brian, 1955–
II. Title.   [DNLM: 1. Doping in Sports.   2. Substance
Abuse—diagnosis.   QT 260 W123d]
RC1230.W33 1989   362.2′9   88-33612
ISBN 0-8036-9008-8   Hardbound Edition
ISBN 0-8036-9009-6   Paperback Edition

To Nancy, David and Erika,
Pascale, Clotilde and Arthur,
Whose love and support
We embrace.

Foreword

In *Drugs and the Athlete*, Wadler and Hainline have produced a trailblazing book that for the first time addresses in a comprehensive, balanced, well-researched, yet candid way, one of the saddest and most unsavory topics of our time. Sad is the tale, because it sets out the enormity of a blight that is damaging or destroying the lives of increasing numbers of young persons. Unsavory it has become, because it necessarily implicates either the neglect or willful greed of trainers, managers, owners, university powers, and media purveyors who have exploited sports for their own small gains with little or no regard for the well-being or fulfillment of the athletes. Further, just imagine what all of this says to the inner-city and suburban youths who idolize those athletes. Facing these issues squarely, *Drugs and the Athlete* describes in detail the size, the affected numbers, the many substances, and the difficulties in treating what has become an international scandal.

As this book reminds us, chemical shortcuts designed to enhance the athletic prowess, dissolve the tensions, or sharpen the ecstasy of the performer probably have seduced athletes for as long as peaceful physical competition has existed. Fifty years ago, the heavy-drinking, heavy-smoking, prematurely dead professional athlete was a figure of at least grudgingly admired legend. Today, that illusion has changed to one of pity. The drugs have become harder and exert commensurately more devastating permanent effects on the players. Even the ostensible amateurs are contaminated: muscles bulge unnaturally in overencouraged teenage athletes, and once comparatively innocent collegians now dose themselves. All this, to meet the demands of alumni and coaches in order to outdo their natural talents, fill the stadium, and achieve the beckoning sweepstakes prize of professional sports. Meanwhile, the epidemic enlarges, as do the number and type of available drug agents. More and more, the drugs assume an increasing capacity to enslave—even to kill—their takers.

Wadler and Hainline appropriately begin their book where the problem starts, that is, with the athlete. They clearly and sympathetically delineate the internal and external pressures these young persons feel. These include the enormous and sometimes almost inhuman urgings they receive from their families and trainers, their difficulties with postponing gratification during the early learning years, and, when they achieve success, the problems of alternating between short bursts of competitive concentration and long stretches of lonely waiting for the next event. Increasing the vulnerability that affects athletes are the large amounts of money many of them earn before they possess the education or maturity to spend it well—and the crash that comes when they first lose or, eventually, move completely offstage. The authors then proceed to enumerate, one by one, the substances—hard, soft, and in-between—that tempt the competitors and to describe the acute and residual effects that these agents leave on their bodies. A final section discusses the delicate and often controversial subject of how to suspect drug taking, how to recognize it specifically, and the merit or otherwise of various programs intended to terminate addiction or to counter its continuation or spread. As the last chapter, the book contains an outstanding contribution by the neurologist and lawyer Dr. H. Richard Beresford. This is a fair but straightforward discussion of the multidimensional legal problems that surround all aspects of this painfully difficult, sad, and human-destroying social problem.

Although written primarily for health workers in the field and, to a degree, for the athletes themselves, *Drugs and the Athlete* treats its subject with such thoroughness, candor, and balance that its contents undoubtedly will attract a wider readership and will influence many others involved both directly and indirectly in sports. This is a definitive work that importantly addresses one of the major problems of our troubled times.

Fred Plum, M.D.
Anne Parrish Titzell Professor of Neurology
Cornell University Medical College
Neurologist-in-Chief
The New York Hospital

Preface

Poisons and medicine are oftentimes the same substance given with different intents.

Peter Mere Latham (1789–1875)
General Remarks on the Practice of Medicine, Ch. IV

As we prepared this text, we were ever mindful that sport is the play of the spirit, the challenge of the mind, and the perfection of the body—not a contest in pharmacology. We are convinced that drug abuse in sports has become so widespread that it threatens the safety, health, and longevity of many athletes, while perverting the original intent of sport. Our concerns about drugs and the athlete are not merely technical, but stem from our professional and personal backgrounds. We address this complex subject as an internist/sports medicine physician who treats both amateur and professional athletes and has been a founder and administrator of a drug abuse program, and as a neurologist who has competed extensively in amateur sports. While striving not to be moralistic, we have asked questions and offered recommendations that we hope will serve to protect athletes from self-abuse or exploitation by others.

Drug use has become an accepted aspect of everyday living. Coffee awakens the morning, cigarettes buffer the day, alcohol smooths the edges. Sedatives mellow, cocaine enhances. Psychic and physical aches and pains seek relief in a swallow or injection. Drug use by the athlete is but a part of this intricate and self-perpetuating web.

The pervasiveness of drug abuse in sports, coupled with a seeming disarray of factual information, led us to conclude that a comprehensive resource was required. This text is intended to serve as such a resource for a variety of audiences, including, but not limited to, sports medicine physicians, primary care physicians, athletic trainers, sports program administrators, mental health professionals, attorneys, the media, athletes, and the interested sports fan.

Part I of this text explores the foundations of drug abuse from both a societal and an athlete-specific perspective. Part II provides detailed information about the drugs most commonly used by athletes. Part III addresses the principles of recognizing and managing drug abuse in the athlete and includes a detailed discussion about drug testing in sports. Chapter 20 analyzes comprehensively the multitude of legal considerations involved in this subject.

For the first time ever, the official drug policies of major professional and amateur sports organizations are presented side by side. Similarities, differences, strengths, and weaknesses of each can therefore be readily identified. In addition, the 1988 International Olympic Charter Against Doping in Sports and the Position Stands of the American College of Sports Medicine are included.

We are indebted to many people for their invaluable help. George Vecsey of the *New York Times*, Joe Browne of The National Football League, Manny Topol of *Newsday*, and Len Berman of NBC-TV provided both general guidance and many specific insights. David M. Martin of Psychiatric Diagnostic Laboratories, Inc., helped with the chapter on drug testing. Karen Torello and Irene Morgan provided patient and diligent secretarial services. We are thankful to Patricia A. Volts for her graphic and artistic contributions. The librarians at North Shore University Hospital assisted us greatly in retrieving numerous journal articles, and David Wadler helped in the collection of data.

We are indebted to H. Richard Beresford, M.D., J.D., for contributing Chapter 20, "Legal Considerations," and for providing other support for this project. The encouragement and patience of F. A. Davis's editors Sylvia Fields, Ed.D., and Linda Weinerman facilitated completion of this work, and Fred Plum, M.D., forever our teacher, nourished the core technical and philosophic features of this book.

Gary I. Wadler, M.D.
Brian Hainline, M.D.

Editor's Commentary

The overuse, misuse, and frank abuse of drugs is a major problem in our society today. Thus, it is not surprising that athletes, both recreational and competitive, are involved. The case of the professional athlete who is found to be using illegal drugs receives a great deal of media attention, but little is reported about the much greater number of amateur athletes who are involved, unless a few are disqualified from competition because of positive drug tests. Physicians and others who work with athletes may not even know that drugs are being used unless they are alerted to what drugs may be involved and the effects they may produce. *Drugs and the Athlete,* by Drs. Wadler and Hainline, provides all sports medicine professionals with the thorough information base necessary to communicate to athletes, their families, and coaches the realities about the hoped-for benefits as well as the inherent dangers of specific recreational and therapeutic drugs—information that may prevent athletes from harming themselves.

The drugs with which athletes may be involved include those that are legally manufactured and sold for specific indications—such as ephedrine, anabolic steroids, and human growth hormone; one whose production and sale is under some government control—alcohol; two that are not controlled—caffeine and tobacco; and illegal drugs—such as cocaine and marijuana. All of these drugs, and other drugs related to them according to their composition or uses, are described and discussed by the authors in chapters that analyze their pharmacology and effects. Drugs taken primarily in the hope that they will improve physical performance are clearly distinguished from those consumed principally for their psychic effects. Much of the information contained in these chapters has never before been brought together in such a clear and comprehensive fashion.

Historical antecedents of drug abuse in sports, and the rationalizations offered by athletes and their mentors, are cogently summarized in the early chapters. Techniques of drug testing and other means of diagnosis of abuse are described in the latter chapters. The chapter on management also stresses means of prevention. Legal considerations of control are discussed thoroughly in terms of privacy rights, methods of control, and the role of the sports physician. *There is no constitutional right to use illegal drugs.*

Appendices include the three Position Stands of the American College of Sports Medicine on alcohol, anabolic-androgenic steroids, and blood doping, as well as the drug testing policies of major national and international sports organizations.

This book should be in the library of not only every physician or other professional who works with or supervises competitive athletes but also those who are involved in the care of recreational athletes. The facts that it contains and the principles derived from them are of value to everyone confronted with the massive problem of drug abuse now and in the future.

Allan J. Ryan, M.D.
Editor-in-Chief
Contemporary Exercise and Sports Medicine

Contributor

CHAPTER 20. Legal Considerations

H. Richard Beresford, M.D., J.D.
Professor of Neurology
Cornell University Medical College
Director, Department of Neurology
North Shore University Hospital
Manhasset, New York

Contents

PART I

Foundations of Drug Abuse in Sports

CHAPTER 1

Introduction

Do you wish to win an Olympic victory? So do I, by the gods! for it is a fine thing. But consider the matters which come before that, and those which follow after, and only when you have done that, put your hand to the task. You have to submit to discipline, follow a strict diet, give up sweet cakes, train under compulsion, at a fixed hour, in heat or in cold; you must not drink cold water, nor wine just whenever you feel like it; you must have turned yourself over to your trainer precisely as you would to a physician.

Epictectus (60?–120?)
Encheiridion, 29[1]

HISTORICAL PERSPECTIVES
EPIDEMIOLOGIC APPROACHES
EDUCATION, TESTING, AND TREATMENT
CATEGORIES OF DRUGS USED IN SPORTS
EVALUATING DRUGS ABUSED IN SPORTS
CONTRIBUTING FACTORS

HISTORICAL PERSPECTIVES

The use, misuse, and abuse of drugs have shaken the foundations of both amateur and professional sports in recent years. As Lipsyte has observed:

> There is no argument that drugs pose at least as serious a health problem in major league sports as they do in most high schools. By the time they have made the pros, most athletes have been given so many pills, salves, injections, potions, by amateur and pro coaches, doctors and trainers, to pick them up, cool them down, kill pain, enhance performance, reduce inflammation, and erase anxiety, that there isn't much they won't sniff, spread, stick in or swallow to get bigger or smaller, or to feel goooood.[2]

The problem is not new. History indicates that long ago athletes sought a competitive advantage by using various substances which have been dubbed "ergogenic aids." The 3rd century BC saw the Greeks ingest mushrooms to improve athletic performance[3]; gladiators used stimulants in the famed Circus Maximus (circa 600 BC)[4] to fight

3

despite fatigue and injury. During the 19th century, athletes experimented with caffeine, alcohol, nitroglycerine, opium, and even strychnine.[3,5] The first recorded fatality from a performance-enhancing drug occurred in 1886, when an English cyclist died from an overdose of "trimethyl."[6]

The anabolic effect of androgens, noted in World War II, set the stage for the use of anabolic steroids by athletes in an effort to increase muscular bulk and strength. Reports continue to suggest that anabolic steroids are widely used, particularly in strength and power sports including weightlifting, track and field, and football. In 1983, seven weightlifters from five countries were cited for using anabolic steroids in the IX Pan American Games.[7] By the end of 1986, 21 college football players were banned from bowl games as a result of tests indicating steroid use[8]; and in 1987, 6 percent of the National Football League's 1600 players tested positive for anabolic steroids during the pre-season physical.[9]

The use of drugs to enhance performance has not been limited to anabolic steroids. Despite the tragedy that befell the Olympic movement in 1960 with the death of a world-class cyclist from amphetamines,[3] stimulants such as amphetamines reportedly became widely used in professional football by the late 1960s and early 1970s.[10]

The explosion of drug abuse in Western society over the past two decades[11] added a new dimension to the problem of drug abuse in sports—recreational drug abuse. However, distinctions between recreational and performance-related drug abuse became less clear as cocaine made its way directly onto the field of play. Beginning in the early 1980s, bold headlines began to dominate the media, detailing an increased association between athletes and drug abuse in all its forms[7,8,12–20a] (Table 1–1).

Table 1–1. DRUG ABUSE AND THE ATHLETE: Names in the News

Name	Sport	Year	Drug
No Name Available **(Deceased)**	Weightlifter (England)	1987	Anabolic steroids[21]
Bias, Len **(Deceased)**	Basketball (U Maryland)	1986	Cocaine[21]
Croudip, David **(Deceased)**	Football (Atlanta Falcons)	1988	Cocaine[21a,21b]
Dressel, Birgit **(Deceased)**	Heptathlete (W Germany)	1987	Anabolic steroids, narcotics, multiple drugs[21,21c]
Furlow, Terry **(Deceased)**	Basketball (Utah Jazz)	1980	Cocaine[22,23]
Gordon, Larry **(Deceased)**	Football (Miami Dolphins)	1986	Cocaine[24]
Howard, Dick **(Deceased)**	Track	1960	Amphetamines[25]
Jackson, Hernell **(Deceased)**	Basketball (U Texas-El Paso)	1987	Cocaine[26,27]
Jensen, Knud **(Deceased)**	Cyclist (Denmark)	1960	Amphetamines[25]
Lindbergh, Pelle **(Deceased)**	Hockey (Phila Flyers)	1985	Alcohol[28]
Lipscomb, Big Daddy **(Deceased)**	Football (Balt Colts)	1963	Heroin[24]
Marshall, Rico **(Deceased)**	Football (USC)	1988	Cocaine[29]
Rogers, Don **(Deceased)**	Football (Cleve Browns)	1986	Cocaine[24,29a]
Simpson, Tommy **(Deceased)**	Cyclist	1967	Amphetamines[30]

Table 1-1—*Continued*

Name	Sport	Year	Drug
Singh, David **(Deceased)**	Bodybuilder (British)	1987	Anabolic steroids[30]
Ylvisaker, Billy **(Deceased)**	Polo	1983	Cocaine[31]
Adarmez Paez, Jose	Weightlifter	1983	Anabolic steroids[32]
Aikens, Willie	Baseball (KC Royals)	1983	Cocaine[33]
Andujar, Joaquin	Baseball (St Louis Cards)	1982	Cocaine[34]
Aniston, Steve	Tennis (UC Irvine)	1984	Cocaine/alcohol[35]
Aquino, Lupe	Boxer	1988	Alcohol[35a]
Barbay, Roland	Football (LSU)	1986	Anabolic steroids[36]
Baroudi, Daniel	Bodybuilder	1984	Anabolic steroids[37]
Bedford, William	Basketball (Detroit Pistons)	1988	Cocaine[38]
Bedrosian, Steve	Baseball (Atlanta Braves)	1983	Cocaine[39]
Bennett, Gary	Football (U Oklahoma)	1986	Anabolic steroids[40]
Bennett, Monte	Football (New Orleans Saints)	1981	Cocaine[41]
Berra, Dale	Baseball (Pitts Pirates)	1981	Cocaine[42]
Bethea, Ryan	Football (USC)	1988	Cocaine[29]
Blanco, Alberto	Weightlifter (Cuba)	1983	Anabolic steroids[7]
Blue, Vida	Baseball (KC Royals)	1983	Cocaine[43]
Bollings, Elnes	Basketball (US Virgin Isles)	1987	Phenylpropanolamine[19]
Bonilla, Juan	Baseball (San Diego Padres)	1982	Cocaine/marijuana[44]
Bosworth, Brian	Football (U Oklahoma)	1986	Anabolic steroids[40,45]
Botham, Ian	Cricket (Great Britain)	1986	Marijuana[25]
Branch, Cliff	Football (LA Raiders)	1981	Cocaine[46,47]
Bregel, Jeff	Football (USC)	1986	Anabolic steroids[40]
Brown, Kerrith	Judo (Great Britain)	1988	Diuretic[47a]
Browner, Ross	Football (Cinn Bengals)	1983	Cocaine[48,80]
Burton, Mike	Football (Salisbury State)	1986	Anabolic steroids[49]
Cabell, Enos	Baseball (Houston Astros)	1980	Cocaine[50,51]
Cadigan, Dave	Football (NY Jets)	1988	Anabolic steroids[52-54]
Candelaria, John	Baseball (Calif Angels)	1987	Alcohol[54a]

Table 1-1—*Continued*

Name	Sport	Year	Drug
Carter, James	Football (Georgia Southern)	1986	Anabolic steroids[49]
Collins, Tony	Football (New England Patriots)	1987	Cocaine[55]
Courson, Steve	Football (Pitts Steelers)	1985	Anabolic steroids[56]
Criswell, Kirby	Football (St Louis Cards)	1981	Marijuana/amphetamines[57]
Crowder, Randy	Football (Miami Dolphins)	1977	Cocaine[58]
Csengeri, Kalman	Weightlifter (Hungary)	1988	Anabolic steroids[58a]
Dailey, Quintin	Basketball (Chicago Bulls)	1986	Cocaine[25]
Davis, Dick	Baseball (Milw Brewers)	1981	Cocaine[12]
Davis, Walter	Basketball (Phoenix Suns)	1985	Cocaine/alcohol[55,59]
De La Cruz, Juan	Track & Field (Dom Rep)	1983	Ephedrine[60]
Delgado, Pedro	Cyclist (Spain)	1988	Probenecid[60a]
Dent, Richard	Football (Chicago Bears)	1987	Marijuana[60b]
Dobie, Reggie	Baseball (NY Mets)	1988	Alcohol[61]
Dokes, Michael	Boxing	1987	Cocaine[63,63]
Dolcey, Caballero	Weightlifter (Columbia)	1983	Anabolic steroids[7]
Drew, John	Basketball (Utah Jazz)	1983	Cocaine[64]
Dudley, David	Football (U Arkansas)	1986	Anabolic steroids[40]
Durbano, Steve	Hockey (St Louis Blues)	1979	Cocaine/marijuana[65]
Duren, Ryne	Baseball (NY Yankees)	1968	Alcohol[66]
Eller, Carl	Football (Minn Vikings)	1980	Alcohol/cocaine[67]
Elliot, Tony	Football (New Orleans Saints)	1983	Cocaine[25]
Ellis, Dock	Baseball (Pitts Pirates)	1980	Alcohol/LSD/cocaine/ amphetamines[50,68]
Finger, Lavell	Basketball (United States)	1988	Cocaine[68a]
Fleming, Flint	Football (N Dakota State)	1986	Anabolic steroids[49]
Franks, Elvis	Football (LA Raiders)	1987	Cocaine[46,69]
Frycer, Miroslav	Hockey (Tor Maple Leafs)	1986	Alcohol[69a]
Gasser, Sandra	Track & Field (Switzerland)	1987	Anabolic steroids[21a]
Gogan, Kevin	Football (Dallas Cowboys)	1988	Alcohol/marijuana[69a,69b,69c]
Gooden, Dwight	Baseball (NY Mets)	1987	Cocaine[55,70]

Table 1-1—*Continued*

Name	Sport	Year	Drug
Grablev, Mitko	Weightlifting (Bulgaria)	1988	Furosemide (diuretic)[70b]
Greavette, Guy	Weightlifter (Canada)	1983	Anabolic steroids[7]
Green, Bill	Hammerthrow	1987	Anabolic steroids[19]
Gregg, David	Basketball (U Maryland)	1986	Cocaine[70a]
Griffin, Eric	Basketball (United States)	1988	Marijuana[68a]
Guenchov, Anguel	Weightlifter (Bulgaria)	1988	Furosemide (diuretic)[58a]
Guthrie, William	Basketball (United States)	1988	Cocaine[68a]
Harmon, Clarence	Football (Wash Redskins)	1983	Cocaine[29a,71]
Harris, Leroy	Football (Phila Eagles)	1983	Cocaine[29a,72]
Haywood, Spencer	Basketball (LA Lakers)	1980	Cocaine[72a]
Heaslip, Mark	Hockey (NY Rangers)	1978	Alcohol/cocaine[67]
Hegg, Steve	Cyclist (United States)	1988	Caffeine[72b]
Henderson, Thomas	Football (Dallas Cowboys)	1981	Cocaine[73]
Hernandez, Keith	Baseball (St Louis Cardinals)	1982	Cocaine[25]
Holt, Issaic	Football (Minn Vikings)	1987	Alcohol[74]
Howe, Steve	Baseball (LA Dodgers)	1983	Cocaine[75]
Hoyt, Lamarr	Baseball (San Diego Padres)	1986	Multiple drugs[76]
Hunter, Dave	Hockey (Edmonton Oilers)	1986	Alcohol[69a]
Israelson, Bill	Golf	1988	Alcohol[76a]
Jacobs, Chris	Swimming	1986	Cocaine, marijuana, alcohol[76b]
Jenkins, Ferguson	Baseball (Texas Rangers)	1980	Cocaine/marijuana[77]
Jimenez, Javier	Weightlifter	1987	Anabolic steroids[19]
Johansson, Thomas	Wrestler (Sweden)	1985	Anabolic steroids[37]
Johnson, Ben	Sprinter (Canada)	1988	Anabolic steroids[20a]
Johnson, Eddie	Basketball (Atlanta Hawks)	1980	Cocaine[78]
Johnson, Pete	Football (Cinn Bengals)	1983	Cocaine[48]
Jones, Hassan	Football (Minn Vikings)	1987	Alcohol[79]
Jordan, Steve	Football (Minn Vikings)	1987	Alcohol[74]
Junior, E. J.	Football (St Louis Cards)	1983	Cocaine[80]
Kay, Clarence	Football (Denver Broncos)	1986	Alcohol[29a,81]

Table 1-1—*Continued*

Name	Sport	Year	Drug
Kimball, Bruce	Diving (United States)	1988	Alcohol[81a,81b]
King, Bernard	Basketball (Utah Jazz)	1980	Alcohol/cocaine[22,82,83]
Korte, Steve	Football (New Orleans Saints)	1986	Anabolic steroids[45]
Kramer, Tommy	Football (Minn Vikings)	1987	Alcohol[18]
Krone, Julie	Jockey	1980	Marijuana[83a]
Lacy, Lee	Baseball (Pitts Pirates)	1981	Cocaine[25]
Landreaux, Ken	Baseball (LA Dodgers)	1983	Cocaine[39,82]
Leonard, Jeff	Baseball (SF Giants)	1981	Cocaine[12]
Lilly, Lindon	Football (Nevada-Reno)	1986	Anabolic steroids[49]
Lloyd, Lewis	Basketball (Houston Rockets)	1987	Cocaine[84]
Long, Terry	Basketball (U Maryland)	1986	Cocaine[70a]
Lopez, Guillermo	Weightlifter (Argentina)	1983	Anabolic steroids[7]
Lozada, Jose	Weightlifter (Puerto Rico)	1983	Anabolic steroids[7]
Lucas, John	Basketball (Wash Bullets)	1981	Cocaine[75]
Lynch, Kerry	Nordic Ski (United States)	1987	Blood doping[85]
Macoun, Jamie	Hockey (Calgary Flames)	1987	Alcohol[69a]
MacTavish, Craig	Hockey (Boston Bruins)	1984	Alcohol[69a,86]
Manley, Dexter	Football (Wash Redskins)	1987	Alcohol[87]
Mann, Carol	Golf	1969	Alcohol/amphetamines[88,89]
Mariaca, Fernando	Weightlifter (Spain)	1988	Amphetamine[58a]
Martin, Jerry	Baseball (KC Royals)	1983	Cocaine[90]
Martin, Scott	Football (Nevada-Reno)	1986	Anabolic steroids[49]
Martinez, Dennis	Baseball (Balt Orioles)	1983	Alcohol[91]
Maxwell, Vernon	Basketball (Univ Florida)	1988	Cocaine[92]
McDowell, Sam	Baseball (Pitts Pirates)	1975	Alcohol[91]
McLain, Gary	Basketball (Villanova)	1985	Cocaine[93]
McLaughlin, Lee	Softball (NCAA Div I)	1982	Alcohol/amphetamines/ barbiturates/narcotics[94]
McKegney, Tony	Hockey (St Louis Blues)	1987	Alcohol[69a]
Mennea, Pietro	Sprinter (Italy)	1974	Human growth hormone[30]

Table 1-1—*Continued*

Name	Sport	Year	Drug
Michaels, Jeff	Weightlifter	1983	Anabolic steroids[37]
Milner, Eddie	Baseball (Cinn Reds)	1988	Alcohol/cocaine[67,96]
Milner, John	Baseball (Pitts Pirates)	1981	Cocaine[95]
Mira Jr, George	Football (U Miami)	1987	Diuretic[96a]
Molitor, Paul	Baseball (Milwaukee Brewers)	1982	Cocaine[12]
Montiel, Enrique	Weightlifter (Nicaragua)	1983	Anabolic steroids[32]
Morawiecki, Jaroslaw	Hockey (Polish-Olympics)	1988	Anabolic steroids[97]
Morris, Eugene "Mercury"	Football (Miami Dolphins)	1982	Cocaine[29a,97a,97b]
Mullin, Chris	Basketball (Golden State)	1987	Alcohol[98]
Muncie, Chuck	Football (San Diego Chargers)	1984	Cocaine[99,100]
Murdoch, Don	Hockey (NY Rangers)	1977	Alcohol/cocaine[91]
Myers, Angel	Swimming	1988	Anabolic steroids[100a,100b]
Newcombe, Don	Baseball (Brooklyn Dodgers)	1966	Alcohol[82]
Newton, Bob	Football (Seattle Seahawks)	1987	Alcohol[74]
Newton, Tim	Football (Minn Vikings)	1987	Alcohol[74]
Niemczak, Antoni	Distance Runner (Poland)	1986	Anabolic steroids[101]
Norris, Mike	Baseball (Oakland Athletics)	1985	Cocaine/alcohol[90,102]
Norwood, Lori	Pentathlete	1986	Tranquilizer[103]
Nunez, Daniel	Weightlifter (Cuba)	1983	Anabolic steroids[7]
O'Neill, John	Football (U Miami)	1987	Diuretic[97]
Ocando, Bernardo	Pistol Shooting (Venezuela)	1987	Propranolol[19]
Oliger, Jacques	Weightlifter (Chile)	1983	Anabolic steroids[32]
Oliver, Frank	Football (Salisbury State)	1986	Anabolic steroids[49]
Parker, Dave	Baseball (Pitts Pirates)	1982	Cocaine[104]
Perez, Pascual	Baseball (Atlanta Braves)	1984	Cocaine[39]
Peters, Tony	Football (Wash Redskins)	1983	Cocaine[29a,105]
Pinango, Bernardo	Boxing	1988	Cocaine[105a]
Plucknett, Ben	Discus Thrower	1981	Anabolic steroids[37]
Porter, Darrell	Baseball (St Louis Cards)	1980	Alcohol/cocaine/ amphetamines[82]
Probert, Bob	Hockey (Detroit Red Wings)	1986	Alcohol[18]
Pryor, Aaron	Boxer	1985	Alcohol/cocaine[84,106,107]

Table 1-1—*Continued*

Name	Sport	Year	Drug
Quesada, Jorge	Pentathlete (Spain)	1988	Beta blocker[58a]
Raines, Tim	Baseball (Montreal Expos)	1982	Cocaine[25]
Reaves, John	Football (Minn Vikings)	1979	Alcohol/marijuana/cocaine[29a,82,108,109]
Reese, Don	Football (Miami Dolphins)	1977	Cocaine[75]
Reilly, Mike	Football (LA Rams)	1982	Alcohol[110]
Richard, JR	Baseball (Houston Astros)	1980	Cocaine[111]
Richardson, Micheal Ray	Basketball (NJ Nets)	1986	Cocaine[25]
Ripken Sr, Cal	Baseball (Balt Orioles)	1988	Alcohol[112]
Robinson, Jerry	Football (LA Raiders)	1987	Cocaine[46,113]
Rogers, George	Football (New Orleans Saints)	1981	Cocaine[41,80]
Roy, Kevin	Weightlifter (Canada)	1988	Anabolic steroids[113a]
Scurry, Rod	Baseball (Pitts Pirates)	1983	Cocaine[114]
Salming, Borje	Hockey (Toronto Maple Leafs)	1981	Cocaine[115]
Sanderson, Derek	Hockey (Boston Bruins; NY Rangers	1974–77	Alcohol/cocaine[115a,115b]
Shoemaker, David	Football (U Oklahoma)	1986	Anabolic steroids[40]
Skiles, Scott	Basketball (Michigan State)	1984	Alcohol/marijuana[116]
Smith, Lonnie	Baseball (St Louis Cards)	1982	Cocaine/marijuana[95,117]
Smith, Tom	Football (N Dakota State)	1986	Anabolic steroids[49]
Smith, Willie	Football (Cleve Browns)	1986	Cocaine[24]
Speidel, Robert	Football (Rutgers)	1988	Alcohol[117a]
Steinkuhler, Dean	Football (Houston Oilers)	1984	Anabolic steroids[118]
Stemrick, Greg	Football (New Orleans Saints)	1983	Cocaine[29a]
Szanyi, Andor	Weightlifter (Hungary)	1988	Anabolic steroids[118a]
Tarbi, Ahmed	Weightlifter (Algeria)	1984	Anabolic steroids[119]
Tarha, Mahmoud	Weightlifter (Lebanon)	1984	Anabolic steroids[119]
Taylor, Lawrence	Football (NY Giants)	1985, 1988	Cocaine[120,120a]
Thomas, Calvin	Football (Chicago Bears)	1988	Cocaine/marijuana[120b]
Thompson, David	Basketball (Denver Nuggets)	1983	Cocaine[87,121]

Table 1-1—*Continued*

Name	Sport	Year	Drug
Torres, Pedro	Weightlifter (Venezuela)	1987	Anabolic steroids[19]
Townsend, Greg	Football (LA Raiders)	1988	Alcohol, marijuana[69a,69b,121a]
Upchurch, Rich	Football (Denver Broncos)	1983	Marijuana[122,123]
Vainio, Martii	Distance Runner (Finland)	1984	Anabolic steroids, blood doping[21a,37]
Vasquez-Mendose, Orlando	Weightlifter (Nicaragua)	1987	Diuretic[19]
Verouli, Anna	Javelin (Greece)	1987	Anabolic steroids[124]
Viau, Michel	Weightlifter (Canada)	1983	Anabolic steroids[7]
Washburn, Chris	Basketball (Atlanta Hawks)	1988	Cocaine[124a]
Washington, Claudell	Baseball (Atlanta Braves)	1983	Cocaine[39,90]
Washington, Duane Eddy	Basketball (NJ Nets)	1988	Cocaine[124b]
Watson, Alexander	Pentathlete (Australia)	1988	Caffeine[70b]
Waymer, David	Football (New Orleans Saints)	1981	Cocaine[41]
Weber, Pete	Bowling (Pro Tour)	1984	Alcohol[125]
Welch, Bob	Baseball (LA Dodgers)	1979	Alcohol[66]
White, Charles	Football (Cleveland Browns)	1983	Cocaine[126]
Whittington, Art	Football (Oakland Raiders)	1982	Cocaine[127]
Wiggins, Alan	Baseball (San Diego Padres)	1982	Cocaine[128]
Wiggins, Mitchell	Basketball (Houston Rockets)	1987	Cocaine[84]
Wilson, David	Football (New Orleans Saints)	1981	Cocaine[41]
Wilson, Mario	Epee (Cuba)	1983	Ephedrine[60]
Wilson, Stanley	Football (Cinn Bengals)	1987	Cocaine[129]
Wilson, Willie	Baseball (KC Royals)	1983	Cocaine[130]
Witherspoon, Tim	Boxer	1985	Marijuana[131,132]
Woolridge, Orlando	Basketball (NJ Nets)	1988	Cocaine[133]
Word, Barry	Football (Un Virginia)	1986	Cocaine[14]
Youmans, Floyd	Baseball (Montreal Expos)	1988	Cocaine[133a]
Zentner, John	Football (Stanford)	1986	Anabolic steroids[49]

Scandals, suspensions, fines, and tragedies became, and have remained, commonplace. In the summer of 1986, the problem of drug abuse in sports came under especially close scrutiny as a result of the cocaine-induced deaths of collegiate basketball superstar Len Bias and professional football player Don Rogers.[14,134] In 1988, drug abuse in sports again dominated the headlines as Canadian sprinter Ben Johnson was stripped of his gold medal at the XXIV Olympiad in Seoul for anabolic steroid use.[20a]

Although competitive athletics has a long history of drug abuse problems, less media attention has been specifically directed to alcohol abuse per se. As a legal and readily available substance, alcohol has not usually been included in sports' drug testing protocols. Nonetheless, in just a 9-month period, the New York newspaper *Newsday* printed 100 sports stories that dealt with alcohol.[18] The alcohol-related death of hockey goalie Pelle Lindbergh and the admitted alcoholism problem of professional basketball star Chris Mullin have served to focus attention on this serious problem.

EPIDEMIOLOGIC APPROACHES

During the 1960s, major efforts were undertaken to cope with the increasing national problem of drug abuse. In order to get an overview of the nature and the extent of the drug problem, three types of surveys have been sponsored by the National Institute on Drug Abuse. The first, initiated in 1975—The High School Senior Survey, more formally called *Monitoring the Future: A Continuing Study of Lifestyles and Values of Youth*[135]—is conducted by the University of Michigan's Institute for Social Research. In this study, annual surveys of drug use patterns are taken from a nationally representative sample of 16,000 seniors from about 130 public and private high schools nationwide. Also reported are follow-up surveys of approximately 10,000 graduates beginning with the class of 1975. The second survey, entitled *The National Household Survey on Drug Abuse,*[136] conducted every 2 to 3 years, measures the prevalence and frequency of drug use among the American household population aged 12 and over. The third survey is *The Drug Abuse Warning System*

(DAWN).[137] It is a large-scale drug abuse data collection system that was designed as an early warning indicator of the severity, scope, and nature of the drug abuse problem in the continental United States. Data are derived from emergency room visits and fatalities resulting from drug abuse.

A comparable study of substance abuse habits by athletes was contracted for by the National Collegiate Athletic Association (NCAA) and was conducted by the College of Human Medicine at Michigan State University during the fall of 1984. In this study, entitled *The Substance Use and Abuse Habits of College Student-Athletes,*[138] student athletes from five men's and five women's sports, representing six Division I, three Division II, and two Division III colleges and universities completed a carefully administered, anonymous questionnaire. The questionnaire and the procedure, which was similar to those used in *Monitoring the Future*, were reviewed and approved by the human subjects committees at Michigan State University and the National Institute on Drug Abuse. The drugs surveyed were alcohol, amphetamines, antiinflammatory pain medications, anabolic steroids, barbiturates and tranquilizers, marijuana and hashish, minor pain medications, psychedelic drugs, smokeless tobacco, vitamins, and minerals.

In 1986, Hazelden-Cork, utilizing a questionnaire technique in cooperation with the Womens Sports Foundation, conducted a survey of alcohol and other drug use patterns, attitudes, and behaviors of women involved in athletic competition at various levels—college varsity, Olympic, other amateur, professional, senior/masters, and retired.[139] Relevant results of the above studies are given in subsequent chapters.

EDUCATION, TESTING, AND TREATMENT

Educational and treatment programs proliferated during the 1970s and the 1980s. By 1986, 1.6 billion dollars were spent for the treatment and prevention of drug and alcohol abuse.[140] But the problem continued to grow,[141] so that by 1986, in a National Institute on Drug Abuse (NIDA) survey of 1,001 Americans age 18 and older, "73% described drug use as one of the most serious problems facing the country" while only 2 percent considered it not important.[142] During the 1980s, both the public and private sectors introduced drug testing on a large scale in an attempt to gain some control over the burgeoning problem.[141,143,144] Similarly, as the problem of drug abuse by athletes increased, the use of drug testing in amateur and professional sports surfaced as an important, yet controversial issue.[14,145–152]

CATEGORIES OF DRUGS USED IN SPORTS

The origins of drug abuse in sports are rooted in efforts to pharmacologically enhance athletic performance—by using ergogenic drugs—while the origins of drug testing in sports relate to efforts to eliminate any ergogenic advantage that might accrue from the unapproved use of drugs. Three major categories of drugs used by athletes today include:

1. *Performance Enhancement (Ergogenic) Drugs.* This category represents the use of drugs (e.g., amphetamines) or methods (e.g., "blood doping") for the purpose of gaining athletic advantage.

2. *Therapeutic Drugs.* This category represents the use of drugs for specific medical indications in accordance with standards of good medical practice.

3. *"Street" / "Entertainment" / "Pleasure" Drugs.* This category applies to those drugs

Table 1–2. REPRESENTATIVE POTENTIAL BENEFITS OF ERGOGENIC DRUGS

Increase in strength and power
Increase in endurance
Increase in aggressiveness
Increase in speed and acceleration
Enhancement of competitive attitude
Enhancement of concentration
Enhancement of fine motor coordination
Enhancement of eye/hand coordination
Diminishment of pain perception
Diminishment of anxiety
Diminishment of tremor
Delay in the onset of fatigue
Weight control

Table 1–3. REPRESENTATIVE POTENTIAL COSTS OF ERGOGENIC DRUGS

Impaired judgment
Impaired reaction time
Impaired muscular coordination
Impaired balance
Impaired eye/hand coordination
Deterioration in the performance of complex motor tasks
Decreased strength
Decreased flexibility
Decreased accuracy
Decreased speed and acceleration

that are taken either illicitly or in greater than prescribed quantities to alter mood and perceptions.

These categories are by no means mutually exclusive. For example, a therapeutic drug such as propranolol may both control migraine headaches and improve hand steadiness in riflery.

The benefits that the athlete seeks from ergogenic drugs relate primarily to the physical and emotional demands of competitive athletics (Table 1–2). However, in performance terms, the potential benefit of any drug must be weighed against any potential cost (Table 1–3).

EVALUATING DRUGS ABUSED IN SPORTS

The evaluation of the effect of an unapproved drug, particularly an illicit drug, on athletic performance is necessarily complicated by the failure to evaluate the effect of the drug in accordance with basic pharmacologic principles. Drug purity, route of administration, dose response, and the relation of drug usage to the time of the event are but some of the variables to be considered.

Practical, ethical, and legal impediments necessarily will leave many of the questions regarding the effects of drugs on athletic performance unanswered. Nonetheless, the 1959 and 1960 classic studies by Smith and Beecher[153–155] on the effects of amphetamines on the athletic performance of world class athletes represent a pharmacologic gold standard for such investigations. This study is discussed in Chapter 6.

CONTRIBUTING FACTORS

The prevalence of drug abuse in the athletic community has necessarily and increasingly stimulated debate in both the lay and the professional communities as to "Why?" Athletes are at least as vulnerable to drug abuse as other members of society.[156,157] Outstanding athletes may suffer a particular vulnerability.[14] Outstanding professional athletes are highly visible and often wealthy. Both they and their amateur counterparts are in a susceptible age group with extended periods of free time. In an effort to excel competitively, often beginning in his or her teens, the skilled athlete is often subject to unusual degrees of stress—both internal and external. For many, drug abuse has become a method of trying to lessen that stress.

Any discussion regarding drug abuse in the athlete cannot view the athlete apart from the whole of society. Family; childhood and adolescent development; genetics; psychological, psychiatric, and cultural issues; peers; economics; and education, as well as the nature of the drug itself, are all factors that impact on drug abuse in all of society, as well as in the athlete. An understanding of this matrix of interacting elements is essential to the prevention, recognition, and management of drug abuse in general and in the athlete in particular.

REFERENCES

1. Strauss, MB (ed): Familiar Medical Quotations. Little, Brown & Co, Boston, 1968, p 487.
2. Lipsyte, R: Baseball & drugs. The Nation, May 25, 1985, p 613.
3. Puffer, J: The use of drugs in swimming. Clin Sports Med 5:77, 1986.
4. Meer, J: Drugs and sports. In Snyder, SH (ed): The Encyclopedia of Psychoactive Drugs. Chelsea House, New York, 1987, p 19.
5. Burks, TF: Drug use in athletics. Fed Proc 40:2680, 1981.
6. Dyment, PG: Drugs and the adolescent athlete. Ped Ann 13:602, 1984.
7. Jeansonne, J: 7 lifters named as drug users. Newsday, August 23, 1983.
8. Wilbon, M: Number of banned players reaches 21. Washington Post, December 28, 1986.
9. Steroid use in the NFL. The New York Times. October 8, 1988.
10. Mandell, AJ, Stewart, KD, and Russo, PV: The

Sunday Syndrome: from kinetics to altered consciousness. Fed Proc 40:2693, 1981.
11. Thomas, E: America's crusade: What is behind the latest war on drugs? Time, September 15, 1986, p 60.
12. Goodwin, M: Baseball and cocaine: A deepening problem. The New York Times, August 19, 1985.
13. Goodwin, M: Baseball orders suspension of 11 drug users. The New York Times, March 1, 1986.
14. Lamar, JV, Jr: Scoring off the field. Time, August 25, 1986, p 52.
15. Neff, C: Caracas: A scandal and a warning. Sports Illustrated, July 11, 1983.
16. Markus, D: Cocaine reported common among players in the NBA. Newsday, August 20, 1980.
17. Durso, J: Kuhn bans 4 players for a year for drug use. The New York Times, December 16, 1983.
18. Sullivan, J: Unrestricted Drug. Leagues just say no to alcohol-abuse sanctions. Newsday, December 22, 1987.
19. Janofsky, M: 6 disqualified from Pan Am games for drug use. The New York Times, August 18, 1987.
20. Jeansonne, J: Drug use heavy, track stars say. Newsday, April 4, 1988.
20a. Johnson, WO and Moore, K: The loser. Sports Illustrated, October 3, 1988, p 20.
21. Voy, RO: Education as a means against doping. The Olympian, December, 1987.
21a. Schwartz, J: Falcon player, 29, dies after seizure. The New York Times, October 11, 1988.
21b. Sports People: Clearly an overdose. The New York Times, October 13, 1988.
21c. Johns, M: The inside dope. Runners World, September, 1988, p 78.
22. Douchant, M: NBA probes drug use. The Sporting News, August 2, 1980.
23. Gould, D: Cocaine scandal threatening NBA. The New York Post, August 19, 1980.
24. Reilly, R: When the cheers turned to tears. Sports Illustrated, July 14, 1986, p 28.
25. Meer, J: Drugs and Sports. In Snyder, SH (ed): The Encyclopedia of Psychoactive Drugs. Chelsea House, New York, 1987.
26. The death of another star. Time, May 25, 1987, p 44.
27. Wulf, S: Jeep Jackson, RIP. Sports Illustrated, May 18, 1987, p 20.
28. Cornwell, B: Alcoholic athletes losing anonymity. The San Jose Mercury News, December 17, 1987.
29. Cocaine death rocks South Carolina grid program. The Bershire Eagle, February 16, 1988.
29a. LaMarre, T: League, player's union can't agree on drug plan. The Los Angeles Times, January 18, 1987.
30. Penycate, J: How athletes stay one jump ahead of drug-testers. The Listener, September 24, 1987, p 4.
31. Axthelm, P: Throwing it all away. Newsweek, April 11, 1983.
32. Litsky, F: Some U.S. athletes leave games at Caracas amid stiff drug tests. The New York Times, August 24, 1983.
33. Berkow, I: It can't happen to me. The New York Times, June 26, 1986.
34. Topol, M: Herndez linked to use of cocaine. Newsday, September 6, 1985.

35. Pentz, L: Drugs and tennis: One player's toughest match. World Tennis, July 1985, p 32.
35a. Two highway deaths charged to Aquino. Newsday, August 15, 1988.
36. Barbay, R: Steroid ruling upheld. The New York Times, January 1, 1987.
37. Baroudi, D: A response to soviets. USA Today, January 23, 1987.
38. Brown, C: Pistons sub Bedford goes into drug rehab. Detroit Free Press, March 31, 1988.
39. The bittersweet 16. Sports Illustrated, May 28, 1984, p 45.
40. Wolff, C: Bosworth barred from bowl for steroids. The New York Times, December 26, 1987.
41. Taubman, P: 2 Saints reported to admit drug use. The New York Times, June 25, 1982.
42. Goodwin, M: Baseball orders suspension of 11 drug users. The New York Times, March 1, 1986.
43. 3 from Royals get 3-month terms in drug case. The New York Times, November 18, 1983.
44. Verducci, T: Bonilla grateful for second chance. Newsday, April 8, 1985.
45. Brubaker, B: Players close eyes to steroids' risks. The Washington Post, February 1, 1987.
46. Cossell, H: NFL must reverse field on drugs. The New York Daily News, July 29, 1987.
47. Cliff Branch's bout with drugs. The San Francisco Examiner, June 5, 1981.
47a. Test won't cost sprinter his medal. Newsday, October 1, 1988.
48. Press Release, the National Football League, July 25, 1983.
49. Several others have been suspended. USA Today, December 26, 1986.
50. Lessem, D: "Hits" as errors—or losing by a nose. The Boston Globe, September 30, 1985.
51. Topol, M: Berra testifies Stargell was drug supplier. Newsday, September 11, 1985.
52. Eskenazi, G: Jets' top pick says he took steroids. The New York Times, April 27, 1988.
53. Logan, G: Jets' Cadigan: I'll do anything to succeed. Newsday, April 27, 1988.
54. Logan, G: Cadigan's account disputed. Newsday, May 1, 1988.
54a. Lupica, M: Candelaria recovers from hell. The New York Daily News, May 20, 1988.
55. Goodwin, M: In sports, cocaine's here to stay. The New York Times, May 3, 1987.
56. Ex-user sounds warning. USA Today, January 23, 1987.
57. Rains, R: A new beginning behind bars. UPI, July 3, 1983.
58. Williams, V: Ex-Dolphin gets 5 year term, no record. The Miami News, August 10, 1977.
58a. Bulgarian lifters exit games. Newsday, September 25, 1988.
59. Shapell, L: Davis' mom dies a week after father. Arizona Republic, May 27, 1987.
60. Litsky, F: Two more athletes cited for drug use. The New York Times, August 26, 1983.
60a. Abt, S: Delgado wins amid cheers, criticism. The New York Times, July 25, 1988.
60b. Forbes, G: Dent accepts drug testing, will play. USA Today, September 16, 1988.
61. Jacobsen, S: Straight pitch saved doc. Newsday, March 16, 1988.
62. Dokes re-arrested on cocaine count. Newsday, April 16, 1987.
63. Matthews, W: For Dokes, coke party finally ends. Newsday, December 12, 1987.
64. Johnson, RS: An athlete, a cocaine addict: John Drew fights for his life. The New York Times, February 27, 1983.
65. Steve Durbano serving a 7-year major penalty. Newsday, February 20, 1983.
66. Cornwell, B: Alcoholic athletes losing anonymity. San Jose Mercury News, December 17, 1987.
67. Coffey, W: The temptations to booze it up. The New York Daily News, July 13, 1987.
68. Dock Ellis: No-hitter while on LSD. Newsday, April 8, 1984.
68a. Berkow, I: What happened to Eric Griffin? The New York Times, July 17, 1988.
69. Raider Franks in coke bust. New York Daily News, July 22, 1987.
69a. Lener, J: Faceoff or standoff? The Main Event, May, 1988.
69b. NFL suspends four. The New York Times, August 8, 1988.
69c. Miklasz, B: Cowboys suspend Gogan. Dallas Morning News, August 5, 1988.
70. Verducci, T: The doctor is out. Newsday, April 2, 1987.
70a. Associated Press, July 22, 1987.
70b. Mifflin, L: 123-pound gold medalist fails drug test. The New York Times, September 22, 1988.
71. Headlines again. The New York Times, October 14, 1985.
72. Coakley, MB and Longman, J: Eagles back says he is a "junkie." The Philadelphia Inquirer, March 4, 1983.
72a. Seduced and betrayed by cocaine, a basketball star rebuilds his life and earns the ring of a champion. People, June 13, 1988.
72b. Cyclist disqualified. The New York Times, September 11, 1988.
73. Weisman, L: 2 NFL players: Drugs no secret. USA Today, July 24, 1987.
74. Cowart, V: Alcohol and athletics don't mix: Can the players now say nix? JAMA 258:1571, 1987.
75. Gross, J: Drug addiction: The threat to sports keeps growing. The New York Times, July 23, 1983.
76. Friend, T: A trip down a twisting road . . . without sleep. The Los Angeles Times, July 12, 1987.
76a. Newsday, September 22, 1988.
76b. Litsky, F: Swimmer outraces his past. The New York Times, September 18, 1988.
77. Brubaker, B: There's a narc at 410 Park. The New York Daily News, October 29, 1980.
78. Cunningham, G: Johnson optimistic—"I know it's going to be rough." The Atlanta Constitution, September 12, 1980.
79. Alcohol awareness. The New York Times, November 11, 1987.
80. Rozelle suspends four for cocaine use. The New York Times, July 26, 1983.
81. Hewitt, B: Case of the missing Kay: A misunderstanding. The Los Angeles Times, January 29, 1988.
81a. Sports People. The New York Times, August 9, 1988.
81b. Berkow, I: Should Bruce Kimball compete in

Seoul Olympics? The New York Times, August 16, 1988.

82. Jacobs, B: Cheers! Here's to the players who have bid farewell to booze and drugs. Family Weekly, August 7, 1983.

83. O'Brien: I'll banish cocaine users. New York Post, August 20, 1980.

83a. Virshup, A: Hitting the track with jockey Julie Krone. New York Magazine, June 13, 1988.

84. Goldaper, S: Lloyd and Wiggins. The New York Times, January 14, 1987.

85. Jeansonne, J: The controversy surrounding blood doping. Newsday, April 5, 1988.

86. Bock, H: Alcohol abuse is rooted in sports lifestyle. San Antonio Express News, December 21, 1987.

87. Bunn, CG: Drugs: The toughest rebound in sports. Newsday, July 19, 1987.

88. Delahanty, H: Let's talk about drugs—honestly. Women's Sports & Fitness, June 1986.

89. Duda, M: Female athletes: Targets for drug abuse. Phys Sportsmed 14:142, 1986.

90. Angell, R: Reflections: Three cheers for Keith. The New Yorker, May 5, 1986.

91. Coffey, W: Everything to lose in booze. The New York Daily News, July 12, 1987.

92. Drug use revealed. The New York Times, April 16, 1988.

93. Vecsey, P: For McLain, things go better with coke. New York Post, March 13, 1987.

94. McLaughlin, L: How my quick fix turned to a bad dream. Women's Sports & Fitness, November, 1986.

95. Goodwin, M: Ueberroth asks all players to undergo tests for drugs. The New York Times, September 25, 1985.

96. Reds' Milner suspended for year. Newsday, March 31, 1988.

96a. Moran, M: Banned Miami players still on sideline. The New York Times, December 31, 1987.

97. Litsky, F: Polish hockey star is banned. The New York Times, February 22, 1988.

97a. Morris, E: Behavior, not cocaine, is the problem. The New York Times, September 4, 1988.

97b. Logan, G: Mercury Morris' longest yard. Newsday, November 28, 1982.

98. Moran, M and Rhoden, WC: Mullin's downfall: Signs were there. The New York Times, December 20, 1987.

99. Bisheff, S: Chargers rip Reese's "coke" story. The San Diego Tribune, June 10, 1982.

100. Another prospective Dolphin fails drug test. The Arizona Republic, September 16, 1984.

100a. U.S. closes book on Myers. The New York Times, September 18, 1988.

100b. Myers appeal fails. The New York Times, September 3, 1988.

101. Marathoner's drug test positive, friends say. Newsday, November 26, 1986.

102. Furthermore.... Newsday, January 25, 1987.

103. Francis, S: Did she or didn't she? Women's Sports & Fitness, April 22, 1987.

104. Kirkman, D: Experts: Coke even hurts best athletes. Newsday, April 24, 1986.

105. Peters of Redskins seized in drug case. The New York Times, August 4, 1983.

105a. Ex-champ faces new drug charges. Newsday, September 15, 1988.

106. Axthelm, P: The Hawk's toughest fight. Newsweek, August 3, 1987.

107. Matthews, W: IBF strips title from Pryor. Newsday, December 11, 1985.

108. Smith, J: The transformation of John Reaves. Newsday, March 16, 1983.

109. St. John, B: For Reaves, life begins at 31. The Dallas Morning News, August 8, 1981.

110. Hoffer, R: The new sober life of Reilly. The Los Angeles Times, January 12, 1988.

111. Creamer, RW: Who hurt J.R.? Sports Illustrated, September 9, 1985, p 9.

112. Ripken gets fine for DWI. USA Today, April 13, 1988.

113. Raider arrested. The New York Times, July 17, 1987.

113a. Janofsky, M: Samaranch calls drug users "the thieves of performance." The New York Times, September 13, 1988.

114. Maisel, I: "The stuff I did was enough to kill you." Sports Illustrated, May 28, 1984, p 38.

115. Sullivan, R: Putting logic on ice. Sports Illustrated, June 2, 1986, p 15.

115a. The Associated Press, September 30, 1987.

115b. The Associated Press, August 8, 1987.

116. Maisel, I: Shooting to even up the score. Sports Illustrated, February 10, 1986, p 168.

117. Chase, M: Cocaine disrupts baseball from field to front office. The New York Times, August 20, 1985.

117a. Sports People. The New York Times, August 21, 1988.

118. Keteyian, A: A former Huskie fesses up. Sports Illustrated, January 5, 1987, p 24.

118a. Hungarian lifter stripped of silver. Newsday, September 28, 1988.

119. Associated Press, August 4, 1984.

120. Taylor, L and Falkner, D: LT: Living off the edge. In Sport, September 1987.

120a. King, P: LT "I'll pay the price." Newsday, September 1, 1988.

120b. Johnson, WO: Hit for a loss. Sports Illustrated, September 19, 1988.

121. Sullivan, J: Knicks' Stirling unaware. Newsday, August 19, 1986.

121a. Dianey, J: Townsend suspended for 30 days for testing positive for marijuana. Los Angeles Herald Examiner, August 5, 1988.

122. Upchurch rehabilitated. USA Today, July 20, 1983.

123. Litsky, F: NFL teams split on use of drug tests. The New York Times, July 18, 1982.

124. Harvey, R: Greek is 5th disqualified by drug test. The Los Angeles Times, August 12, 1987.

124a. Washburn suspended. The New York Times, September 27, 1988.

124b. Goldaper, S: Nets guard banned for drugs. The New York Times, October 1, 1988.

125. Friedman, J and Shaw, B: Young, gifted, and reckless: Bowler Pete Weber tries to keep his life out of the gutter. People Magazine, February 22, 1988.

126. Burwell, B: White, Eller made it back. The New York Daily News, August 15, 1983.

127. Newhouse, D: High that was low. The Oakland Tribune, March 29, 1983.

128. Adler, A: The Associated Press, October 29, 1986.

129. UPI, April 20, 1988.

130. Berkow, I: "It can't happen to me." The New York Times, June 26, 1986.

131. New champ Witherspoon could lose his WBA title. Jet, February 24, 1986, p 45.

132. WBA title goes to pot, Witherspoon fined $25,000, must fight Tubbs again. Jet, March 31, 1986, p 46.

133. Goldaper, S: Woolridge admits to cocaine problem. The New York Times, February 24, 1988.

133a. Sports People. The New York Times, August 13, 1988.

134. Cantwell, JD and Rose, FD: Cocaine and cardiovascular events. Phys Sportsmed 14:77, 1986.

135. Monitoring the Future: A Continuing Study of the Lifestyles and Values of Youth. NIDA, Rockville, Maryland, 1987.

136. Alcohol, Drug Abuse, and Mental Health Administration: National Household Survey on Drug Abuse: Population Estimates 1985. National Institute on Drug Abuse. DHHS Pub. No. (ADM) 87-1539, 1987.

137. Alcohol, Drug Abuse, and Mental Health Administration: Data from the Drug Abuse Warning Network (DAWN). National Institute on Drug Abuse Statistical Series. DHHS Pub No. (ADM) 87-1530, 1987.

138. Anderson, WA and McKeag, DB: The Substance Use and Abuse Habits of College Student-Athletes. College of Human Medicine, Michigan State University. East Lansing, Michigan, June 1985.

139. Elite Women Athletes Survey. Hazelden Health Promotion Services, Minneapolis, Minnesota, 1987.

140. Gunby, P: Nation's expenditures for alcohol, other drugs, in terms of therapy, prevention, now exceeds $1.6 billion. JAMA 258:2023, 1987.

141. Castro, J: Battling the enemy within. Time, March 17, 1986, p 52.

142. Highlights of an attitude and knowledge survey about illegal drug use. NIDA Capsules, C-86-12, November, 1986.

143. Chapman, FS: The ruckus over medical testing. Fortune, August 19, 1985, p 57.

144. Brinkley, J: U.S. panel urges testing workers for use of drugs. The New York Times, March 3, 1986.

145. Breo, DL: Teams MDs call for mandatory drug tests. American Medical News, March 14, 1986, p 1.

146. Duda, M: Drug testing in professional sports. Phys Sportsmed 13(12):46, 1985.

147. Duda, M: Drug testing challenges college and pro athletes. Phys Sportsmed 12(11):109, 1984.

148. Topol, M: Drug testing gaining foothold. Newsday, July 9, 1985.

149. Rust, M: Drug deaths heat up testing debate. American Medical News, July 18, 1986, p 1.

150. Ryan, AJ: Drug testing in athletics: Is it worth the trouble? In Drug Test for Athletes—Pros and Cons. Phys Sportsmed 11(8):131, 1983.

151. Murray, TH: Drug testing and moral responsibility. Phys Sportsmed 14(11):47, 1986.

152. Begel, D: Medical problems of random drug test. The New York Times, May 26, 1985.

153. Smith, GM, Beecher, HK: Amphetamine sulfate and athletic performance: I. Objective effects. JAMA 170:542, 1959.

154. Smith, GM and Beecher, HK: Amphetamine, secobarbital and athletic performance: II. Subjective evaluations of performances, mood states, and physical stress. JAMA 172:1502, 1960.

155. Smith, GM and Beecher, HK: Amphetamine, secobarbital and athletic performance: III. Quantitative effects on judgment. JAMA 172:1623, 1960.

156. Ryan, AJ: Causes and remedies of drug misuse and abuse by athletes. JAMA 252:517, 1984.

157. Bell, J and Doege, TC: Athlete's use and abuse of drugs. Phys Sportsmed 15(3):99, 1987.

CHAPTER 2

Antecedents

It was not very many years ago, in the 1950s, that the illicit use of drugs was viewed as a smoldering phenomenon of the urban ghetto, removed from the mainstream of society's consciousness. While college students may have occasionally experimented with marijuana, suburban America acted as though it was immune to the worry, frustration, and ravages of drug abuse.

The 1960s witnessed a dramatic change in the sociology of drug abuse in the United States. It was a time of social upheaval and crisis—a period characterized by the struggle for civil rights, the Black Power movement, and the assassination of Martin Luther King, John F. Kennedy, and Robert Kennedy. Protests over the war in Vietnam and riots in the cities dominated the headlines. College campuses became the foci for challenging traditional values and attitudes. Psychoactive and psychedelic drugs became a vehicle of altered consciousness and of escape advocated by the likes of Harvard's Timothy Leary. From the streets of Greenwich Village in New York and Haight Ashbury in San Francisco, drug abuse—from marijuana to heroin, from LSD to mescaline, from amphetamine to cocaine—found its way to suburbia, to the middle class, and flourished.

Surveys detailing the incidence and prevalence of drug abuse have been reported over the past 2 decades. The most notable of these are the two on-going surveys sponsored by the National Institute on Drug Abuse. The first, *Monitoring the Future*, initiated in 1975 by the University of Michigan, examines samples of high school seniors annually, while continuing to follow-up on subsets of these seniors since their graduation. The second, the *National Household Sur-*

vey, analyzes drug abuse in general household populations annually and bi-annually. Differences in research design account for data that at times seem conflicting, contradictory, and confusing. Nonetheless, several factors remain clear:

1. Drug abuse, both licit and illicit, remains a major public health problem. It has been estimated that 24 million Americans use illicit drugs every month.[1]

2. Stereotypic images of drug abusers are inappropriate.

3. Drug abuse increased at an alarming rate during the late 1970s and early 1980s. Recent data from high school seniors suggest that the prevalence of licit and illicit drug use may be decreasing.[2]

4. Alcohol continues to be the most abused drug in the United States. Three million teenagers are problem drinkers.[3] As many as 30 to 40 percent of the 80 to 90 percent of the United States population that drink develop some temporary alcohol-related problem at some time during their lives. An additional 8 to 10 percent of men and 3 to 5 percent of women actually fulfill the criteria for the diagnosis of alcoholism.[4]

WHO IS AT RISK?

A vast body of literature addresses the question, "Who is at risk of drug abuse?" but provides no simplistic answers. As noted by Beschner,[5] "No one factor—whether it be pursuit of pleasure, relief from boredom or psychic distress, peer influence, or family problems such as a broken home—can adequately explain why a youngster becomes involved with drugs." According to Newcomb and associates,[6] researchers have suggested that ". . . there are probably many diverse paths to drug use and that looking for the definitive path or cause is doomed to failure since this may very well not exist." However, an understanding of many of the antecedents and risk factors of drug abuse is possible, and facilitates early identification and management of this problem.

AGE

Adolescence

Drug abuse before age 15 appears to predict future serious abuse disorders.[7] Thus, it is disconcerting that drug abuse has been starting at increasingly younger ages.[8] As an example, in 1978, approximately 20 percent of eighth-grade students reported the use of illicit drugs, whereas in 1971, the number stood at only 8 percent.[9]

The widespread use of drugs among adolescents is well known, and adolescence per se may be construed as a risk factor. Adolescent drug use has been documented in all populations of teenagers without respect for ethnic, social, racial, or economic lines. For many adolescents, drug use is a rite of passage.[10]

The 1987 survey of more than 16,000 high school seniors, sponsored by the National Institute on Drug Abuse, revealed disconcerting prevalence rates but some encouraging trends relative to adolescent drug abuse (Table 2–1). Reported marijuana and alcohol usage decreased between 1980 and 1987. However, nearly 57 percent of the surveyed high school seniors admitted trying an illicit drug at some time. Ten percent of the seniors reported that they had tried cocaine, as contrasted with 12 percent in 1980 and 6 percent in 1975.[2]

In 1985, 2.7 million adolescents between ages 12 and 17 reported using marijuana in the 30 days prior to a national survey, and 7.1 million people between ages 18 and 25 reported using marijuana in the same period. Thus, 9.8 million young people between ages 12 and 25 reported using marijuana in the 30-day period, whereas 8.4 million individuals age 26 or older reported using the agent during the same time-frame.[11]

Not all alcohol and drug use should be construed as representing problem behavior. For many, limited experimentation with alcohol and drugs represents a part of the process of developing independence as one begins to approach adulthood. Care must be exercised, according to Baumrind,[12] in distinguishing between health-compromising risk-taking behavior, which is ultimately harmful, and growth-enhancing limit-testing behavior, which is ultimately positive and contributes to optimal competence. Although the majority of adolescents use one or more drugs at some time, only a minority become considerably involved with drug abuse.[13] As emphasized by Jessor and Jessor,[14] adolescent experimentation with drugs is so omni-

Table 2–1. TRENDS IN DRUG USE AMONG HIGH SCHOOL SENIORS,
1975 TO 1987

Drugs Used	Percent Reported Using Drug		
	Class of 1975	Class of 1980	Class of 1987
Marijuana			
Used in past year	40	49	36
Used in past month	27	34	21
Daily use	6	9	3
Alcohol			
Used in past year	85	88	86
Used in past month	68	72	66
Daily use	6	6	5
5+ drinks in a row/last 2 weeks	37	41	38
Cigarettes			
Used in past year	NA*	NA*	NA*
Used in past month	37	31	29
Daily use	27	21	19
Cocaine			
Used in past year	6	12	10
Used in past month	2	5	4
Daily use	0.1	0.2	0.3
Illicit Drugs			
Ever used	55	65	57
Used in past year	45	53	42

*Data not available.
From Johnston and Bachman.[2]

present that the need to come to terms with oneself in relation to abusive substances is a major developmental task of adolescence. With this in mind, health care professionals must come to terms with themselves to avoid diagnosing psychopathology in normal adolescents.

Problem adolescent drug abuse tends to be sequential. Experimentation with and use of alcohol and tobacco in early adolescence tend to progress to experimentation with and use of marijuana and other illicit drugs in later adolescence, and eventually to the use of prescribed psychoactive drugs in young adulthood.[15,16] So significant is the sequential process of initiation into drug abuse that "the probability that individuals who never use marijuana will initiate the use of other illicit drugs is very low."[17] Men and women are similar with respect to this sequential process, with one notable exception: Tobacco appears to play a particularly important role for women in the progression of their drug involvement.[16]

Young Adulthood

The sequential process of initiation into drug abuse peaks at age 18 and subsequently declines, so that by the mid 20s there is essentially no new initiation into the use of alcohol and tobacco.[18] Similarly, during the mid to late 20s, there is essentially no initiation into the use of illicit drugs such as heroin and psychedelics. The most important predictor of drug use in early adulthood, particularly in the first 3 years following high school, is the individual's drug use habits in high school.[19]

Specifically with respect to alcohol, a follow-up study of "problem" drinkers in adolescence and 7 years later revealed interesting findings.[20] In the initial study, when the subjects were adolescents, problem drinking was defined as being drunk more than 6 times in the past year, or having experienced negative consequences owing to drinking 2 or more times in the past year, in 3 or more of the 6 following areas:

1. Trouble with teachers
2. Difficulties with friends
3. Criticism from dates
4. Driving under the influence of alcohol
5. Trouble with parents
6. Trouble with the police

At the end of 7 years, in the follow-up study, problem drinking was defined as being drunk 6 or more times in the past 6 months or experiencing 3 or more of the following consequences as a result of drinking in the same period:

1. Interpersonal problems (criticism from friends and family about their drinking)
2. Job-related problems (missing work or calling in sick owing to drinking; being told that drinking was creating problems on the job)
3. Trouble with the police
4. Financial problems
5. Accidents caused by drinking
6. Problems with spouse or person living with the drinker
7. Driving under the influence

The findings revealed that 53 percent of the men and 70 percent of the women previously identified as problem drinkers were no longer so categorized. However, the remainder did persist as problem drinkers—a sizable minority. Interestingly, women were much more likely to abandon problem drinking as they entered adulthood.

The antecedents of continued problem drinking as measured by personality-system measures included a lower value on academic achievement, a lower expectation of academic achievement, and a higher value on independence relative to achievement. Other indicators of continued problem drinking into young adulthood included fewer controls over other problem behaviors such as higher acceptance of socially unacceptable behavior, more positive reasons for marijuana use, and less religiosity.

Young adulthood represents a period of transition in three major areas—living arrangements/marital status, employment status, and educational status. Of the three, it has been reported that post–high school living arrangements/marital status seem to have the greatest influence on drug usage patterns in this age group. Those who continued to live with their parents showed no significant change in their drug usage patterns. Those who married and moved out decreased their drug usage; those who moved away from their parents to live with a member of the opposite sex or in some other living arrangement increased their drug usage.[19]

Earlier data indicated an apparent exception to the sequential patterns of drug abuse by young adults—the initiation into cocaine use.[16] Up to 90 percent began using cocaine, without significant prior drug usage, between ages 26 and 29.[18] However, patterns of cocaine usage are changing considerably; initiation into cocaine usage is beginning at a much younger age, and despite the reported decrease in cocaine use among high school students, the incidence of adolescent cocaine abuse has increased faster than that for any other drug.[9] Data reported in 1984 from the national telephone helpline, "800-COCAINE," has provided insight into the adolescent cocaine abuser.[9] Males outnumber females 2 to 1; 83 percent are white; and the average age of the user is approximately 16. Most are in the 11th or 12th grade. Thirty-eight percent come from families with an annual income greater than $25,000, with many coming from middle- and upper-class backgrounds. Consumption ranged from 1 to 4 grams per week, with a weekly expenditure averaging $95. Eighty-eight percent used cocaine intranasally; 10 percent freebased the drug. Undoubtedly, the data will change considerably with the ready availability of the very powerful and less expensive form of cocaine, crack.

GENETICS

Alcohol

Epidemiology

The role of genetics in drug abuse has been a subject of increased interest in recent decades. However, the observation that alcoholism runs in families dates back thousands of years and was the subject of commentary by the likes of Aristotle and Plutarch, who noted "drunkards beget drunkards."[21]

Over the past 2 decades, many studies have been undertaken to define to what extent alcoholism is, in fact, heritable. Such studies have been prompted by the observation that "about one of every four or five sons of alcoholics (in North America and Western Europe) became alcoholic; about five percent to ten percent of the daughters became alcoholic."[21] To date, far fewer studies have addressed the issue of familial transmission in other forms of drug abuse and addiction. An analysis of the genetic contribution to drug abuse requires that the contribution of environmental factors be eliminated or minimized. Put differently, a distinction must be made between the word "familial" and the word "genetic." This is particularly important in the analysis of the genetics of drug abuse because of the important role the biologic parents play in the environment of a drug abuser.

The issue of "nature" versus "nurture" has been addressed most substantively with respect to alcohol abuse and addiction.[22] Both twin studies and adoption studies have shed considerable light on the contribution of genetics to alcohol abuse and addiction.[21-26]

The study of twins has been considered a good way to assess the genetic versus the environmental contribution of a given behavioral trait. If a given behavior, such as the tendency to alcoholism, has a genetic component, then there should be a substantially higher concordance rate in identical twins than in fraternal twins. Although not all the twin studies of alcoholism are in agreement, the evidence appears to indicate that the likelihood of alcohol abuse and alcoholism is substantially greater in an identical twin of an alcoholic than in a fraternal twin. Specifically, if one twin is alcoholic, then the likelihood of an identical twin being alcoholic approximates 60 percent or more. On the other hand, if one twin is an alcoholic, the likelihood of a fraternal twin being alcoholic is 30 percent or less.[23]

The genetic contribution to alcoholism is even more impressive when adoption studies are considered. These studies, which began in the early 1970s, were conducted in Sweden, Denmark, and the United States.[21,23] The purpose of the studies was to assess the incidence of alcohol-related problems in children who were removed from their alcoholic biologic parents at the time of birth. Sons of alcoholic parents were three to four times more likely to be alcoholic than the sons of nonalcoholic parents; being raised by an alcoholic adoptive parent did not further in-

crease the risk.[3,21,27] This observation refuted the notion that alcoholics took up drinking simply because they learned it at home.

Cloninger and colleagues[25] employed adoption studies in an attempt to assess the relative contribution of "nature and nurture" to alcoholism. They noted ". . . that the susceptibility to alcoholism is neither entirely genetic, nor entirely environmental, nor simply the sum of separate genetic and environmental contributions. Rather, specific combinations of predisposing genetic factors and environmental stressors appear to interact before alcoholism develops in most persons."[25]

Cloninger and colleagues[25] identified two types of alcohol abuse that have different genetic and environmental causes (Table 2-2). One group, which is only found in men, they called "male-limited" (Type II) alcoholism, which represents a particularly severe form of alcoholism. In Cloninger and Bohman's study, about 25 percent of all male alcoholic subjects fit this category, and their alcoholism did not appear to be affected by the environment. As a group, these alcoholics tended to drink heavily before age 25, tended to have poor work records, had extensive criminal records, and had many attempts at treatment. Their course seems to be more severe and more fulminating. Alcoholism apppeared to occur nine times more frequently in the male sons of these alcoholics than in the general population.

The other group, which they called "milieu-limited" (Type I) alcoholism, accounted for approximately 75 percent of their subjects. This group, which was composed of both men and women, appeared to require both a genetic predisposition as well as certain environmental stressors to bring out their alcoholism. As a group, they tended to drink chronically after age 25, had relatively few problems with the law, and frequently were able to stop drinking. The offspring of these alcoholics were only twice as likely to have trouble with alcohol as the general population. The severity of alcoholism in the "milieu-limited" group ranged from mild to severe, with environmental factors being an important determinant of severity.

Having established a genetic contribution to most forms of alcoholism, there are many nonfamilial, sporadic cases of alcoholism in which neither parent has a clinically appar-

Table 2–2. PROFILE OF PROMINENT FEATURES DISTINGUISHING
TWO TYPES OF ALCOHOLISM

	Type 1 (Milieu-Limited)	Type 2 (Male-Limited)
Prevalence in adopted men, %	13	4
Biologic father's characteristics	Mild alcohol abuse, minimal criminality, no treatment	Severe alcohol abuse, severe criminality, extensive treatment
Biologic mother's characteristics	Mild alcohol abuse, minimal criminality	Normal
Postnatal environment	Determines both frequency and severity of alcoholism in susceptible sons	No effect on frequency (may influence severity)
Severity of alcoholism	Usually isolated or mild problems, but may be severe	Usually recurrent or moderate problems, but may be severe
Relative risk in congenitally predisposed sons*	Two with postnatal provocation; 1 without postnatal provocation	Nine regardless of postnatal milieu

*This relative risk is the ratio of the risk of alcoholism in congenitally predisposed sons to that in others. Thus, a relative risk of 1 indicates no difference.
From Cloninger, Bohman, and Sigvardsson,[25] with permission.

ent alcohol abuse disorder. However, even within this group there may exist individuals whose parents carry the genetic make-up for alcoholism, but who, because of environmental reasons, do not become alcoholics. As a group, nonfamilial alcoholics tend to show signs of alcohol dependence at a later age than familial alcoholics and tend to have a less severe form of dependence.[21] Recent estimates suggest that as many as 30 percent of alcoholics have no family history of the disease.[28]

Although alcoholism and major affective disorders are genetically influenced and often co-exist, it appears from adoption and other studies that the genetic component of alcoholism is inherited independent of psychopathology such as depression and sociopathy.[3,21]

There have been fewer studies of the genetic contribution to female alcoholism, but there does appear to be a genetic component as well.[29] Parenthetically, although women begin the early stages of alcohol abuse at a later age than men, they reach the later stages of alcoholism at about the same time as men.[30] Although no specific sex linkage has been demonstrated with respect to the genetics of alcoholism, it has been observed in a Swedish adoption study that alcoholism in the biologic mother predicted alcohol abuse in the daughters, but alcoholism in the

fathers did not.[31] Adoption studies have suggested that, as a rule, the drinking patterns of adoptees parallel those of their biologic parent of like gender—so-called gender-mediated alcoholism.[25,26,31]

Biologic Markers

With respect to genetic vulnerability to alcoholism, a number of hypotheses have been put forward; but to date, no clear-cut genetic pattern has been established. A number of attempts also have been made to identify biologic markers that could be used to identify individuals at risk of alcoholism prior to the development of the disease. In this regard, several clinical, biologic, and electrophysiologic observations are noteworthy.[23,32,33] In the research laboratory, individuals with a genetic risk of alcoholism appear to experience less subjective intoxication, as well as less body sway, from a given amount of alcohol than individuals with a negative family history of alcoholism.[34] Additionally, studies of cognitive and psychomotor performance have been suggestive of a greater degree of impairment from alcohol in the genetically low-risk group.[33] These observations have suggested the presence of some genetically determined "protective" factor in the high-risk individuals that appears to insulate them from many of the adverse reactions of modest doses of alcohol.

One specific population group appears to have a rather distinct inherited response to alcohol, which, in effect, acts as a biologic deterrent to alcoholism. Over 80 percent of a group of 82 Asian (Japanese, Taiwanese, and Korean) adults have been reported to experience a cutaneous flush, particularly of the upper body, after consuming very small amounts of alcohol.[35] This flush is accompanied by other physiologic reactions, including feelings of warmth and queasiness, an increase in heart rate, and a drop in blood pressure. Japanese and Taiwanese infants have been shown to have a similar flushing reaction to tiny amounts of alcohol. In the United States, American Indians have similarly exhibited a sensitivity to alcohol manifested by facial flushing and other vasomotor symptoms.[32]

Aldehyde dehydrogenase (ALDH) is a key enzyme required for the metabolism of alcohol. Alcohol is initially metabolized in the liver by alcohol dehydrogenase to acetaldehyde. The acetaldehyde in turn is metabolized in the liver by ALDH. Approximately 50 percent of Asian populations of Mongoloid extraction lack an isoenzyme of ALDH, which is referred to as ALDH I. It appears that this lack of ALDH I has resulted from a mutation of human chromosome 12, which is genetically transmitted. The deficiency of ALDH I and the consequent increased levels of acetaldehyde are, in part, responsible for the adverse vasomotor reactions to alcohol in the aforementioned populations.[32,36] In addition to acetaldehyde, prostaglandins, catecholamines, and histamine have been implicated in producing the flushing reaction in this population.[37]

Three biologic markers associated with alcoholism that have genetic overtones are: (1) plasma cortisol levels after ingestion of alcohol, (2) alterations in platelet enzyme activity, and (3) alterations in adenosine receptor-stimulated cAMP signal transduction. With respect to cortisol levels, Schuckit and colleagues[34] have demonstrated that the sons of alcoholics consistently have lower cortisol levels after drinking than the sons of nonalcoholics. With respect to platelet enzyme activity, Tabakoff[38] has shown that the inhibition of monoamine oxidase by ethanol is significantly higher in the platelets of alcoholics than in those of controls, and that stimulation of platelet adenylate cyclase activity by guanine nucleotide, cesium fluoride, and prostaglandin E_1 is significantly reduced. The results are too preliminary to conclude whether these changes were due to alcoholism or were present prior to the abuse of alcohol.[38,39] Nagy and colleagues[39a] demonstrated an independent genetically determined alteration in cAMP signal transduction, in addition to the previously shown suppression of adenosine receptor-stimulated cAMP levels in lymphocytes exposed to ethanol. Their findings may have important implications in the development of dependence and tolerance since adenosine mediates some of the effects of ethanol in the brain.

Electrophysiologic studies have similarly opened up new areas of research into the genetics of alcoholism.[23] Brainstem evoked-response studies of both high-risk and low-risk pre-adolescents have revealed a difference in the response in the two groups. Specifically, there is a diminished response in the P300 wave in pre-adolescents who are in the genetic high-risk group. Other than being a marker of genetic vulnerability to alcoholism, however, the significance of this observation remains speculative. A parallel observation is the decrease in alpha (8 to 13 Hz) and slow theta and delta waves (<8 Hz) and an increase in beta (>13 Hz) waves, the significance of which is also speculative.

Other Drugs

Genetic studies of drug abuse and addiction are almost nonexistent. Although there have been no reported twin studies of drug abusers, a Danish adoption study suggested that two separate genetic pathways influence drug abuse and addiction. The first pathway relates to the inheritability of antisocial behavior from the biologic parents and the consequent abuse of drugs as a manifestation of the inherited antisocial behavior (a factor in alcoholism as well).[40]

The second pathway, although statistically less sound, suggests that the offspring of alcoholic parents carry an increased tendency toward drug abuse independent of any antisocial behavior. Furthermore, the multiplicity of abused drugs found in this study suggests the existence of some inherited common biochemical or psychosocial mechanism that is independent of the metabolism of any specific drug. With respect to this second pathway, Goodwin,[21] citing a Danish adoption study, concluded that familial alcoholism does not increase the possibility the person will abuse other substances. However, before definitive conclusions can be drawn regarding the heritability of drug abuse, detailed studies will need to be done, similar to those performed for alcohol. Given the multiple classes of abused drugs and their varied pharmacologic properties, scientific studies must replace the often used term "other substances" by identifying the specific drugs of abuse.

FAMILY FACTORS (NONGENETIC)

Americans have undergone a substantial change in family life over the past 50 years. Economic and educational opportunities, together with the modernization of transportation, have decentralized the family. Closely knit extended families of aunts, uncles, grandparents, brothers, and sisters increasingly have become the exception rather than the rule. The increased accessibility to social institutions has resulted in a weakening of support structures within the family unit.

Divorce, working mothers, and single-parent families have compounded the above changes. Changes have also occurred in parenting styles, the implications of which remain unclear, particularly as they relate to the initiation of adolescent drug abuse.[41,42]

Over the past quarter century, adolescent drug experimentation in and of itself can no longer be classified officially as pathologic behavior.[12,43] The adolescent years represent a particularly important stage in the developmental process, during which drug abusing behaviors do or do not become established.[44] During these years of adolescence, both parents and siblings have been identified as important influences on the young person's future drug abusing behavior.

It has been consistently reported that adolescents from families in which one or more members smoke, drink, or take other drugs are more likely to use mind-altering substances than adolescents whose families do not use such drugs.[45] Children of alcoholics have been reported to have not only high incidences of abusing alcohol and other drugs,

but to have higher than normal incidences of psychiatric disorders as well. The latter include anorexia nervosa, neuroses, antisocial behavioral disorders, hyperactivity, and psychosomatic disorders.[46] Family instability has been associated with an excess incidence of substance abuse, whereas parental religious involvement has been associated with a low incidence of substance abuse.[43]

Poor family management and interactions contribute to substance abuse behaviors.[46] Included in such behaviors are poor communication patterns, inconsistent rules, excessive demands, persistent family strife, lack of praise, and negative parental feedback fostering low self-esteem. Conversely, positive family communication patterns appear to be associated with a lowered incidence of drug abuse, particularly when these positive family patterns were developed before adolescence began.

When considering parental influence on adolescent drug abuse behavior, one must be specific about which substance is being abused. Parental alcohol abuse and adolescent alcohol abuse correlate directly; little or no relationship shows up between the initiation into adolescent marijuana use and any other type of drug use by the parents.[26,41,45,47] With respect to the initiation into the use of other illicit drugs by the adolescent, it appears that poor parent-child relationships play a much stronger role.[41] Additionally, parental reliance on drugs to deal with life crises has been proposed as a role-model coping mechanism that contributes to adolescent drug abuse.[47]

Any consideration of the role of the family on a youngster's drug abusing behavior must consider the influence of siblings in addition to that of the parents.[45] Although research in the area has been limited, several observations suggest that at least for alcohol, cigarette, and marijuana use, the behavior of an older sibling produces a stronger influence than that of the parents. When an older sibling uses alcohol, cigarettes, or marijuana, the younger sibling tends to use these drugs at an earlier age than do adolescents without older siblings. Conversely, adolescents with older siblings who used drugs either not at all or sparingly tended to use these drugs less frequently and to initiate their usage at a later age. Older siblings often serve as a source of these drugs. Similar observations with respect to older sibling influences on an adolescent have also been noted for a broader range of abused drugs.

PEERS

Peers have long been considered to be the most important influence in determining an individual's drug abusing attitudes and behaviors.[45] It has been suggested that drug use represents a way of belonging to, identifying with, and being accepted by a particular peer group.[4] Some, however, also hold that the concept of "peer pressure" has been both oversimplified[43] and understudied.[41]

Over the past 3 decades, the reliance on one's peer group has assumed increasing importance for the adolescent as parental involvement has diminished.[42] Even the relatively autonomous adolescent will comply with the standards of his or her peer group to a degree so as to achieve status within the group.[12]

Although the term adolescence was first used in 1904, it remains imprecisely defined. It is a period that generally begins by age 12 and ends by age 22. All agree that adolescence is a time of transition, a time of change—biologic, emotional, social, intellectual. The peer group has been dubbed "the lifeline for adolescents."[42] The peer group has a greater influence than do parents on an adolescent's drug abusing behavior except in alcohol abuse, where, as noted already, parental patterns appear to be the strongest influence.

There is no precise age when parental influence diminishes and peer influence increases. Rather, adolescence is an evolutionary process, during which young persons derive progressively less protection and information from their parents and, at the same time, seek increasing support from and choose more interaction with their peers.[13] The relative influence of family and peers does not affect all areas of life equally. In some areas, such as educational objectives, moral and social values, and vocational plans, parental influence appears to dominate. With respect to shorter term issues, such as dress styles, leisure time activities, language, and the use and nonuse of alcohol and drugs, peer group influences appear stronger. Peer group dynamics can represent a positive support structure during adolescence by offering opportunities for advice, exploration, and dialogue. On the other hand, peer group dynamics can undermine the spirit by manipulation and coercion and stifle individuality through the pressures of conformity.

With respect to drug use, peer marijuana use appears to be the strongest predictor of an adolescent's marijuana use.[17,41,48] With respect to alcohol, parental drinking patterns, particularly the father's, appear to be the strongest interpersonal predictor of alcohol abuse, although the behavior of peers is also a factor.[47] The use of other illicit drugs by an adolescent seems to be influenced by a combination of both family and peer usage of these drugs. The actual initiation into drug use most often occurs through the influences of close friends or best friends, rather than through drugs being offered by strangers.[49] Yet, the adolescent at risk of drug abuse has a particular vulnerability manifested by an inability to develop intimate and meaningful relationships with peers.[41]

EDUCATION

Although a large body of literature addresses the adverse effects of drug abuse on academic performance, few hard data deal with the question of education as a predictor of future drug abuse. In 1978, Kandel and associates[47] assessed degree of academic orientation as an antecedent of adolescent initiation (first experience) into drug abuse in New York State high school students. The variables of academic orientation that were studied were: number of classes cut, grade-point average, number of days absent, and educational expectations. For the purposes of this study, drug abuse was divided into three categories: hard liquor, marijuana, and other illicit drugs. The investigators found significant correlations between the number of classes cut and the initiation into hard liquor or marijuana, whereas low grades in school correlated only weakly with initiation into marijuana use. It is noteworthy that academic orientation did not differentiate those who began using other illicit drugs from those who did not. Jessor and colleagues[50] have noted that proneness to marijuana usage correlates with a greater value on independence than on academic achievement, and with lower expectations for academic achievement.

The initiation phase of drug abuse aside, it has been observed that high school seniors who have aspirations of completing college have lower rates of alcohol and illicit drug abuse than those who do not expect to complete college.[2] Similarly, individuals who quit school prematurely carry a significantly increased risk of drug abuse.[51] A 7-year follow-up study of high school students who were considered to have "problem drinking" in high school, which continued in young adulthood, revealed that the persistent problem drinking correlated with lower academic achievement and with lower academic expectations.[20]

The use of standard IQ tests as a predictor of future drug abuse has been of limited value and has been influenced by the demographics of the populations that were studied. One such study[26] analyzed 524 primarily Caucasian working-class children from a child guidance clinic in the St. Louis area. The subjects were followed over a 30-year period, beginning in the 1920s and early 1930s. A large percentage subsequently became alcoholic. When compared with a control group, the individuals who subsequently became alcoholic not only tended to have antisocial traits, but also had had, as children, lower IQ scores, as well as greater tendencies toward truancy. The fact that these children were initially referred to a child guidance program for various behavioral problems obviously biased the sample and limits conclusions derived from the study.

Contrary results with respect to the predictive value of IQ scores were reported in a prospective study of 1,242 first-grade students from a predominantly black, relatively poor section of Chicago. Initially studied in 1966 and 1967, 705 students were re-evaluated 10 years later at ages 16 and 17. Drug abuse was common, with 61.3 percent using marijuana or hashish and 8 percent using alcohol. It was noted that high first-grade IQ scores correlated with high rates of drug use during adolescence for both males and females. Conversely, low first-grade IQ scores correlated with low rates of adolescent drug use.[52]

With respect to drug abuse and higher education, the findings also have been contradictory, with some reports indicating higher drug use in college students than in nonstudents, others reporting lower drug use, and still others finding no difference.[53] Given the complex sociology of substance abuse, the significance of any statistical analysis requires that it be contemporary and address precisely the extent of the substance abuse as well as the specific substance abused, for example, snorted cocaine versus crack, beer versus hard liquor, etc.

MENTAL HEALTH

A considerable literature has been developed over the years assessing the psychodynamic, psychopharmacologic, and behavioral aspects of alcohol and drug abuse. Even a brief survey of this literature is beyond the scope of this book; however, a number of concepts and observations deserve highlighting. Most of this research has focused on two drugs, alcohol and heroin, with an emphasis on addiction and dependency. Less emphasis has been placed on the broader issue of drug abuse in the absence of addiction and dependency.

Psychodynamics

Psychodynamics, the systematized knowledge and theory of human behavior and its motivations,[54] views the personality organization or the character development of an individual, that is, how he or she interacts with the environment. In general terms, there appears to be a high degree of correlation between the severity of a personality disorder and the extent of drug abuse. Certain elements of character development have been specifically associated with the development of drug dependency. These include problems with affect management, problems with closeness to others and with self-esteem, and problems with judgment and self-care as manifested by an inability to anticipate harm and avoid danger.[55]

Affect, or emotion, can be described as the feeling, whether pleasurable or painful, that accompanies an idea. Affects serve as subjective signals. They serve as a feedback mechanism, indicating the approach of satisfaction or satiation and the relaxation of tension, or they serve as subjective signals warning of threat or the lack of satisfaction.[54] When an affective state is maintained for a reasonable period of time, it is referred to as a *mood*. Psychoactive drugs alter the affect or the feeling state. Furthermore, the preference or selection of a specific drug category by a drug-dependent individual appears to be, at least in part, determined by the dominant painful affective state with which an individual struggles.[56,57]

Dominant affects reported in drug-dependent individuals include aggression, rage, fear, anxiety, loneliness, depression, dysphoria or unpleasant feelings, restlessness, and hyperactivity. In reviewing the work of numerous authors with respect to drug abuse and disorders of affect management, Treece and Khantzian[55] concluded ". . . that the substances are used by the individual to bolster, support, and compensate for inadequate internal regulatory mechanisms including those for defense, self-soothing, and modulation of affect."

The drug-dependent individual often exhibits defects in character development, manifested by difficulties in forming close and intimate relationships. Coupled with this characterologic defect goes a defect or disturbance in self-esteem and narcissism, that is, the satisfaction of inner needs and the preservation of a sense of well being. With respect to these defects, Treece and Khantzian[55] noted: "Narcissistic vulnerabilities and the disturbances in relationships that they engender are presumed also to predispose to drug dependence . . . via the need to ameliorate the rage, shame, loneliness, anxiety, and depression that are a consequence."

Lastly, drug dependency appears to correlate with a characterologic defect whereby the drug-dependent individual fails to anticipate harm and to avoid danger. Treece and Khantzian[55] dubbed this quality as a "self-care deficit." The failure to experience fear, where fear is a normal protective response, leads to inappropriate risk taking and impulsivity. The use of illicit drugs in and of itself may be viewed as such an expression of a defect in judgment.

Self-Medication Concept

Initial studies of drug addiction focused almost exclusively on narcotics. Explanations for self-selecting narcotics ranged from pleasure seeking to relief from anxiety, pain, and stress. Wurmser,[56] in his classic paper, "Psychoanalytic Considerations of the Etiology of Compulsive Drug Use," stated: "I consider all compulsive drug use as an attempt at self treatment." In the same paper, Wurmser quotes Wieder and Kaplan, who in 1969, noted: "The dominant conscious motive for drug use is not the seeking of 'kicks', but the wish to produce pharmacologically a reduction in distress that the individual cannot achieve by his own psychic efforts."

Research in psychodynamic theory and in psychopharmacology has attempted to dissect the concept of self-medication with respect to drug abuse. Khantzian[57] hypothesized that narcotic and cocaine addicts do not randomly choose their drug of addiction. Rather, following experimentation with a number of drugs, they choose the one whose action best meets their needs. Stated differently, addicts, in their choice of a drug, are attempting to treat themselves with a drug that will provide relief from a psychiatric problem or a painful emotional state. Khantzian thus postulates that the choice of a drug class or of a specific drug is related to its psychopharmacologic properties. For example, opiates are chosen because they exhibit anti-rage and anti-aggression properties, whereas, in the same individual, alcohol and sedatives may actually precipitate feelings of rage and aggression. Cocaine, on the other hand, may be selected through a trial-and-error process in individuals with chronic depression or in individuals who suffer low self-esteem or lack assertiveness.[58] The increased use of physician-prescribed psychoactive drugs by young adults who used illicit drugs during adolescence is consistent with this formulation.[15]

Classification of Psychiatric Disorders

Psychiatrists classify psychiatric disorders in accordance with a very specific and official classification format that is published in a text entitled: Diagnostic and Statistical Manual of Mental Disorders, DSM-III-R, 1987 Revised Third Edition.[74] For the most part, each person's psychiatric disorder is viewed from three separate perspectives, with each perspective referred to as an *Axis*.

Axis I: Clinical Syndromes

Axis II: Developmental Disorders and Personality Disorders

Axis III: Physical Disorders and Conditions

With respect to Axis I and Axis II, a typical diagnosis might read:

Axis I: Alcohol Dependence
Axis II: Borderline Personality Disorder

or

Axis I: Psychoactive Substance Dependence
Axis II: Antisocial Personality Disorder

Psychopathology

Depression

One form of psychopathology that appears to be highly correlated with many forms of drug abuse is depression.[59,60] The association of alcoholism and depression is well known,[60,61] although the nature of the association remains a subject of investigation. As Nace[62] has noted: "The alcoholic patient is very vulnerable to depression, but the risk of alcoholism for the primary depressed patient is less clear." Recently it has been reported that college males, ages 16 to 19, with a history of alcohol abuse were at least four times more likely to have a history of a major depressive disorder than similar young men who did not abuse alcohol. Similarly, college female adolescents were at least six times more likely to have had a major depressive disorder if they were alcohol abusers than those who were not. More often than not, the major depressive disorder preceded the onset of alcohol abuse.[60]

Hesselbrock and associates' study[63] of hospitalized alcoholics revealed that a major depression preceded severe alcohol abuse 65 percent of the time in women and 41 percent of the time in men. In Cadoret and Winokur's study[64] of 259 hospitalized alcoholics, 39 percent met diagnostic criteria for either a major or a minor primary or secondary depression. In a community survey of alcoholism, 65 percent of diagnosed alcoholics were diagnosed as having had a depression at some point in their lives, in addition to 18 percent who were diagnosed as having a depressive personality disorder.[61] Behar and colleagues' study[65] of 72 alcoholics who had

abstained for a mean of 64 months revealed that 15 percent had serious debilitating depressive symptoms, which began after a mean of 35 months of sobriety.

These correlations between depression and alcoholism have inspired studies of the familial transmission of depression and alcoholism, from which it has been concluded that alcoholism and depression are not alternate manifestations of the same underlying disorder.[66]

Similar correlations have been made between narcotic addiction and depression.[67-69] One-third or more of narcotic addicts were found at some point to suffer from moderate to severe depression. With respect to lifetime vulnerability to depression, Rounsaville reported that nearly 50 percent of 157 opiate addicts under age 30 studied had had at least 1 major depressive episode.[67] However, these major depressive episodes tended to be mild and of relatively short duration and appeared to be related to specific finite stresses such as legal and social problems.

Weiss and Mirin[70] have noted that the signs and symptoms of depression are evident in many cocaine abusers who are seeking treatment. He emphasized: "The clinician's task is to determine whether these are the result of cocaine withdrawal (crashing), a response to adverse life events engendered by chronic drug abuse, or an underlying primary affective disorder."

In assessing the role of depression in adolescent drug abuse among 424 college students between ages 16 and 19, Deykin and colleagues[60] noted that drug abusers, primarily marijuana abusers, were 3.3 times as likely as nonabusers to have a history of a major depressive disorder, with the depression preceding or occurring concurrently with drug abuse in the majority. The use of marijuana and subsequently other illicit drugs has been associated with a decrease in depressive mood symptoms during the course of a school year.[71,72]

Antisocial Personality Disorder

The association between drug abuse and antisocial behavior has long been recognized.[69,73] As defined in DSM-III-R,[74] an antisocial personality disorder "is a pattern of irresponsible and antisocial behavior beginning in childhood or early adolescence and continuing into adulthood." The individual must be at least age 18 and have had a conduct disorder before age 15. Examples of antisocial behaviors include repeated fights and assaults, spouse and child beating, reckless behavior without regard to others, promiscuity, unemployment when work is available, failure to honor financial obligations, failure to form significant attachments to others, disregard for truth, lack of remorse, and a great capacity to rationalize one's behavior. Previously, individuals with antisocial personality disorders carried the diagnosis of psychopath.

That there is a genetic pattern to the development of an antisocial personality is evidenced by the observation that, compared with the general population, this personality disorder is 5 times more common among first-degree biologic relatives of males with an antisocial personality disorder and 10 times more common in the first-degree biologic relatives of females with an antisocial personality disorder.[74] Mechanism aside, both men and women with a diagnosis of antisocial personality disorder suffer a high risk for alcoholism.[30,73] They are more likely to be exposed to alcoholism and, once exposed, are more susceptible to developing the full-blown syndrome.

Alcoholics with an antisocial personality tend to begin heavy drinking at an earlier age than their non-antisocial counterparts.[73] Similar observations have been made with respect to the relation of an antisocial personality disorder to other forms of drug abuse and addiction.[40,75,76] In fact, incidence reports of an antisocial personality disorder in as high as 29.3 percent of opiate addicts in therapeutic community treatment programs[76] and 26.5 percent for opiate addicts in a mix of therapeutic programs[75] are considered underestimates because of the insufficiently precise definitions of the diagnosis. Increasingly, former heroin addicts are turning to cocaine as their primary drug, at least in part because of the ready availability of cocaine. Weiss and Minin[70] have noted that many of these individuals have antisocial personality disorders. Adolescent drug abusers[77] tend to have similar characterologic traits, although the technical definition of an antisocial personality disorder requires a minimum age of 18. The specific association between so-called conduct disorders (under age 18) and

drug abuse remains a fertile area for future research.

Borderline Personality Disorder

A personality disorder akin to a childhood conduct disorder and to adult antisocial personality disorder is called a *borderline personality disorder*.[69,74] The condition can be diagnosed in childhood and adolescence, if it appears that the disturbance is pervasive and persistent and if it seems unlikely that it will change with time. Characteristic of the personality disorder is an instability of self-image, poor interpersonal relationships, and fluctuating mood. An instability of self-image is manifested by a marked and persistent identity disturbance, accompanied by chronic feelings of emptiness and boredom. Interpersonal relationships are often unstable or intense, and individuals with a borderline personality disorder have difficulty tolerating being alone. Mood swings are common, as evidenced by periods of depression, anxiety, and temper tantrums. Impulsivity may be evidenced by potentially self-damaging activities such as gambling, overeating, casual sex, and even self-mutilation. Another manifestation of impulsivity relates to a proclivity toward drug abuse. It has been suggested that drug abuse in individuals with borderline personality disorders represents a method of discharging anger, overcoming boredom, and warding off painful affect.[77]

Attention-Deficit Hyperactivity Disorder

Attention-deficit hyperactivity disorder (ADHD)[74] refers to a pediatric neuropsychiatric disorder, affecting 5 to 10 percent of children, characterized developmentally by inappropriate inattention, impulsivity, and hyperactivity. Associated features include low self-esteem and academic underachievement. Most children outgrow ADHD as they enter adolescence. However, about one third of the children continue to show signs of the condition into adulthood but without hyperactivity, leaving them with problems of inattention and impulsivity. Longitudinal studies have suggested that there is an association between childhood ADHD and subsequent adolescent and adult psychopathology, particularly antisocial behavior.[78] In adulthood, the disorder, which was referred to in DSM-III[79] as an Attention Deficit Disorder (ADD), residual type, currently falls under the rubric of undifferentiated attention-deficit disorder in DSM-III-R.[74]

A catecholamine-deficient state—in particular, a dopamine-deficient state—in ADHD has been postulated.[78] For this reason, dopamine agonists have been utilized in the treatment of this disorder. The central nervous system (CNS) stimulant most commonly used for this purpose is methylphenidate (Ritalin). In fact, many consider a response to methylphenidate to be diagnostic of this syndrome. However, using responsiveness to this drug as a basis for the diagnosis of ADD may lead to an inaccurate conclusion because the pharmacokinetics of the drug in a given patient may not have been considered.[80]

The stimulant effects of methylphenidate, *d*-amphetamine, and cocaine are mediated primarily through central dopaminergic pathways.[81] Thus, adults with ADD, residual type, in keeping with Khantzian's theory of self-medication, may self-select the central nervous system stimulant, cocaine.[70,81-84] However, cocaine abuse may further deplete dopamine stores (depletion of presynaptic dopamine consequent to a re-uptake blockade), and consequently cocaine withdrawal can produce marked ADHD symptomatology. Cocores and associates[84] have emphasized the need to distinguish between adult ADHD, bipolar disorder, and cocaine abuse, all of which can share many similar features—restlessness or hyperactivity, rapid or racing thoughts, impulsivity, and mood instability.

An unsettled question is the possible relationship between attention-deficit disorders and alcoholism. Wood[85] has speculated that attention-deficit disorders in childhood and adulthood may be associated with an increased risk for the development of alcoholism, suggesting that such a relationship may be partially mediated by genetic factors, whereby alcoholic parents have an increased likelihood of having hyperactive children. Recent work by Schuckit and colleagues,[86] however, has failed to substantiate that symptoms or syndromes involving hyperactivity relate closely to alcoholism.

Other Psychiatric Disorders

Numerous studies have documented an array of other psychiatric disorders that have been associated with drug abuse. Included are affective disorders other than depression, schizophrenia, anxiety disorders (including phobias), personality disorders other than antisocial personality, borderline personality disorders, and eating disorders.[60,68,69,76,87] Although the cited studies pertain primarily to the psychiatric diagnoses in adult alcoholics and opiate addicts, it is clear that psychiatric illnesses in adolescents frequently precede or occur concurrently with alcohol and drug abuse. In a study of 424 college students, of the 8.2 percent who met criteria for alcohol abuse and the 9.4 percent for other drug abuse, 79 percent had another primary psychiatric disorder anteceding the alcohol or drug abuse.[56]

Stress

In the 1920s, Harvard physiologist Walter Cannon began experimenting with the physiologic effect of stress on cats and dogs. In the 1940s and 1950s, Hans Selye, an endocrinologist at Montreal's Institute of Experimental Medicine and Surgery, demonstrated the importance of the concept of stress relative to the human condition. Selye defined two important terms—stressor and stress. A *stressor* referred to the external cause or stimulus, and *stress* referred to the state of bodily disequilibrium produced by the stressor.[88,89] He emphasized that "Stress does not necessarily imply a morbid change; normal life, especially intense pleasure and ecstasy of fulfillment, also causes some wear and tear in the body. Indeed, stress can even have curative value, as in shock therapy, bloodletting, and sports."[90] Thus, specific stressors, whether physical or psychological, can be either constructive or destructive. Similarly, the bodily disequilibrium, or the stress produced as the body attempts to adapt to a specific stressor, can be either favorable or unfavorable. The stressor and resultant stress can be either acute or chronic.

In an attempt to quantitate human stress, psychiatrists Thomas Holmes and Richard Rahe[91] developed a Social Readjustment Rating Scale (Table 2-3). Although the eco-

Table 2–3. SOCIAL READJUSTMENT RATING SCALE

Rank	Life Event	Mean Value
1	Death of spouse	100
2	Divorce	73
3	Marital separation	65
4	Jail term	63
5	Death of close family member	63
6	Personal injury or illness	53
7	Marriage	50
8	Fired at work	47
9	Marital reconciliation	45
10	Retirement	45
11	Change in health of family member	44
12	Pregnancy	40
13	Sex difficulties	39
14	Gain of new family member	39
15	Business readjustment	39
16	Change in financial state	38
17	Death of close friend	37
18	Change to different line of work	36
19	Change in number of arguments with spouse	35
20	Mortgage over $10,000	31
21	Foreclosure of mortgage or loan	30
22	Change in responsibilities at work	29
23	Son or daughter leaving home	29
24	Trouble with in-laws	29
25	Outstanding personal achievement	28
26	Wife begin or stop work	26
27	Begin or end school	26
28	Change in living conditions	25
29	Revision of personal habits	24
30	Trouble with boss	23
31	Change in work hours or conditions	20
32	Change in residence	20
33	Change in schools	20
34	Change in recreation	19
35	Change in church activities	19
36	Change in social activities	18
37	Mortgage or loan less than $10,000	17
38	Change in sleeping habits	16
39	Change in number of family get-togethers	15
40	Change in eating habits	15
41	Vacation	13
42	Christmas	12
43	Minor violations of the law	11

From Holmes and Rahe,[91] with permission.

nomic figures in Table 2–3 are outdated, the life events, which are listed in order of maximal to minimal stress, remain relevant.

Many chemical mediators of stress have been identified, including catecholamines, endorphins, prolactin, and serotonin, to name but a few. Although the discipline of psychopharmacology is new, physicians have long prescribed alcohol and other psychoactive drugs for the amelioration of excess stress. Indeed, chemicals have been used by humans throughout history as a means of coping with stress. It is therefore not surprising that the reduction of stress, tension, and anxiety have long been linked to drug abuse. Stated differently, drug abuse may be viewed as a method of "emotional self-regulation which requires little effort and ability, promises instant effects and provides a sense of control."[92]

As noted earlier, adolescence is a period during which persons develop coping skills to deal with the stresses associated with life's events. Coping may be defined "as the set of behavioral or cognitive responses that people use to deal with problematic events."[93] The manifestations of stress during adolescence peak twice, the first prepubertally between ages 11 and 13 and the second between ages 18 and 19.[77] By abusing alcohol and other drugs, the adolescent blunts the development of the coping skills necessary to deal with these stresses,[77] thereby prolonging adolescent behavior. In this regard, Labouvie's observations[92] regarding the use of alcohol and marijuana by teenagers to cope with stress are pertinent. In his study of adolescents from all but 5 counties in New Jersey, he noted that of all the users of alcohol, 44 percent relied on it at least sometimes as a reactive coping means. Similarly, of those who used alcohol and marijuana, 36 percent utilized drugs at least sometimes as a reactive coping means. These observations, together with an assessment of other mechanisms, led Labouvie to conclude that ". . . alcohol and drug use do not constitute one of the more common and more frequently used reactive coping behaviors and that the link between substance use and emotional self-regulation in adolescence is generally a weak one." On the other hand, he noted that adolescents who were regularly involved with the heavy use of alcohol and marijuana employed the use of these substances to a greater extent as a coping behavior.

The pervasiveness of stress in the United States is evidenced by the estimate that 70 percent of the population between ages 18 and 60 are under moderate to heavy stress.[94] Albeit an indirect measure, the medical use of benzodiazepine compounds in the United States is further evidence of the extent of stress-related disorders. In 1975, approximately 100 million prescriptions were written for benzodiazepines. In 1981, the number fell to 65 million and leveled off.[95] Viewed differently, household survey data for the United States in 1979 and 1981 showed that 11 to 13 percent of the adult population had taken an anxiolytic 1 or more times in the preceding year and that 2.3 to 2.5 percent of the population had taken anxiolytics on a daily basis for 4 months or longer. These statistics take into account neither other prescriptive psychoactive drugs for stress-related disorders nor the use of illicitly obtained drugs.

REFERENCES

1. Koroch, M: Group fights to keep alcohol, drug problems in forefront. Amer Med News, October 16, 1987, p 33.
2. Johnston, L and Bachman, J: The Monitoring the Future Study. Institute for Social Research, The University of Michigan, Ann Arbor, 1988.
3. MacDonald, DI: Patterns of alcohol and drug use among adolescents. Pediatr Clin North Am 34:275, 1987.
4. Schuckit, MA: Genetic and clinical implications of alcoholism and affective disorder. Am J Psychiatry 143:140, 1986.
5. Beschner, GM and Friedman, AS: Introduction. In Beschner, GM, Friedman, AS (eds): Youth Drug Abuse. DC Heath & Co, Washington, D.C., 1979, p 1.
6. Newcomb, MD, Maddahian, E, and Bentler, PM: Risk factors for drug use among adolescents: Concurrent and longitudinal analyses. Am J Public Health 76:525, 1986.
7. Robins, LN and Pryzbeck, TR: Age of onset of drug use as a factor in drug and other disorders. In Jones, CL and Battjes, RJ (eds): Etiology of Drug Abuse: Implications for Prevention. NIDA Research Monograph 56, Rockville, Maryland: NIDA, 1985, p 178.
8. Hawkins, JD, Lishner, DM, and Catalano, RF, Jr: Childhood predictors and the prevention of adolescent substance abuse. In Jones, CL and Battjes, RF (eds): Etiology of Drug Abuse: Implications for Prevention. NIDA Research Monograph 56, Rockville, Maryland: NIDA, p 75.
9. Semlitz, L and Gold, MS: Adolescent drug abuse: Diagnosis, treatment, and prevention. Psychiatr Clin North Am 9:455, 1986.
10. MacKenzie, RG and Jacobs, EA: Recognizing the adolescent drug abuser. Prim Care 14:225, 1987.
11. Schuster, CR: Substance abuse. JAMA 258:2269, 1987.
12. Baumrind, D: Familial antecedents of adolescent drug use: A developmental perspective. In Jones, CL and Battjes, RD (eds): Etiology of Drug Abuse: Implications for Prevention. NIDA Research Monograph 56, Rockville, Maryland: NIDA, 1985, p 13.
13. Norem-Hebeisen, A and Hedin, DP: II. Influences on adolescent problem behavior: Causes, connections, and contexts. In Adolescent Peer Pressure: Theory, Correlates, and Program Implications for Drug Abuse Prevention. DHHS Pub. No. (ADM) 81-1152, Rockville, Maryland, 1981, p 21.
14. Jessor, R and Jessor, SL: Adolescent development

and the onset of drinking. J Stud Alcohol 36:27, 1975.

15. Kandel, DB and Logan, JA: Patterns of drug use from adolescence to young adulthood: I. Periods for initiation, continued use and discontinuation. Am J Public Health 74:660, 1984.

16. Yamaguchi, K and Kandel, DB: Patterns of drug use from adolescence to young adulthood: II. Sequences of progression. Am J Public Health 74:668, 1984.

17. Yamaguchi, K and Kandel, DB: Patterns of drug use from adolescence to young adulthood: III. Predictors of progression. Am J Public Health 74:673, 1984.

18. Ravies, VH and Kandel, DB: Changes in drug behavior from the middle to the late twenties: Initiation, persistence, and cessation of use. Am J Public Health 77:607, 1987.

19. Bachman, JG, O'Malley, PM, and Johnston LD: Drug use among young adults: The impacts of role status and social environment. J Pers Soc Psychol 47:629, 1984.

20. Donovan, JE, Jessor, R, and Jessor L: Problem drinking in adolescence and young adulthood. J Stud Alcohol 44:109, 1983.

21. Goodwin, DW: Alcoholism and genetics. Arch Gen Psychiatry 42:171, 1985.

22. Goodwin, DW, et al: Alcohol problems in adoptees raised apart from alcoholic biologic parents. Arch Gen Psychiatry 28:238, 1973.

23. Schuckit, MA: Genetics and the risk of alcoholism. JAMA 254:2614, 1985.

24. Goodwin, DW, et al: Drinking problems in adopted and nonadopted sons of alcoholics. Arch Gen Psychiatry 31:164, 1974.

25. Cloninger, CR, Bohman, M, and Sigvardsson, S: Inheritance of alcohol abuse. Arch Gen Psychiatry 38:861, 1981.

26. Wilcox, JA: Adolescent alcoholism. J Psychoactive Drugs 17:77, 1985.

27. Schulsinger, F, et al: A prospective study of young men at high risk for alcoholism. Arch Gen Psychiatry 43:755, 1986.

28. Desmond, EW: Out in the open. Time Magazine, November 30, 1987, p 80.

29. Blume, S: Women and alcohol. JAMA 256:1467, 1986.

30. Stabenau, JR: Implications of family history of alcoholism, antisocial personality, and sex differences in alcohol dependence. Am J Psychiatry 141:1178, 1984.

31. Bohman, M, Sigvardsson, S, and Cloninger, R: Maternal inheritance of adopted women. Arch Gen Psychiatry 38:965, 1981.

32. Goedde, HW and Agarwal, DP: Genetics and alcoholism: Problems and perspectives. In Goedde, HW and Agarwal, DP (eds): Genetics and Alcoholism. Alan R. Liss, Inc, New York, 1987, p 3.

33. Schuckit, MA: Studies of populations at high risk for future development of alcoholism. In Goedde, HW and Agarwal, DP (eds): Genetics and Alcoholism. Alan R. Liss, Inc, New York, 1987, p 83.

34. Schuckit, MA, Gold, E, and Risch C: Plasma cortisol levels following ethanol in sons of alcoholics and controls. Arch Gen Psychiatry 44:942, 1987.

35. Wolff, PH: Ethnic differences in alcohol sensitivity. Science 175:449, 1972.

36. Harada, S, Agarwal, DP, and Goedde, HW: Aldehyde dehydrogenase deficiency as cause of facial flushing reaction to alcohol in Japanese. Lancet 2:982, 1981.

37. Miller, NS, et al: Histamine receptor antagonism of intolerance to alcohol in the Oriental population. J Nerv Ment Dis 175:661, 1987.

38. Tabakoff, B, et al: Differences in platelet enzyme activity between alcoholics and nonalcoholics. N Engl J Med 318:134, 1988.

39. Reich, T: Biologic marker studies in alcoholism. N Engl J Med 318:180, 1988.

39a. Nagy, LE, Diamond, I, and Gordon, A: Cultured lymphocytes from alcoholic subjects have altered cAMP signal transduction. Proc Natl Acad Sci USA 85:6973, 1988.

40. Cadoret, RJ, et al: An adoption study of genetic and environmental factors in drug abuse. Arch Gen Psychiatry 43:1131, 1986.

41. Glynn, TJ: From Family to Peer: Transitions of influence among drug-using youth. In Lettiere, DJ and Ludford, JP (eds): Drug Abuse and the American Adolescent. NIDA Research Monograph 38, Rockville, Maryland: NIDA, 1981, p 57.

42. Varenhorst, B: 1. The adolescent society. In Adolescent Peer Pressure: Theory, Correlates, and Program Implications for Drug Abuse Prevention. DHHS Publication No. (ADM) 81-1152. Rockville, Maryland: 1981, p 1.

43. Blum, RW: Adolescent substance abuse: Diagnostic and treatment issues. Pediatr Clin North Am 34:523, 1987.

44. Johnston, LD: The etiology and prevention of substance use: What can we learn from recent historical changes? In Jones, CL and Battjes, RJ (eds): Etiology of Drug Abuse: Implications for Prevention. NIDA Research Monograph 56. Rockville, Maryland: NIDA, 1985, p 155.

45. Needle, R, et al: Interpersonal influences in adolescent drug use: The role of older siblings, parents and peers. Int J Addict 21:739, 1986.

46. Zarek, D, Hawkins, JD, and Rogers, PH: Risk factors for adolescent substance abuse. Pediatr Clin North Am 34:481, 1987.

47. Kandel, DB, Kessler, RC, and Margulies, RZ: Antecedents of adolescent initiation into stages of drug use: A developmental analysis. Journal of Youth and Adolescence 7:13, 1978.

48. Robinson, TN, Killen, JD, and Taylor CB: Perspectives on adolescent substance use: A defined population study. JAMA 258:2072, 1987.

49. Kandel, DB, Simcha-Fagan, O, and Davies, M: Risk factors for delinquency and illicit drug use from adolescence to young adulthood. Journal of Drug Issues 60:67, 1986.

50. Jessor, R, and Chase, JA, and Donovan, JE: Psychosocial correlates of marijuana use and problem drinking in a national sample of adolescents. Am J Public Health 70:604, 1980.

51. Anglin, TM: Interviewing guidelines for the clinical evaluation of adolescent substance abuse. Pediatr Clin North Am 34:381, 1987.

52. Kellam, SG, Ensminger, ME, and Simon, MB: Mental health in first grade and teenage drug, alcohol, and cigarette use. Drug Alcohol Depend 5:273, 1980.

53. Kandel, DB: Drug use by youth: An overview. In

Lettiere, DJ and Ludford, JP (eds): Drug Abuse and the American Adolescent. NIDA Research Monograph 38, Rockville, Maryland: NIDA, 1981, p 1.

54. Kolb, LC: Modern Clinical Psychiatry, ed 9. WB Saunders, Philadelphia, 1977, p 11.

55. Treece, C and Khantzian, EJ: Psychodynamic factors in the development of drug dependence. Psychiatr Clin North Am 9:399, 1986.

56. Wurmser, L: Psychoanalytic considerations of the etiology of compulsive drug use. J Am Psychoanal Assoc 22:820, 1974.

57. Khantzian, EJ: The self-medication hypothesis of addictive disorders: Focus on heroin and cocaine dependence. Am J Psychiatry 142:1259, 1987.

58. Khantzian, EJ and Khantzian, NJ: Cocaine addiction: Is there a psychological disposition? Psychiatric Annals 14:753, 1984.

59. Nicholl, AM, Jr: The nontherapeutic use of psychoactive drugs. N Engl J Med 308:925, 1983.

60. Deykin, EY, Levy, JC, and Wells, V: Adolescent depression, alcohol and drug abuse. Am J Public Health 77:178, 1987.

61. Weissman, MW and Myers, JK: Clinical depression in alcoholism. Am J Psychiatry 137:372, 1980.

62. Nace, EP: The Treatment of Alcoholism. Brunner/Mazel, New York, 1987, p 47.

63. Hesselbrock, MN, Meyer, RE, and Keener, JJ: Psychopathology in hospitalized patients. Arch Gen Psychiatry 42:1050, 1985.

64. Cadoret, R and Winokur, G: Depression in alcoholism. In Seixas, FA, Cadoret, R, and Eggleston, S (eds): The Person with Alcoholism. Ann NY Acad Sci 233:34, 1974.

65. Behar, D, Winokur, G, and Berg, CJ: Depression in the abstinent alcoholic. Am J Psychiatry 141:1105, 1984.

66. Merikangas, KR, Leckman, JF, and Prusoff, BA: Familial transmission of depression and alcoholism. Arch Gen Psychiatry 42:367, 1985.

67. Rounsaville, BJ, et al: Diagnosis and symptoms of depression in addicts. Arch Gen Psychiatry 39:151, 1982.

68. Rounsaville, BJ, et al: Heterogeneity of psychiatric diagnosis in treated opiate addicts. Arch Gen Psychiatry 39:161, 1982.

69. Khantzian, EJ and Treece, C: DSM-III psychiatric diagnosis of narcotic addicts. Arch Gen Psychiatry 42:1067, 1985.

70. Weiss, R and Mirin, SM: Subtypes of cocaine abusers. Psychiatr Clin North Am 9:491, 1986.

71. Paton, S, Kessler, R, and Kandel, DB: Depressive mood and illegal drug use: A longitudinal analysis. J Genet Psychol 131:267, 1977.

72. Kandel, DB: Epidemiological and psychosocial perspectives on adolescent drug use. J Am Acad Child Psychiat 121:328, 1982.

73. Lewis, CE, Rice, J, and Helzer, JE: Diagnostic interactions: Alcoholism and antisocial personality. J Nerv Ment Dis 171:105, 1983.

74. American Psychiatric Association: Diagnostic and Statistical Manual of Mental Disorders. 3rd Ed., Revised. American Psychiatric Association, Washington, DC, 1987.

75. Rounsaville, BJ, et al: Psychiatric disorders in treated opiate addicts. In Serban, G (ed): The Social and Medical Aspects of Drug Abuse. Spectrum Publications, New York, 1984, p 135.

76. Jainchill, N, DeLeon, G, and Pinkham, L: Psychiatric diagnoses among substance abusers in therapeutic community treatment. J Psychoactive Drugs 18:209, 1986.

77. Morrison, MA and Smith, QT: Psychiatric issues of adolescent chemical dependence. Ped Clin North Am 34:461, 1987.

78. Garfinkel, BD: Recent developments in attention deficit disorder. Psychiatric Annals 16:11, 1986.

79. American Psychiatric Association: Diagnostic and Statistical Manual of Mental Disorders. 3rd Edition. American Psychiatric Association, Washington DC, 1980.

80. Patrick, KS, et al: Pharmacokinetics and actions of methylphenidate. In Meltzer, HY (ed): Psychopharmacology: The Third Generation of Progress. Raven Press, New York, 1987, p 1387.

81. Cocores, JA, Davies, RK, and Mueller, PS: Cocaine abuse and adult attention deficit disorder. J Clin Psychiatry 48:376, 1987.

82. Khantzian, EJ: The self-medication hypothesis of addictive disorders: Focus on heroin and cocaine dependence. Am J Psychiatry 142:1259, 1987.

83. Gawin, F and Kleber, H: Pharmacologic treatments of cocaine abuse. Psychiatr Clin North Am 9:573, 1986.

84. Cocores, JA, et al: Cocaine abuse, attention deficit disorder and bipolar disorder. J Nerv Ment Dis 175:431, 1987.

85. Wood, D, Wender, PH, and Reimherr, FW: The prevalence of attention deficit disorder, residual type, of minimal brain dysfunction, in a population of male alcoholic patients. Am J Psychiatry 140:95, 1983.

86. Shuckit, MA, Sweeney, S, and Huey L: Hyperactivity and the risk of alcoholism. J Clin Psychiatry 48:275, 1987.

87. Kosten, TR and Rounsaville, BJ: Psychopathology in opioid addicts. Psychiatr Clin North Am 9:515, 1986.

88. Wilder, FJ and Plutchik, R: Stress and psychiatry. In Kaplan, HI and Sadock, BJ (eds): Comprehensive Textbook of Psychiatry IV, Vol 2, ed. 7. Williams & Wilkins, Baltimore, 1985, p 1198.

89. McNeil, C: The dimensions of stress: Introduction. Perspectives on Prevention 2:6, 1988.

90. Murphy, P: Stress and the athlete: Coping with exercise. Phys Sportsmed 14(4):141, 1986.

91. Holmes, TH and Rahe, RH: The social readjustment rating scale. J Psychosom Res 2:213, 1967.

92. Labouvie, EW: Alcohol and marijuana use in relation to adolescent stress. Int J Addict 21:333, 1986.

93. Wills, TA: Stress and coping in adolescence: Relationships to substance use in urban school samples. Health Psychol 5:503, 1986.

94. Serban, G: Social stress and drug abuse. In Serban, G (ed): The Social and Medical Aspects of Drug Abuse. Spectrum Publications, New York, 1984, p 125.

95. Griffiths, RR and Sannerud, CA: Abuse of and dependence on benzodiazepines and other anxiolytic/sedative drugs. In Meltzer, HY: Psychopharmacology: The Third Generation of Progress. Raven Press, New York, 1987, p 1535.

CHAPTER 3

The Athlete

Being an athlete provides no special immunity to drug abuse. Genetic predisposition, familial influences, and peer relationships affect everyone. Although much has been written about drug abuse and sports, particularly collegiate and professional sports, no scientific data provide definitive conclusions regarding the athlete's vulnerability to drug abuse. While anecdotes abound, not even the incidence and prevalence of drug abuse in amateur and professional athletics are known accurately. The Michigan State study of 1984 represented a significant step in the quantification of drug abuse in collegiate athletics,[1] while the 1986 Hazelden-Cork study, performed in cooperation with the Women's Sports Foundation, addressed alcohol and drug use patterns in women athletes.[2] The drug-testing programs of the United States Olympic Committee (USOC), the International Olympic Committee (IOC), and the National Collegiate Athletic Association (NCAA) have, and continue to, shed some light regarding the incidence of drug abuse among athletes in select circumstances (see Chapter 18 and Appendices).

To better understand any special vulnerabilities to drug abuse that the athlete may have, one must have an understanding of some of the psychological and physical issues pertinent to sports and performance.

The discipline of sports psychology became accepted as a scientific field in Europe during the 1920s and the 1930s, although World War II interrupted momentum in the field. Stimulated by government institutions, sports psychology developed as a scientific discipline, primarily in Eastern Europe and in the Soviet Union, between World War II and 1965. In 1965, the first International Congress of Sport Psychology met in Rome.[3]

Coleman Griffith, the father of sports psychology in this country, established the first sports psychology laboratory in the United States at the University of Illinois. Like exercise physiology, sports psychology in this country initially attracted interest primarily from physical education departments. As contrasted with Eastern Europe, interest in sports psychology lagged in the United States. Not until 1986 did the American Psychological Association formally recognize sports psychology with a division of its own: Division 47, Exercise and Sport Psychology.[4] Given its relative infancy as a discipline, the term "sports psychologist" in this country remains open to broad interpretation and issues of credentials. Nonetheless, in 1977, the United States Olympic Committee (USOC) appointed a part-time director of sports psychology; and, in 1984, the USOC inaugurated the Sports Psychology Registry, which, in 1987, listed 47 persons with competencies in sports psychology. Originally focused on social-psychological theories and their relationship to exercise and sport, sport psychology has expanded to include such areas as the child in sports, psychophysiology, exercise, the regulation of sports behavior, the effects of sports and exercise upon mental health, and the psychological rehabilitation of physical illness and injury.[5]

ENTERING COMPETITIVE SPORTS

It has been estimated that over 20 million North Americans participate in organized sports.[6] Fifty-nine percent of second-through fifth-grade children spend an average of 5.13 hours per week in organized sports.[7] Peak participation occurs between ages 11 and 13, following which there appears to be a sharp and steady decline. What dynamics lead a youngster into the world of competitive athletics? The specifics of a given sport aside, the child engages in sport for a variety of reasons, both intrinsic and extrinsic. Thoughts of college scholarships and a professional career, needless to say, appear much later on, if at all.

Perhaps first and foremost, young athletes engage in athletics to have fun. Second, athletics represent a vehicle for relating to one's peers. Third, athletic participation enables the young athlete to test and to improve his or her skills. Fourth, athletics creates a climate for enhancing one's physical fitness.[6,8] The relative importance of each factor varies from individual to individual, from sport to sport, and from time to time.

A variety of reasons have been advanced to explain the achievement behavior of the young athlete, that is, why does a given athlete strive to perform at a higher level?[8]

1. For some, athletic excellence provides the young athlete with an opportunity to demonstrate a high level of ability in a well-defined area. This premise implies the likelihood that the athlete would self-select a sport which would most likely "showcase" his or her athletic ability.

2. Some young athletes appear to be particularly motivated by the inner challenge of acquiring new skills required by a certain sport. For them, demonstrating specific athletic skills to others assumes a secondary importance.

3. For some, sports participation represents a vehicle for gaining approval from individuals such as important friends, parents, siblings, peers, physical education teachers, and coaches.

4. For some, it has been postulated that the pursuit of athletic achievement represents a form of risk taking. Examples cited of such risks include performing in front of a crowd or being asked to play at higher levels of competition.

THE ELITE ATHLETE— "THE PRIVILEGED FEW"

Contrary to what might be expected, scant literature addresses the psychological characteristics of the young elite athlete—"the privileged few"[9]—as distinct from young athletes in general. Specifically, only nine studies have been reported that assess the psychological characteristics of elite young athletes[8] who range in age from 7 to 19. The specific sports studied were wrestling, hockey, gymnastics, running, and speed skating. Table 3–1 summarizes the demographic data from these studies.

Even fewer data address the elite athlete's motives for participating in competitive sports. Specifically, only two sports were

Table 3–1. DEMOGRAPHIC DATA FROM STUDIES ON ELITE YOUNG ATHLETES

Variable	Sport Study					
	Wrestling	Hockey	Gymnastics	Gymnastics	Running	Speed Skating
Age range	13–19	15–19	7–18	7–13	9–15	14–27
Mean age (year)	16.74	17.23	12.40	*	12.63	19.90
Mean age began competing	11.48	5.80	7.00	6.50	8.82	*
Mean year involved	5.45	11.65	3.60	*	3.36	5.80
Mean number of competitions/year	67.64	*	*	*	24.38	*
Mean number of workouts/week	*	*	6.00	5.00	4.30	6.50
Mean number of hours training/day	*	*	3.98	5.50	0.50	4.00
Number in study	464	121	43	46	28	32

*Information was not reported in the study.
From Feltz and Ewing,[8] with permission.

studied in this regard—hockey and gymnastics.[8,10] Reasons put forth for the participation in these sports by the elite athlete included improving one's skills, enjoying the competition, maintaining fitness, demonstrating one's ability so as to enable competition at higher levels, and wanting to please others. With such limited data on the psychological assessment of the elite athlete in general, what role, if any, drug abuse plays in the elite athlete's success-oriented efforts remains speculative.

It has been estimated[11] that fewer than 2 percent of the athletes recruited into the "major" college sports programs ever play professional sports (football or basketball). As Underwood[11] reported in 1980:

> According to the National Federation of State High School Associations, every year close to 700,000 boys play high school basketball and one million play high school football. On the varsities of NCAA institutions, those numbers are reduced to 15,000 in basketball and 41,000 in football. In the NFL, about 320 college-draft choices come to camp each year; roughly 150 make it. On the average, those rookies who succeed play pro ball for 4.2 seasons. About 4000 players complete their college basketball careers each year; approximately 200 get drafted by the 22 NBA teams; around 50 actually make a team. The average NBA career lasts 3.4 seasons.

Nonetheless, for the gifted or elite athlete, the lure of professional athletics may significantly influence his or her life during early adulthood. Vallerand notes: "The instant fame and enormous wealth that accrue to athletes who make a great play in front of millions of television viewers lead participants, parents, and coaches alike to covet making the big time."[6] College sports is often essential for the elite athlete to showcase his or her athletic abilities. However, the price is high and often extends into later years.

From the outset, the college athlete is asked to perform in two completely different spheres—the academic and the athletic. In many ways, a career choice for the gifted collegiate athlete is an "and/or" decision. Will he or she make it to the professional ranks, and for how long? "And/or" should his or her participation in sports, even though paid for by an athletic scholarship, come second to academic pursuits? For many, an athletic scholarship represents a precious passport to higher education. For most, the lure of a career in professional sports may be nothing but fool's gold. For other college athletes, albeit a very small percentage, a career in professional sports may represent a realistic goal. Unfortunately, most college athletes never realize that professional career goal, leaving them with the question: "Did I prepare myself adequately in college for a career after sports, or did I let an educational opportunity irretrievably pass me by?"

Depending on the sport, there may be disruptions of formal education even at the elementary and junior high school levels, resulting in the failure to develop proper study and time management skills. Training with world-renowned coaches often requires relocating alone to other parts of the country, where the focus is on training, not academics. Tremendous time demands leave few hours for nonstructured educational activities. By age 15 or 16, some elite athletes in sports such as gymnastics, swimming, and diving have trained for nearly a decade.[12] Actual competition frequently requires extensive national and international travel, particularly in individual sports such as tennis or gymnastics. This, in turn, may necessitate the use of tutors or instruction by mail.

The young elite athlete is not immune to the developmental problems of nonathletic youth. In addition to those problems, stardom brings still other problems. Spare time is consumed during much of the year in sports-related activities, and thus relationships with students outside sports are often limited, as is relaxation time. As Kirshenbaum has noted: "The attempt to perform effectively in any sport, even in the most intricate team sport, can be a very solitary endeavor."[13] This may result in a failure to learn how to socialize with peers. Furthermore, the peer relationships and friendships that are formed are frequently restricted to athletes in the same sport.[9] Yet, within these friendships and relationships, there exists either an overt or covert competitiveness.

From early childhood, the gifted athlete has been singled out by friends, relatives, teachers, and the community as being someone special. Local recognition soon becomes regional recognition, and depending on the sport, international recognition may appear in the early teens. Soon promoters, agents, scouts, recruiters, coaches, entrepreneurs, and others become involved at various levels, all reinforcing the notion—"winning counts." As Wadler has noted: "The pressures increase tremendously when child-athletes realize that more and more people have something invested in them. It becomes much harder to pull back and change directions. The web has become too complicated."[14]

Self-esteem can be enhanced with repeated success in competitive athletics. As Lanning[9] has observed, "The majority of skilled athletes have been rewarded all their life for their success as athletes." As they successfully move up the competitive ladder, their self-esteem is further enhanced. However, as the competition toughens, and it rises to a level of excellence not previously encountered, the chances for continued success begin to diminish. In a sport such as tennis, for example, being number 1 in national competition in the 16-year-old age division can be very enhancing to one's self-esteem. However, competing repeatedly and unsuccessfully against "number 1s" from other countries can be devastating, as the realization of one's limitations sets in. The experience can engender feelings of unworthiness and social isolation,[15] and the absence of viable career alternatives can increase the athlete's vulnerability to drug abuse. Career-ending injuries can leave the athlete equally vulnerable, if career alternatives were not planned for earlier in their lives.

STRESS

Stress—an integral part of competitive sports—should be considered in terms of acute and chronic stress and in terms of negative and positive effect.

From an athletic perspective, chronic stress relates to the tremendous time investment; the repetition and monotony of training; and the narrowing of physical, intellectual, and social activities.[16] One manifestation of chronic stress has been referred to as "overtraining," a phenomenon in which peak performance is impaired. Overtraining should be considered when an inexplicable fall-off in performance is associated with an increasing intolerance to training.[17] What was a pleasure becomes a burden; anticipation turns to resignation. Sleep patterns become disturbed, as reflected by retiring later, difficulty falling asleep, and repeated awakening during the night. Depression may cloud the day, associated with a loss of appetite. Increased thirst may be noted during the evening hours. A sense of heaviness and of being run down may accompany feelings of chronic fatigue. Overtraining thus represents a condition with both psychological and physiologic overtones. Currently there are no specific data to evaluate what role chronic stress and overtraining play in athletic drug abuse.

Although acute stress may be present during periods of intensive training prior to an athletic competition, the term when applied to sports is generally limited to perceived stresses at or about the time of actual competition. Within the competitive setting, the process of acute stress may be either a positive *(eustress)* or a negative *(distress)* phenomenon. What is eustress for one athlete may be distress for another. What is distress at one time may be eustress at another. Acute stress is a manifestation of a dynamic process involving one's self and one's environment. Stress is often manifested by feelings of anxiety. It is noteworthy that of all the psychiatric disorders, anxiety appears to be the one most intimately concerned with motivation. Anxiety is the internal energizer that supports persistent goal-directed behavior such as that required in sports performance. From a clinical perspective, individuals who suffer from anxiety are typically intense, ambitious individuals who drive themselves beyond ordinary limits.[18]

Despite the almost universal tension felt by competitive athletes, it has been estimated that fewer than half of high-level young athletes complain of competitive stress.[19] In his review of stress in competitive sport, Dishman[19] concludes: ". . . that both physiologic and psychometric measures of acute anxiety are elevated above resting levels immediately prior to sport competition and are most pronounced when critical competitive situations are approached. These elevations are believed to result from apprehension over social evaluation and performance outcomes which can be a function of personality and perceived threat." Dishman[19] further notes: "Although youth athletes also report elevations in anxiety following competitive failures (losing), the magnitude of both pre- and post-game anxiety levels typically remains within a clinically normal range. They are no greater than those that accompany non-sport performance when evaluative outcomes are expected by the participant. . . ." Measurements of both the physiologic and the psychological manifestations of stress during competition indicate that the physiologic expressions of stress, such as increased muscle tension and heart rate, may well exceed psychologic expressions of stress, such as nervousness and anxiety, and that these stresses may be akin to those seen in spectating and recreational sport.[20]

In specifically addressing the issue of psychological stress or anxiety levels in elite young athletes, Feltz and Ewing[8] reviewed four studies involving elite and nonelite male wrestlers, male and female elite and nonelite gymnasts, and distance runners. There appeared to be no difference between the elite and the nonelite young athletes with the exception of 13- to 15-year-old female gymnasts. In this group, anxiety levels were higher among elite athletes; they had as their goal making the Olympic team, facing odds of 7 out of 3163, or 0.2 percent.

The data are relatively scant with respect to the quantification and characterization of stress in amateur youth elite athletes. By contrast, no definitive scientific studies address this issue in professional sports.

PERFORMANCE AND STRESS

It has long been known that the relationship between stress and performance is not linear but curvilinear. As shown graphically in Figure 3–1, increased arousal improves performance up to a point, beyond which, performance begins to deteriorate.

What is arousal? From a neurologic perspective, there are two components that govern conscious behavior—content and arousal. *Content* represents the sum of cognitive and affective mental functions, and *arousal* relates to degrees, or levels, of wakefulness.[21] However, the term arousal, as used

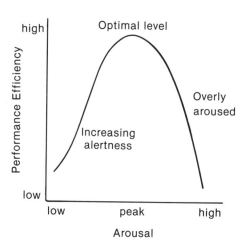

Figure 3–1. *Performance-arousal curve. Increased arousal is associated with enhanced performance up to a point, beyond which performance deteriorates.*

by sports psychologists, represents an amalgam of both content and arousal and can be thought to encompass such terms as alertness, stress, wakefulness, excitement, concentration, attention, and motivation.[22] Arousal may also be viewed as a measure of the intensity level of focused behavior, and as such, it encompasses such terms as drive and tension.[23] There are various physiologic indicators of arousal, including electroencephalographic changes, heart rate and blood pressure levels, and muscle tension.[24]

Low levels of arousal which are associated with poor performance might include feelings of apathy, boredom, malaise, and sluggishness, and may account, in part, for the so-called "upset" in a sporting event. On the other hand, levels of overarousal might be associated with feelings of tension, anger, frustration, and even panic. There may be a loss of focused attention and concentration with an increase in distractability. Often, individuals may be aware of the fall-off in performance associated with excessive drive or arousal, and the drive to achieve optimal performance may continue long after the peak of efficiency is reached.[25] Optimal arousal is a subjective feeling or mindset that coincides with maximal performance.

Recognizing the delicate balance between arousal and performance, sports psychologists and coaches have increasingly attempted to bring the athlete to a recognizable level of optimal arousal so as to maximize his or her competitive performance. Browne and Mahoney[3] have summarized some of the subjective feelings that athletes have reported coincident with peak performance: "a. dissociation and intense concentration, often being unaware of their surroundings during these times; b. feeling neither fatigue nor pain, the body performing on its own; c. perceptual changes which include time-slowing and object enlargement; and d. feeling unusual power and control."

It has long been recognized through experimental, correlational, and anecdotal evidence that patterns of thought can influence athletic performance.[26,27] Numerous non-pharmacologic psychological, behavioral, and coping techniques and interventions, some controversial, have been advocated and used in efforts to enhance performance in a consistent manner. The need for such techniques and interventions has arisen from the observation that: "Athletes simply do not lose or gain skill and stamina over the course of a single game in a manner that explains their fluctuation in performance! In the final analysis, with all other things being equal . . . it is the psychological skill that will determine the degree of success in competition."[28] However, in considering the use of psychological, behavioral, and coping techniques and interventions, Dishman's[29] admonition is worth heeding: "Present-day claims for success in sports exceed empirical data that satisfy conventional standards for internal (results are best attributable to the intervention) and external (results are reproducible with other athletes in other sports settings) validity."[29]

Although not all-inclusive, the concepts, techniques, and interventions that follow reflect those that have been employed to enhance performance and to decrease stress and anxiety by psychological means. We do not judge the relative merit but simply survey them to demonstrate the variety of psychological approaches that have been employed. The approaches primarily utilize principles associated with the so-called cognitive-behavioral approach to human psychology. They focus on: (1) identifying patterns of cognition ("self-talk," thinking, expectations, perceptions, attributions) and behavior that aggravate and maintain stress responses; and (2) utilizing strategies for coping with the adverse effects of stress.[30–33]

Inherent in cognitive-behavioral therapy is the recognition that the individual's cognitive, behavioral, somatic/physiologic, and emotional systems interrelate.[34] In recent years, there has been an increased emphasis on actually quantitating the effect of these psychological interventions on athletic performance by the use of psychometric inventories, rating scales, behavioral observations, and, most recently, by psychophysiologic measures.[24,35] In the laboratory setting, cognitive strategies have been shown to facilitate endurance performance such as marathon running by enabling subjects to tolerate a greater amount of discomfort for a longer period of time. This cognitive or coping strategy has been referred to as a dissociative strategy. Using this strategy the athlete ignores pain by focusing on something else, but by so doing, runs the risk of injury. This is in contrast to an associative strategy, in which the athlete monitors his or her physical sensations, which enables him or her to modulate the pace of the endurance activity. This approach minimizes the risk of injury.[36-38]

Psychological Approaches to Performance Enhancement

Biofeedback

Biofeedback employs electronic instrumentation to teach the athlete how to control the physiologic components of the stress response, such as muscle tension or heart rate. However, if an athlete is unaware, for example, that his or her muscle tension or that his or her heart rate is increasing, then there is no way he or she can consciously prevent such an increase. By learning how to recognize and to control these stress responses in the laboratory, it is intended that the athlete can subsequently reproduce a desired level of relaxation at will during competition without equipment. Questions have been raised regarding the efficacy of biofeedback outside the laboratory setting, and more specifically in enhancing athletic performance during competition.[29,31,39] Zaichkowsky and Fuchs[40] recently reported that over 80 percent of studies found biofeedback procedures to be highly successful in facilitating sport and athletic performance, and beneficial for the athletes' well-being.

Goal Setting

Simply stated, a goal is what an individual is trying to accomplish, whereas the task represents the necessary work to accomplish the goal. Harder goals, like harder tasks, require more knowledge and skill than easier goals and easier tasks. The literature is replete with evidence that setting goals is beneficial to the performance of a task, provided that the task is commensurate with the individual's ability. There are certain conditions or circumstances under which the setting of goals is particularly beneficial to performance. For example, difficult, challenging, and specific goals enhance performance more than easy "do your best" goals. Setting intermediate goals appears beneficial to the attainment of longer term goals.

Feedback or knowledge of one's performance in relation to a goal appears to be necessary for performance enhancement. In this regard, supportiveness by others, such as a coach, also appears to be beneficial, particularly when the coach interpolates some negative feedback along with positive feedback.[41] Goal setting in athletic competition has an especially enhancing effect on task performance.[42]

Short, intermediate, and long-range goal setting is an integral part of an athlete's career. Goal setting impacts on matters as diverse as training, practice, specific competitions, season objectives, and career objectives.

Relaxation Training

Various types of relaxation techniques have been developed, some of which date back to the classic work of Jacobsen[43] in 1929. These techniques include progressive relaxation, electromyogram feedback training, hypnosis, and meditation (Zen and Transcendental Meditation).

Most forms of relaxation training relate to muscle relaxation. The term *relaxation* refers to the lengthening of skeletal muscle fibers, and the term *tension* refers to the contraction or shortening of skeletal muscle fibers. In progressive relaxation, the individual learns to recognize tension states. Individual muscle groups are tensed, and then they are slowly relaxed. In one approach that has been applied to athletes, the body is arbitrarily divided into 16 muscle groups. The individual directs attention to one muscle group at a time, developing tension in that muscle group for up to 7 seconds, then releasing it. While that muscle group is in the relaxed state, the individual directs attention to it for an additional 20 to 30 seconds. Deep breathing is also used to facilitate the relaxation response. Feelings of tingling or warmth may arise during the relaxation phase.

To be valuable in stressful or competitive settings, the athlete must practice the relaxation response regularly and frequently, from 10 to 15 minutes daily. With sufficient practice one can bring back in moments the relaxed sensations of warmth and tingling by closing one's eyes and mentally going through each of the muscle groups.[22,44,45]

Assertiveness Training

Assertiveness requires thinking positively, being self-controlled, and being goal-oriented, all in a self-confident frame of reference. Assertive behavior has been defined by Wolpe[46] as "the proper expression of any emotions other than anxiety toward another person." Assertiveness training is a technique often used in psychology for the treatment of anxieties related to interpersonal relationships.[47] This technique focuses on the behavioral as well as the cognitive aspects of the stress response. Assertiveness training has been used to bolster athletes who, for fear of disapproval or anger, tend to be shy and who may experience anxiety when interacting with teammates and coaches. Such individuals may feel uncomfortable in the competitive setting primarily because of the fear of losing.

Assertiveness training has also been used to help individuals who respond with inappropriate anger when faced with situations in which they cannot control the outcome. In contact sports such as football or boxing, assertiveness training has been used to emphasize that anger and rage impulses directed at an opponent are counterproductive and are poor motivators for consistent performance.[45]

Imagery and Mental Practice

Imagery and mental practice refers to the ability to visualize or to imagine emotional states and physical events in the mind. Other terms used in the literature to describe this process include imaginary rehearsal, symbolic rehearsal, implicit practice, mental rehearsal, and conceptualizing practice.[26] Studies have clearly demonstrated psychophysiologic and neurophysiologic alterations in response to such imagery.[29] For example, consistent changes in both systolic and diastolic blood pressure as well as in pulse rate have been produced with imagery associated with feelings of happiness, sadness, anger, and fear.[48] It has also been demonstrated, as far back as 1931, that the imagery of voluntary movement of a body part without the actual movement of that body part has been associated with electromyographic (EMG) activity.[49]

These types of observations, together with anecdotal reports by athletes, have led to the use of imagery and mental practice in attempts to enhance athletic performance.[50] Imagery and mental practice is not restricted to visual constructions. All of the senses, as well as the feeling of movement (kinesthetics), may be involved in imagery. For athletes, kinesthetic imagery would appear to be particularly important, as they can "see" and "feel" themselves, in their "mind's eye," performing a specific athletic activity. Utilizing this technique, the athlete can mentally rehearse specific athletic activities, causing low-level activation of the neurologic and physiologic pathways associated with those activities.[27]

Imagery and mental practice would appear to be a more effective training method for highly skilled individuals whose sport is an individual sport, rather than a team sport where the actions of others cannot be controlled or consistently predicted. Individual performers, such as gymnasts, can mentally prepare and practice entire routines in anticipation of competition.

Although from the 1930s to the mid-1980s, there have been more than 100 research studies discussing the efficacy of imagery and mental practice on athletic performance, questions still exist regarding its efficacy. In 1983, Feltz and Landers[51] extensively reviewed the literature utilizing a statistical technique called meta-analysis, whereby the results of multiple studies are compared, contrasted, analyzed, and integrated.[52] They concluded that "mentally practicing a motor skill influences performance somewhat better than no practice at all," and that "employing cognitive tasks had larger average effect sizes than motor or strength tasks." Their analysis also called into question the significance of Jacobsen's observation[53] regarding electrical activation of the specific muscles by mental practice. They concluded from their analysis that there is a more generalized increase in muscle tension, suggesting that this increase may be a manifestation of a generalized increase in one's pre-performance arousal level.

A recent variation of the technique of mental imagery has been termed visuo-motor behavior rehearsal (VMBR). This technique, originally described by Suinn in 1972, combines both visual imagery and relaxation. VMBR consists of "(a) an initial relaxation phase, (b) visualizing performance during a specific stressful situation, and (c) performing the skill during a simulated stressful situation."[54]

Self-Talk and Thought

Athletes can be assisted in developing mental self-statements that serve "to challenge and repudiate self-defeating thoughts that elicit stress, and to give self-instructions that direct attention and enhance performance."[55] By ruminating or dwelling on negative past situations, past performances, and past outcomes, or by becoming preoccupied with potential negative outcomes in anticipation of an event, the athlete decreases focused attention in current competitive situations.

On the other hand, reflection on positive past situations, past performances, and past outcomes can serve to reinforce expectations of positive performances and outcomes. Although not limited to the concept of self-talk and thought, Bandura's model of self-efficacy has relevance in this regard.[56] Bandura noted that one of the factors that determines the expectation of personal efficacy is prior performance accomplishment:

> Successes raise mastery expectations; repeated failures lower them, particularly if the mishaps occur early in the course of events. After strong efficacy expectations are developed through repeated success, the negative impact of occasional failures is likely to be reduced. Indeed, occasional failures that are later overcome by determined effort can strengthen self-motivated persistence if one finds through experience that even the most difficult obstacles can be mastered by sustained efforts."[56]

He further states: "Once established, enhanced self-efficacy tends to generalize to other situations in which performance was self-debilitated by preoccupation with personal inadequacies."[56] A number of studies have shown a statistically significant relationship, although not necessarily a causal one, between self-efficacy and athletic performance.[57]

Athletes have also employed two related procedures to enhance performance—cognitive restructuring and self-instructional training.[58] In cognitive restructuring, one first identifies the thoughts evidently responsible for inappropriate behavior or inadequate athletic performance. Once these have been identified, attitudinal changes are fostered. Thus, in cognitive restructuring, stress-producing thoughts such as "I'll be benched if I miss this . . ." are analyzed and challenged and are replaced by thoughts such as "I'll give it my best shot!" By identifying those thoughts that increase anxiety or that serve as negative reinforcements, the athlete can develop strategies for changing such thoughts into positive ones, for it is well recognized that self-fulfilling prophecies can affect performance in sports.

Cognitive restructuring is, in essence, an adaptation of the "power of positive thinking." It is also akin to the strategy of "psyching-up," which has been shown to have some degree of task specificity. For example, Weinberg[59] has noted that "psyching-up" enhanced the performance of a task measuring isokinetic leg strength but failed to enhance the performance of specific tasks designed to measure speed and balance. The term "psyching-up" can mean any type of mental preparation that the athlete believes enhances performance. These include preparatory arousal, imagery, and attention focus.[26]

Once a cognitive problem has been identified that results in poor performance, and once it has been restructured or changed, the next step is self-instructional training. Self-instructional training emphasizes "specific task-relevant self-commands that can be used in relevant situations."[55] In self-instructional training, a word or several words are linked to the restructured or changed attitude. During competition, these words serve to recall changes that were made in the practice setting. A phrase such as "stick to the ice" may remind the hockey player to avoid the penalty box by avoiding useless penalties.[58] For some athletes, self-talk may be beneficial even in the absence of cognitive restructuring. Self-talk may include comments such as: "Keep calm," "pay attention to the game," and "take a deep breath and relax."

Concentration and Attentional Focus

Every elite athlete is aware of the importance of concentration in competition. It is not uncommon to hear an athlete muttering: "Concentrate, concentrate!" Concentration reflects the ability to sustain a maximal level of attention over a period of time. Failure to concentrate is a prime cause of performance inconsistency. Concentration requires the athlete to become completely focused on a task to the exclusion of any distractions, either internal or external. The ability to concentrate is a skill that can be enhanced by regular practice.

The notion of attentional focus[28] is intimately related to the concept of concentration. Attentional focus refers to the scope of the relevant cues upon which the athlete must concentrate while ignoring irrelevant stimuli. The cues may be external (environmental) as well as internal (thoughts, feelings), and they may change rapidly during competition as circumstances change.[60] For example, the external cues for a quarterback are numerous and might include such diverse actions as reading the defensive alignment while judging the wind conditions. For a baseball batter, the external cues become narrowly focused as he watches the ball leave the pitcher's hand, watches the action of the ball in flight, and ultimately watches the bat make contact with the ball.

Internal cues principally relate to thoughts and emotions such as worry and anxiety. Preoccupation with previous errors can interfere with the requisite concentration on external cues. Similarly, looking ahead beyond the immediate task at hand can significantly impair performance by interfering with concentration.

PERFORMANCE AND PHYSICAL FACTORS

"In top flight competition, the difference between winning and placing may very often be measured in tenths, or even hundredths, of a second. The athlete who is striving for excellence attempts to gain every possible edge over the competition."[61]

Whereas sports psychology deals primarily with the psychological aspects of sports, sports medicine deals primarily with the physical aspects of sport. In the United States, sports medicine is going through an evolutionary process and the sports medicine community is quite heterogeneous. This heterogeneity is evidenced by the diverse professional backgrounds of the membership of the American College of Sports Medicine, which was founded as recently as 1955, and by the fact that there are more than 75 other national groups that deal with sports medicine. Even the United States Olympic Committee (USOC) had a minimal involvement with sports medicine until Congressional passage of the Amateur Sports Act of 1978.

As a result of the Amateur Sports Act, three goals referable to sports medicine have been established by the USOC[62]:

1. To achieve optimal health and superior performance in athletes
2. To provide and to coordinate sports medicine services for United States teams, sports organizations, and National Governing Bodies and the United States Olympic Committee
3. To promote the benefits of Olympic sports medicine and Olympic ideals for all

Given this history of sports medicine, it is not surprising that there has been great inconsistency in the United States with regard to the application of sports medicine principles to organized sports, whether amateur or professional. However, great strides have been made in recent years to apply the principles of medicine and science to the athlete in his or her pursuit of excellence.

Specifically, with respect to performance enhancement from a physical perspective, as contrasted with a psychological perspective, there are a number of disciplines under the rubric of sports medicine that have a direct bearing on athletic performance. Any classification is necessarily arbitrary, because all of these disciplines have areas of overlap. Those enumerated here serve to highlight what the athlete can do physically to enhance his or her athletic performance without drugs.

Physical Approaches to Performance Enhancement

General Health

Athletes have no special immunity to, or protection from, the gamut of conditions, illnesses, and injuries that might befall individuals of like age who are not involved in organized competitive athletics. Although the pre-participation or pre-season examination may detect many of these conditions, these examinations do not take the place of a sustained relationship between the athlete and his or her primary care physician. The preseason or pre-participation examination is generally a more specific, sports-oriented examination that is primarily intended to identify medical conditions that would preclude safe athletic participation and to identify musculoskeletal abnormalities or physical inadequacies that might result in injury. Additionally, the recognition, detection, and treatment of specific sports-related ailments, such as exercise-induced asthma, have played a substantial role in enhancing athletic performance.

Advances in the early diagnosis and management of sports injuries, together with advances in rehabilitative techniques, have minimized the adverse effects of injury on athletic performance, Further, these advances in orthopedics and rehabilitative medicine have decreased the athlete's reliance on pain-relieving drugs.

Biomechanics

Biomechanics is the study of the structure and function of biologic systems by using the methods of mechanics.[63] Although the study of the mechanical aspects of sports began in the 1920s in the United States, it wasn't until the 1960s that this discipline began to flourish. Furthermore, it has only been during the last decade that the observations from the sports biomechanics research laboratories were translated into methodologies that could actually be employed by coaches and athletes.

In addressing the question of performance enhancement, the sports biomechanics researcher specifically addresses the following issues[63]:

1. The determination of optimum techniques for performance in sports events
2. The investigation of stresses placed upon the body during the performance of sports activities
3. The design of sports equipment

Exercise Physiology

The understanding of the physiologic principles of exercise and fitness, with all their diversity, has had a considerable impact on enhancing performance. For example, understanding such issues as aerobic and anaerobic metabolism, and their relative contributions to various sports activities, has fostered the development of training techniques and schedules to optimize energy utilization during competition.

The application of physiologic principles to minimize the development of heat illness or to prevent problems associated with failure to permit acclimatization are specific examples of how exercise physiology can have a direct bearing on athletic performance. In recent years, the study of chronobiology has resulted in recommendations relative to the effect of travel across time zones on athletic performance.

The physiologic testing of athletes has become increasingly sophisticated, particularly that done under the aegis of the United States Olympic Committee. Activities designed to overcome specific deficits in physiologic function as related to the demands of a given sport can then be incorporated into an individual's training program.

Physical Conditioning and Training

Figure 3–2 illustrates the respective roles of conditioning and training as physical tools used to enhance athletic performance. Within this conceptual framework, conditioning produces the general fitness that is required before one embarks upon a training program, which, in turn, then focuses on the specific endurance and strength requirements of a particular sport. Inherent in any general conditioning program are the qualitative elements of cardiovascular and mus-

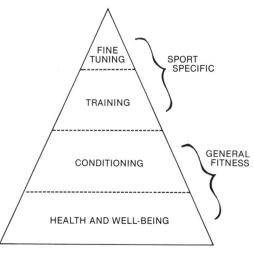

Figure 3–2. The relative contribution of various physical factors in athletic performance. (From Clarke,[64] p. 4, with permission.)

cular endurance; strength and flexibility; and the quantitative elements of frequency, intensity, and duration. The intent of the training program is to optimize performance by coordinating the athlete's physical and skill development with training-induced adaptations so that he or she achieves maximum results during competition.[65] Finally, "fine tuning is what separates athletes of equivalent skill and training—getting the extra edge reliably (consistently) through an athlete's fullest 'reading' and use of his or her body's resources for that sport at the time of competition."[64]

Building on the principles of exercise physiology and physical conditioning, training programs have become increasingly scientifically based. Detailed investigations into the specific physiologic demands of a given sports activity has resulted in the development of highly sophisticated training techniques directed at addressing these demands. For example, gymnastic events are of high intensity and short duration and require specialized training to adapt to the metabolic, strength, and power demands of that sport.

It is thus clear that proper and effective physical conditioning of the athlete requires long-range planning with specific goals and objectives.

Nutrition

As early as the 3rd century BC, the Greeks ingested mushrooms in an attempt to enhance athletic performance.[66] Athletes still continue to search for that magical nutritional ingredient that will give them that extra edge over opponents. "Ergogenic aids classified as nutritional are hypothesized to increase performance either by renewing or increasing energy stores in the body, facilitating the biochemical reactions that yield energy, modifying the biochemical changes contributing to fatigue, or maintaining optimal body weight."[67]

Whereas diet and dietary manipulation cannot replace physical conditioning and training, they can contribute to enhanced athletic performance. Specific examples of such performance-enhancing dietary manipulations include carbohydrate loading, proper fluid intake, and proper selection of precompetition meals.

However, like physical conditioning and training, proper nutrition requires long-term planning with specific goals and objectives. Performance enhancement through dietary manipulation cannot be achieved by first addressing this issue 1 or 2 days prior to competition.

Practice and Competitive Experience

Practice and drills permit the acquisition, development, and refinement of sport-specific skills. In individual endeavor sports, as in team sports, practice enables the individual athlete to develop proficiency and confidence in the performance of that skill. In team sports, which require coordinated efforts between teammates, practice permits the athletes to develop proper timing so that specific athletic maneuvers can be performed with precision. During practice athletes test plans and strategies in anticipation of actual competition. Properly planned practices should enable the athlete to peak from a performance perspective at the time of actual competition.

Of course, the ultimate test of performance takes place during actual competition. Ideally, competition represents the culmination of a process in which both general athletic ability and sport-specific skills have been honed to perfection.

PERFORMANCE AND DRUG ABUSE

Given the extent to which the disciplines of exercise physiology, sports medicine, and sports psychology have gone to enhance athletic performance, it is not surprising that the pharmacologic manipulation of athletic performance has found its way into competitive athletics in order to provide "that extra edge." Ethics, morality, and legality aside, athletes have used pharmacologic substances as an extension of the psychological and physical principles enumerated above. Consequently, studies have increasingly reported the effects of various pharmacologic substances on athletic performance. These substances span the spectrum of effects on performance—from the purely psychologic to the purely physical—with some drugs, such as amphetamines, affecting multiple aspects of athletic performance. Detailed discussions of the most commonly used drugs are presented in subsequent chapters. Below is an overview of the major objectives associated with the use of performance enhancing drugs in competitive athletics.

Stress

Drug abuse in the athlete may be viewed, in part, from the perspective that it represents still another coping method for enhancing performance by reducing stress. The Michigan State study did not specifically address the question of whether or not an athlete used alcohol or drugs as a coping mechanism to deal with stress and anxiety.[1] However, a review of the Michigan State data derived from the question, "Where do you usually get your *(name of drug)?*" at least suggests that student athletes were disturbed enough by stress to seek stress- and anxiety-reducing medications, for example, barbiturates and tranquilizers, from physicians and trainers/coaches. Eight percent received them from a team physician; 21 percent from another physician; and 8 percent from a trainer or coach.

The lack of quantitative data on the role of stress on performance in amateur and professional sports coincides with the lack of any firm data on drug abuse as a coping methodology for enhancing performance in organized sports.

Physical Factors

The use of performance-enhancing drugs has been unquestionably tied to the achievement goals of the competitive athlete. When the Michigan State study[1] asked why college-student athletes used specific drugs, 69 percent indicated they used anabolic steroids to improve performance. Additionally, 37 percent used amphetamines, and 8 percent used barbiturates and tranquilizers for the same purpose. As will be discussed in subsequent chapters, very few controlled scientific studies address the *net* effect of performance-enhancing drugs on actual athletic performance. For drugs such as anabolic steroids, it is unlikely that the FDA will approve testing their effects on overall performance, particularly at the massive dosages in which they are often used by athletes.

Athletes continue to use drugs as ergogenic aids despite the general lack of scientific evidence that such drugs are efficacious.

Such use would appear to be, for them, an extension of the principles developed earlier in this chapter relative to enhancing performance by physical means such as training, nutrition, and practice. Although the data are lacking, anecdotal information suggests that athletes who may be particularly at risk of utilizing pharmacologic means to enhance physical performance include, but are not limited to:

1. Athletes who are at risk of not making the team, or "the cut"
2. Athletes who are approaching the end of their career and are trying to "hang on"
3. Athletes who are having weight problems, either because they are too heavy or too light
4. Athletes who are attempting to play despite injuries
5. Athletes who are responding to "external pressures" from a variety of sources to use performance-enhancing drugs

Examples of some physical effects sought by athletes using pharmacologic substances include: hand steadiness with beta blockers, increased muscle bulk and power with anabolic steroids, increased speed and the delay in onset of fatigue with amphetamines, weight control with diuretics and amphetamines, and pain relief with narcotics.

THE ATHLETE AND NON-PERFORMANCE-RELATED DRUG ABUSE

The factors contributory to drug abuse in the general population considered in the preceding chapter apply equally to the athlete. In addition, competitive athletics presents additional vulnerabilities for the athlete. For the adolescent, participation in competitive athletics can be an anxiety-producing experience, and thus can be labeled a stressful life event.[68] According to one study, the stress of failing to make a junior or senior high school team rated above experiences such as the death of a grandparent, suspension from school, and the loss of a job by a parent.[69,70] Failure to realize such an athletic goal not only has the potential for producing significant stress and anxiety; it can also adversely affect one's self-esteem.[71] Although the use of alcohol and marijuana may not be one of the more common coping behaviors for the stressed (distressed) adolescent, it is not an infrequent coping behavior. Smilkstein[71] has identified two groups of young people who are most likely to experience repeated failure and suffer the psychological trauma of high levels of anxiety in sports:

1. Individuals "who demonstrate a low level of competence, relative to their peer group, due to inexperience, lack of innate ability, or late maturation"
2. Individuals "who perceive that they are not meeting the expectations of their peer group, coach, or parents"

At the elite level, it has been noted that depression is one of the most common emotional problems among athletes.[72,73] As noted previously, depression, particularly in the adolescent, appears to correlate positively with many forms of drug abuse.[74]

Aside from the stress associated with performance, or the fear of the termination of a career, athletes are not immune to the stresses that are associated with being in the public eye. The role of stress and drug abuse in individuals in the public eye was highlighted by the disclosure of diazepam (Valium) and alcohol abuse of former senior White House aide Michael K. Deaver and former national security adviser Robert C. McFarlane. As Sharfstein has noted: "I don't think it (tranquilizer and alcohol use) is any different for high political figures than for business leaders or professional athletes."[75]

Dr. Arnold M. Nicholl, Jr., consultant psychiatrist to the New England Patriots professional football team, addressed some mental health issues in professional football. Although his observations pertained only to a limited number of players on one professional team, and in only one sport, they do have a bearing on the coping behaviors of professional athletes in general. He notes[73]: "... because of their outstanding talent, some of the players have been indulged for most of their lives. Parents and teachers have bent the rules and moved boundaries to accommodate them. Consequently, a few players have failed to internalize the controls that most people acquire before reaching late adolescence and early adulthood. In one sense, athletic development has proceeded at the expense of emotional development." He further notes[73]: "... many players come out of

college in limited financial circumstances, and then, at a very young age, begin to earn huge sums of money. They also find themselves with a great deal of public recognition. ... This sudden access to money, recognition and an excess of free time imposes considerable stress on a person just out of college."

Outstanding athletes are at least as vulnerable to drug abuse as are other members of society. High visibility, extended periods of free time, and considerable wealth may create an increased susceptibility for the outstanding athlete. Like others in the public eye—politicians, media stars or actors—some athletes have come to believe that they are exempt from the everyday obligations that society imposes.[76] This sense of entitlement too often extends to drug abuse.

REFERENCES

1. Anderson, WA and McKeag, DB: The Substance Use and Abuse Habits of College Student-Athletes. College of Human Medicine, Michigan State University, East Lansing, Michigan, June 1985.
2. Elite Women Athletes Survey. Hazelden Health Promotion Services, Minneapolis, Minnesota, 1987.
3. Browne, MA and Mahoney, MJ: Sport psychology. Ann Rev Psychol 35:605, 1984.
4. Monahan, T: Sports psychology: A crisis of identity. Phys Sportsmed 15(9):203, 1987.
5. McCauley, E: Sport psychology in the eighties: Some current developments. Med Sci Sports Exerc 19:S95, 1987.
6. Vallerand, RJ, Deci, EL, and Ryan, RM: Intrinsic motivation in sport. Exerc Sports Sci Rev 15:389, 1987.
7. Gill, DL, Gross, JB, and Huddleston, S: Participation motivation in youth sports. International Journal of Sports Psychology 14:1, 1983.
8. Feltz, DL and Ewing, ME: Psychological characteristics of elite young athletes. Med Sci Sports Exerc 19:S98, 1987.
9. Lanning, W: The privileged few: Special counseling needs of athletes. J Sports Psychol 4:19, 1982.
10. Klint, KA and Weiss, MR: Dropping in and dropping out: Participation motives of current and former youth gymnasts. Can J Appl Sport Sci 11:106, 1986.
11. Underwood, J: Student-athletes: The sham, the shame. Sports Illustrated, May 19, 1980.
12. Feigley, DA: Psychological burnout in high level athletes. Phys Sportsmed 12(10):108, 1984.
13. Kirshenbaum, DS: Self-regulation and sport psychology: Nurturing an emerging symbiosis. J Sports Psychol 6:159, 1984.
14. Nash, HL: Elite child-athletes: How much does victory cost? Psy Sportsmed 15(8):128, 1987.
15. Orlick, TD: The athletic drop out. A high price for inefficiency. Can Assoc Health, Phys Ed and Recreat 41:21, 1974.
16. Gutman, MC, et al: Training stress in Olympic

speed skaters: A psychological perspective. Phys Sportsmed 12(12):45, 1984.

17. Wadler, G: Too much, too soon—Overtraining. Inside Women's Tennis 10:12, 1986.

18. Malmo, RB: Motivation. In Kaplan, HI and Sadock, BJ (eds): Comprehensive Textbook of Psychiatry IV, vol I, ed 4. Williams & Wilkins, Baltimore, 1985, p 198.

19. Dishman, RK: Medical psychology in exercise and sport. Med Clin North Am 69:123, 1985.

20. Skubic, V and Hilgendorf, J: Anticipatory, exercise, and recovery heart rates of girls as affected by four running events. J App Physiol 19:853, 1964.

21. Plum, F and Posner, JB: The Diagnosis of Stupor and Coma, ed 3. FA Davis, Philadelphia, 1982, p 1.

22. May, JR: Psychological aspects of athletic performance: An overview. In Butts, NK and Gushiken, TT (eds): The Elite Athlete. Spectrum Publications, New York, 1985, p 119.

23. Landers, DM: The arousal-performance relationship revisited. Research Quarterly in Exercise and Sport 51:77, 1980.

24. Hatfield, BD and Landers, DM: Psychophysiology in exercise and sport research: An overview. Exerc Sports Sci Rev 15:351, 1987.

25. Mills, IH: Arousal of the brain and coping mechanisms. In McGuigan, FJ, Sime, WE, and Wallace, JM (eds): Stress and Tension Control, Plenum Press, New York, 1980, p 7.

26. Weinberg, RS: The relationship between mental preparation strategies and motor performance: A review and critique. Quest 33:195, 1982.

27. Myers, AW and Schlesser, R: A cognitive behavioral intervention for improving basketball performance. J Sport Psych 2:69, 1980.

28. Harris, DV: Cognitive skills and strategies for maximizing performance. In Butts, NK, Gushiken, TT, and Zarin, B (eds): The Elite Athlete. Spectrum Publications, New York, 1985, p 145.

29. Dishman, RD: Psychological aids to performance. In Strauss, RH (ed): Drugs and Performance in Sports. WB Saunders, Philadelphia, 1987, p 121.

30. Meichenbaum, D and Turk, D: The cognitive-behavioral management of anxiety, anger. In Davidson, PO (ed): The Behavioral Management of Anxiety, Depression and Pain. Brunner/Mazel, New York, 1976, p 1.

31. Holroyd, KA and Lazarus, RG: Stress, coping and somatic adaptation. In Goldberger, L and Breznitz, T (eds): Handbook of Stress—Theoretical and Clinical Aspects. The Free Press, New York, 1982, p 21.

32. Coates, TJ and Polonsky, WH: Behavior therapy. In Michels R, et al (eds): Psychiatry, vol 2. JB Lippincott, Philadelphia, 1987 (rev), chap 77, p 1.

33. Ramirez, SZ, Kratochwill, TR, and Morris, RJ: Childhood anxiety disorders. In Michelson, L and Ascher, LM (eds): Anxiety and Stress Disorders—Cognitive and Behavioral Assessment and Treatment. The Guilford Press, New York, 1987, p 149.

34. Emery, G and Tracy NL: Theoretical issues in the cognitive behavioral treatment of anxiety disorders. In Michelson, L and Ascher, LM (eds): Anxiety and Stress Disorders—Cognitive and Behavioral Assessment and Treatment. The Guilford Press, New York, 1987, p 3.

35. Ziegler, SG, Klinzing, J, and Williamson, K: The effects of two stress managment training programs on

cardiorespiratory efficiency. J Sports Psychol 4:280, 1982.

36. Morgan, WP, et al: Facilitation of physical performance by means of a cognitive strategy. Cognitive Therapy and Research 7:251, 1983.

37. Morgan, WP: The trait controversy. Research Quarterly in Exercise and Sport 51:50, 1980.

38. Morgan, WP and Pollock, ML: Psychologic characterization of the elite distance runner. In Milvey, P: The Marathon: Physiological, Medical, Epidemiological, and Psychological Studies. Ann NY Acad Sci 301:382, 1983.

39. Lynn, SJ and Freedman, R: Biofeedback and stress-related disorders: Enhancing transfer and gain maintenance. In McGuigan, FJ, Sime, WE, and Wallace, JM (eds): Stress and Tension Control. Plenum Press, New York, 1980, p 187.

40. Zaichkowsky, L and Fuchs, CZ: Biofeedback applications in exercise and athletic performance. In Pandolf, KB (ed): Exercise and Sport Sciences Reviews, American College of Sports Medicine Series. Macmillan, New York, 1988, p 381.

41. Kirschenbaum, DS and Smith, RJ: A preliminary study of sequencing effects in simulated coach feedback. J Sports Psychol 5:332, 1983.

42. Locke, EA, et al: Goal setting and task performance: 1969–1980. Psychol Bull 90:125, 1981.

43. Jacobsen, E: Progressive Relaxation, ed 2. University of Chicago Press, Chicago, 1938.

44. McGuigan, FJ: Principles of scientific relaxation. In McGuigan, FJ, Sime, WE, and Wallace JM (eds): Stress and Tension Control. Plenum Press, New York, 1980, p 209.

45. Stoyva, J and Anderson, C: A coping-rest model of relaxation and stress management. In Goldberger, L and Breznitz, S (eds): Handbook of Stress—Theoretical and Clinical Aspects. The Free Press, New York, 1982, p 745.

46. Wolpe, J: The Practice of Behavior Therapy, ed 2. Pergamon Press, New York, 1973, p 81.

47. Prochaska, JO: Systems of Psychotherapy—A Transtheoretical Analysis. The Dorsey Press, Chicago, Illinois, 1984, p 274.

48. Schwartz, GE, Weinberger, DA, and Singer, JA: Cardiovascular differentiation of happiness, sadness, anger and fear following imagery and exercise. Psychosom Med 43:343, 1981.

49. Jacobsen, E: Electrical measurements of neuromuscular states during mental activities. Am J Physiol 96:115, 1931.

50. Woolfolk, RL, Parrish, MW, and Murphy SM: The effects of positive and negative imagery on motor skill performance. Cognitive Therapy and Research 9:335, 1985.

51. Feltz, DL and Landers, DM: The effects of mental practice on motor skill learning and performance: A meta-analysis. J Sport Psychol 5:25, 1983.

52. Thacker, SB: Meta-analysis. JAMA 259:1685, 1988.

53. Jacobsen, E: Electrical measurements of neuromuscular states during mental activities. Am J Physiol 96:115, 1931.

54. Hall, E and Erffmeyer, ES: The effect of visuo-motor behavior rehearsal with videotaped modeling on free throw accuracy of intercollegiate female basketball players. J Sports Psychol 5:343, 1983.

55. In Smith, NJ: Sports Medicine: Health Care for

Young Athletes. American Academy of Pediatrics, Evanston, Illinois, 1983, p 203.

56. Bandura, A: Self-efficacy: Toward a unifying theory of behavioral change. Psychol Rev 84:191, 1977.

57. Feltz, DL: Self-confidence and sports performance. In Pandolf, KB (ed): Exercise and Sport Sciences Reviews, American College of Sports Medicine Series. Macmillan, New York, 1988, p 423.

58. Silva, JM: Competitive sports environments. Performance enhancement through cognitive intervention. Behav Modif 6:443, 1982.

59. Weinberg, RS, Gould, D, and Jackson, A: Cognition and motor performance: Effect of psyching-up strategies on three motor tasks. Cognitive Therapy and Research 4:239, 1980.

60. Nideffer, RM: Test of attentional focus and interpersonal style. J Pers Soc Psychol 34:394, 1976.

61. Morris, F: Sports Medicine Handbook. WC Brown Publishers, Dubuque, Iowa, 1985, p 122.

62. Zarins, B: Challenge to sports medicine in the United States. In Butts, NK, Gushiken, TT, and Zarins, B: The Elite Athlete. Spectrum Publications, New York, 1985, Foreword.

63. Dillman, CJ and Ariel, GB: The biomechanical aspects of Olympic sports medicine. Clin Sports Med 2:31, 1983.

64. Clarke, KS: The United States Olympic Committee Sports Medicine Program: An overview. In Butts, NK, Gushiken, TT, and Zarins, B: The Elite Athlete. Spectrum Publications, New York, 1985, p 3.

65. Van Handel, PJ and Puhl, J: Sports physiology: Testing the athlete. Clin Sports Med 2:19, 1983.

66. Coddington, RD: The significance of life events as etiologic factors in the disease of children: Part 1: A survey of professional workers. J Psychosom Res 16:7, 1972a.

67. Coddington, RD: The significance of life events as etiologic factors in the disease of children: Part 2: A study of normal population. J Psychosom Res 16:205, 1972b.

68. Scanlon, TK and Passer, MW: Factors related to competitive stress among male youth sports participants. Med Sci Sports Exerc 10:103, 1978.

69. Puffer, J: The use of drugs in swimming. Clin Sports Med 5:77, 1986.

70. Grandjean, AC: Vitamins, diet, and the athlete. Clin Sports Med 2:105, 1983.

71. Smilkstein, G: Psychological trauma in children and youth in competitive sports. J Fam Pract 10:737, 1980.

72. Roundtable Discussion: The emotionally disturbed athlete. Phys Sportsmed 9(7):67, 1981.

73. Nicholl Jr, AM: Psychiatric consultation in professional football. N Engl J Med 316:1095, 1987.

74. Deykin, EY, Levy, JC, and Wells, V: Adolescent depression, alcohol and drug abuse. Am J Public Health 77:178, 1987.

75. Shabecoff, P: Stress and the lure of harmful remedies. The New York Times, October 14, 1987.

76. Rosecan, JS, Spitz, HI, and Gross, B: Contemporary issues in the treatment of cocaine abuse. In Spitz, HI and Rosecan, JS: Cocaine Abuse—New Directions in Treatment and Research. Brunner/Mazel, New York, 1987, p 299.

PART II

Drugs of Abuse in Sports

CHAPTER 4

Anabolic Steroids

HISTORY

The abuse of anabolic steroids has historic foundations in man's desire to create a body-building "wonder drug." Like other wonder drugs, anabolic steroids occur naturally in the human body—in this case as testosterone and its derivatives. The discovery and isolation of testosterone led to the various formulations of the anabolic steroids. These drugs should more specifically be called "androgenic-anabolic steroids," as they produce both androgenic (masculinizing) and anabolic (tissue-building) effects.

It has long been suspected that the testes were critical for the development of the male phenotype. In 1771, Hunter transplanted testes from the cock to the hen and observed that the hen developed male characteristics.[1] Similarly, Berthold demonstrated in 1849 that testes transplanted into castrated roosters prevented signs of castration.[2]

Brown-Sequard, an English neurologist, believed that chemicals in the testes caused increased physical vigor. He became convinced of this in 1889 after administering testicular extracts to himself. It is now known that these extracts had minimal, if any, active hormone.[3] This historic event should be put in the context of a more recent statement made by Dr. John Ziegler, one of the developers of anabolic steroids in the United States: "I honestly believe that if I'd told people back then that rat manure would make them stronger, they'd have eaten rat manure."[4]

Testosterone was first isolated in crystalline form by Laqueur in 1935 and was synthesized shortly thereafter.[3] Once testosterone was synthesized, the exploitation of

55

naturally occurring anabolic steroids for therapeutic purposes began. Anabolic steroids were employed in the 1930s to promote a positive nitrogen balance in starvation victims.[5] During World War II, German troops employed anabolic steroids in efforts to enhance their muscle strength[6] and increase their aggressiveness.[7]

In 1954, the first reports appeared of male and female Russian athletes using anabolic steroids to increase weight and power.[6-8] The perception that the Russians could dominate the sports world by ingesting a chemical agent led to the development and use of anabolic steroids in the United States. Initially weight lifters were given the drug and, by Dr. Ziegler's account, ingested far more than the recommended dosage in hopes of achieving a greater advantage.[4] Use then quickly spread from weight lifters and throwers to football players and swimmers.[8]

A wave of enthusiasm and suspicion ensued in the sports world. Athletes felt they had discovered a wonder drug, and they perceived themselves to be at a disadvantage if a competitor took anabolic steroids and they did not. As early as 1956, Olga Fikotova Connally said: "There is no way in the world a woman nowadays, in the throwing events—at least the shot put and the discus—I'm not sure about the javelin—can break the record unless she is on steroids. These awful drugs have changed the complexion of track and field."[4]

Responding to the claims of enhanced athletic performance attributable to anabolic steroid usage, a number of clinical investigations were undertaken in the late 1960s and early 1970s.[7] Unfortunately, many questions regarding efficacy and safety still remain unanswered.

By 1976, accurate urine tests became available to detect exogenous anabolic steroid usage.[7] As a result, 7 of 19 athletes were disqualified from the 1983 Pan American games for anabolic steroid use as detected by urine testing, and many more withdrew from competition, presumably over concerns about drug testing and its potential impact on Olympic eligibility. Since then, other athletes have been disqualified or banned from major sporting events because of positive urine tests for anabolic steroids. The most notable of them is the Canadian sprinter Ben Johnson, who was stripped of his gold medal during the 1988 Summer Olympic Games because of the presence of anabolic steroids in his urine.[7a]

The use of anabolic steroids remains an integral part of athletics today, beginning with teenagers and even pre-adolescents.[8] The desire by those taking anabolic steroids to perform superhuman feats remains, coupled with the suspicion of disadvantage among those who abstain. Dave Cadigan, the newly acquired New York Jets offensive lineman, recently explained why he had used anabolic steroids: "I played against a lot of guys that I know for a fact were using steroids. I'd play them one year, and the next year, they'd come back 15 pounds heavier, stronger and they looked different. They played better and hit harder. That was one piece of the pie in my decision. . . . I will do anything to become the best lineman in the NFL. . . . If they [the NFL] don't like it, screw them. This is a business. They're not naive to the situation."[9]

CHEMISTRY AND PHYSIOLOGY

The isolation of testosterone allowed the development of the many synthetic anabolic steroids, whose actions mimic those of endogenous testosterone.[9a] Following the crystallization of testosterone, numerous derivatives of the compound were developed in an effort to dissociate the androgenic or masculinizing effects from the anabolic or tissue-building effects. This may not be entirely possible, however, because the anabolic and androgenic actions of anabolic steroids appear to be mediated through the same receptor complex. The target tissue, rather than the drug, appears to be the important behavioral determinant.[10]

The biosynthetic pathway for testosterone and its derivatives is shown in Figure 4–1. Testosterone is metabolized to both active and inactive compounds (Fig. 4–2). In women and in pre-pubertal boys, plasma testosterone concentrations are much lower than in adult men—15 to 65 ng per dl compared with 300 to 1000 ng per dl (Table 4–1). The biologically active component represents the 2 percent of testosterone which is not plasma protein bound. The testes secrete most testosterone in men, but the adrenal cortex also secretes some.

In men, a sudden and sustained surge in

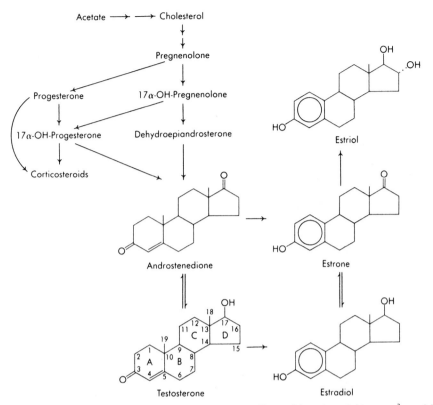

Figure 4–1. The biosynthetic pathway for testosterone. (From Murad and Haynes,[3] p. 1413, with permission.)

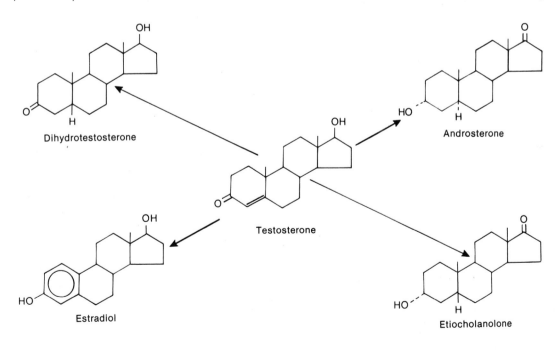

Active Metabolites   **Inactive Metabolites**

Figure 4–2. Metabolism of androgens. (From Murad and Haynes,[3] p. 1440, with permission.)

Table 4–1. TESTOSTERONE CONCENTRATION
AND PRODUCTION

	Pre-Pubertal Boys	Men	Women
Testosterone	<20 ng/dl	300–1000 ng/dl	15–65 ng/dl
Daily rate of testosterone production	<0.25 mg/day	2.5–11 mg/day	0.25 mg/day

testosterone production heralds the onset of puberty. The events which lead to this hormonal change are not completely understood, although the hypothalamus of the brain and the pituitary gland play an integral role. The hypothalamus produces releasing hormones which may inhibit or increase the release of pituitary gonadotropins—follicle-stimulating hormone (FSH) and luteinizing hormone (LH). The pituitary hormones FSH and LH interact in complex ways with the testes and seminiferous tubules, leading to increased spermatogenesis plus testosterone production and release. During puberty, testosterone production increases from less than 0.25 mg per day to 11 mg per day (see Table 4–1). At a certain plasma concentration, testosterone can cause feedback inhibi-

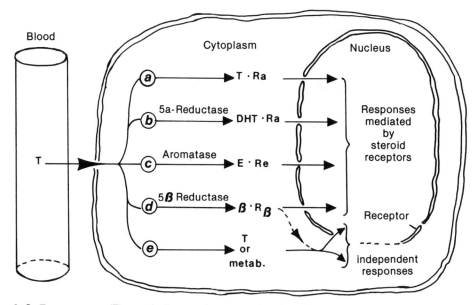

Figure 4–3. Testosterone (T) metabolism and receptor binding. The known pathways of testosterone metabolism that lead to biological activities in various tissues are summarized as though they occurred in a single cell. Testosterone leaves the blood and enters the cell by diffusion. In the cytoplasm, testosterone can react in the following ways: (a) Without being metabolized, in which case testosterone binds directly to the androgen receptor (Ra), and this steroid receptor complex (T·Ra) is then transferred to nuclear acceptor sites in chromatin for initiation of the steroid-specific responses; (b) testosterone is metabolized by 5a-reductase to 5a-dihydrotestosterone (DHT) which then binds to Ra and the steroid receptor complex (DHT·Ra) is bound in the nucleus; (c) testosterone is aromatized to estradiol (E) which binds to estrogen receptor (Re) which is transferred and bound in nuclei as for (a) and (b); (d) testosterone is metabolized to 5b metabolites (b) which bind to the b steroid receptor (Rb) and the steroid receptor complex (b·Rb) presumably acts in the nucleus; and (e) testosterone or one of its metabolites (metab.) acts in the nucleus or cytoplasm by mechanisms which are independent of known receptors (receptor-independent responses). (From Bardin and Catterall: Testosterone: A major determinant of extragenital sexual dimorphism. Science 211:1286, 1981 with permission.)

tion of gonadotropin release. A metabolite of testosterone, estradiol, also appears to play an important role.

In women, the ovaries and adrenal cortex are responsible for testosterone production, either directly or indirectly. At least half of testosterone in women occurs from the metabolic conversion of androstenedione to testosterone in peripheral tissues. Daily testosterone production in women is about 0.25 mg per day (see Table 4–1).

The physiologic effects of testosterone and synthetic anabolic steroids are mediated through a steroid receptor complex[11] (Fig. 4–3). The reduced form of testosterone, dihydrotestosterone (see Fig. 4–2), is the principal intracellular mediator of hormonal action. Androsterone and etiocholanolone are the major urinary metabolites of the naturally occurring anabolic steroids, and they are both physiologically inactive. Estradiol is an active metabolite which inhibits gonadotropin release and in excessive concentrations leads to feminization of the body (see Fig. 4–2).

Intracellular studies of the action of anabolic steroids show that they first become bound to cytoplasmic receptors.[12] In the case of testosterone, free testosterone enters the cell by diffusion and is then converted to dihydrotestosterone in the cytoplasm. The dihydrotestosterone binds to a specific high-affinity cytosol protein receptor. The resulting steroid-receptor complex then undergoes a biochemical transformation. The transformed complex is translocated to the nucleus, where it ultimately binds to chromatin receptor sites resulting in protein synthesis (Fig. 4–4). Separate receptor complexes exist for glucocorticoids, estrogen, and testosterone in skeletal muscle; the effect of the anabolic steroids is mediated through the testosterone (anabolic-androgenic) complex.

In skeletal muscle, the limiting factor with respect to the action of anabolic steroids is the number of existing anabolic steroid receptor complexes. This means that supraphysiologic doses of anabolic steroids have no further effect on skeletal muscle changes. Under normal conditions, the skeletal mus-

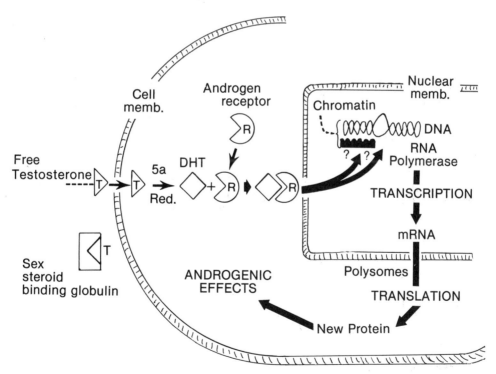

Figure 4–4. Diagrammatic representation of the mechanism of action of testosterone at the target organ. 5-a-Red = 5-a-reductase. DHT = dihydrotestosterone. (From Williams: Textbook of Endocrinology, ed. 6, p. 445, WB Saunders, Philadelphia, 1981, with permission.)

cle anabolic steroid receptors are saturated due to the high-affinity, low-capacity nature of the receptor-drug complex. In the rat, forced muscle hypertrophy leads to a major adaptive response in skeletal muscle. An increased number of unsaturated receptor complex sites exist following forced muscle hypertrophy.[11] This model may provide a rationale for training with anabolic steroids under specified conditions, which will be discussed later in the chapter. Castrated rats and hypogonad men are much more sensitive to exogenous anabolic steroids because of the availability of more receptors. A similar principle is felt to hold true for women.[11]

Anabolic steroid receptors exist not only in skeletal muscle but also in other tissues throughout the body, including the prostate, heart, testes, seminiferous tubules, and probably the brain. It is the abundance of receptors in various tissues which leads to the diverse physiologic effects of anabolic steroids.

Testosterone and its active metabolites (excluding estradiol) are responsible for the development of primary male sexual characteristics in utero and in the neonatal period. The surge in testosterone production at puberty is followed by the development of secondary male characteristics, which include enlarged testes and penis, pubic hair, laryngeal enlargement and a deepened voice, sebaceous gland proliferation and acne, and facial and axillary hair growth. Concomitantly, increases in height and skeletal muscle growth occur, undoubtedly influenced by the testosterone surge, but also influenced by other complex physiologic and hormonal changes.

Aggression and sexual orientation are in part mediated through testosterone. Although not universal, even within a given species, male and female differential behavior is influenced strongly by testosterone production and action. Several authors have demonstrated a link between plasma testosterone levels and aggressive behavior.[13-16] In monkeys, a correlation exists between plasma testosterone level, aggressive behavior, and social rank.[16] These studies imply that brain receptors may be important in mediating psychological effects of anabolic steroids. Testosterone may also exert some of its central nervous system effects through estradiol, a metabolite. Brain catecholamine levels may become elevated secondary to estradiol-induced monoamine oxidase activity reduction.[17]

CLINICAL PHARMACOLOGY

Testosterone, given orally, has no pharmacologic effect because the absorbed agent is rapidly degraded by the liver. Similarly, parenteral testosterone is rapidly metabolized.[18] These considerations led to two principal modifications of the testosterone molecule:

1. Esterification of the 17 beta hydroxyl group with a variety of carboxylic acids to increase lipid solubility, allowing for the development of slow-release injectables;
2. Alkylation of the 17 alpha position to decrease metabolism by the liver, thereby making oral anabolic steroids effective (Table 4-2).

Parenteral steroids require less frequent administration and are less often associated with liver toxicity than oral steroids.

Commonly used anabolic steroids are shown in Table 4-2. The therapeutic dose is the dose recommended to produce pharmacologic responses in well-defined clinical conditions. Doses used by athletes usually greatly exceed the recommended therapeutic dose. For example, some athletes have been reported to have taken up to 6000 mg methandrostenolone (Dianabol) in two weeks during "stacking" periods, in contrast to therapeutic doses of 2.5 to 5 mg daily.

Clinical Uses

Clinically, the parenteral anabolic steroids have been used as hormonal replacement for hypogonadal males during adolescence to accelerate the initiation of a growth spurt when a constitutional delay of growth occurs and also to stimulate erythropoiesis in hematologic disorders such as aplastic anemia, myelofibrosis, and the anemia of renal failure. They also have been used for palliative therapy in breast carcinoma and advanced osteoporosis. The oral preparations are effective in the management of the autosomally dominant hereditary skin condition angioneurotic edema.

USE IN SPORTS

The exact incidence of anabolic steroid use among amateur and professional athletes is not known but is regarded as widespread. In the 1984 Michigan State Study of NCAA athletes, 9 percent of football players polled used anabolic steroids during the prior year. Four percent of athletes from basketball, track, and tennis had similarly used steroids.[19] In the Elite Women Athletes Survey, 3 and 5 percent of Olympic and professional athletes, respectively, admitted to anabolic steroid use during their lifetimes. However, zero percent had used steroids during the prior month.[20] A 15-year study by Dezelsky and colleagues[20a] revealed that 20 percent of intercollegiate athletes reported using anabolic steroids, whereas less than 1 percent of nonathletes used these drugs. In a more recent study,[20b] 17 percent of varsity college athletes who responded to a questionnaire reported using anabolic steroids. Of interest, nonathletes also reported using anabolic steroids to improve personal appearance.

Coupled with the paucity of epidemiologic data is the speculation that anabolic steroid use may be higher than the available data suggest. Marty Liquori recently said: "I doubt whether you'll see very many athletes on our '88 Olympic team who haven't had some steroid use. I don't think anyone will make the team without having been very involved in drugs."[21] Of concern is that an increase in anabolic steroid usage is probably occurring at the high school and even junior high school level.[22,23] Anabolic steroid use remains a subject of considerable controversy in the sports and sports medicine communities[6,8,24,25] because of its known widespread use associated with an uncertain risk versus benefit ratio.

It is estimated that athletes spend $100 million annually for anabolic steroids, about 20 percent through legal prescriptions and the rest through the black market.[26] Health professionals and legitimate drug distributors have been implicated in the legal and black market activity. One physician claims to have prescribed anabolic steroids to over 10,000 athletes.[4] The Food and Drug Administration (FDA) has asked health professionals to report suspected improper use of anabolic steroids to the Health and Fraud staff of the FDA. The FDA, the Federal Bureau of Investigation, and the Department of Justice are cooperating in an effort to clamp down on black market distribution and threaten to bring indictments against alleged violators.[25,27]

Effects on Performance

The exact effects of anabolic steroids on the athlete and athletic performance remain controversial. There appears, however, to be a consensus regarding the effect of anabolic steroids on aerobic metabolism: no beneficial effect of anabolic steroids has ever been shown on aerobic metabolism or on an individual's $\dot{V}O_2max$.[28-37]

Personality changes after anabolic steroid use include an increased sense of well-being, increased energy, and increased aggressiveness, as well as increased sexuality. The actual performance benefit, if any, from the personality changes is uncertain. Associated with these changes is an element of unpredictability and irritability.

Numerous studies have addressed the issue of the effect of anabolic steroids on bulk and strength, but without consistent or definitive conclusions.[28-51] Illustrating the controversy are the opposite conclusions of two investigators reviewing essentially the same reported data. Ryan stated: ". . . there is a substantial body of evidence that will stand very close scrutiny to indicate that anabolic steroids will not contribute significantly to gains in lean muscle bulk or muscle strength in healthy young adults."[5] Haupt and Rovere, by contrast, concluded: ". . . anabolic steroids will consistently result in significant strength increases if all of the following are satisfied:

"1. They are given to athletes who have been intensively trained in weight lifting immediately before the start of the steroid regimen and who continue this intensive weight lift training during the steroid regimen.

"2. The athletes maintain a high-protein diet.

"3. The changes in the athletes' strength are measured by the single repetition–maximal weight technique for those exercises with which the athlete trains."[7]

Much of the controversy regarding ana-

Table 4–2. SOME COMMONLY USED ANABOLIC STEROIDS

GENERIC AND BRAND NAMES	CHEMICAL STRUCTURE	RECOMMENDED DOSAGE

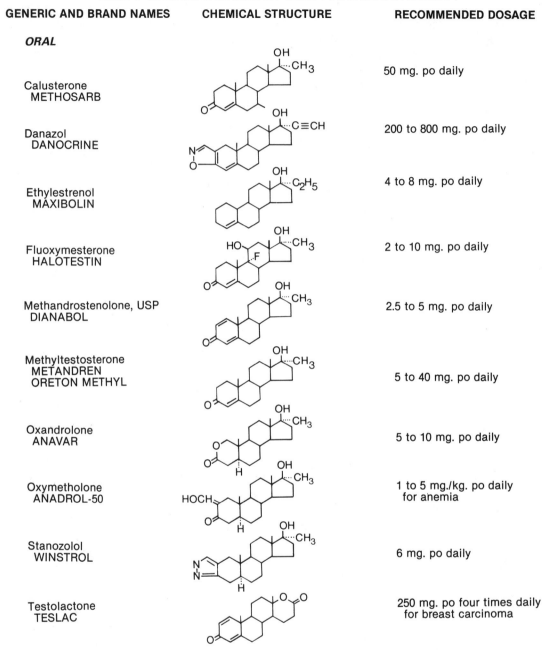

ORAL

Calusterone
METHOSARB — 50 mg. po daily

Danazol
DANOCRINE — 200 to 800 mg. po daily

Ethylestrenol
MAXIBOLIN — 4 to 8 mg. po daily

Fluoxymesterone
HALOTESTIN — 2 to 10 mg. po daily

Methandrostenolone, USP
DIANABOL — 2.5 to 5 mg. po daily

Methyltestosterone
METANDREN
ORETON METHYL — 5 to 40 mg. po daily

Oxandrolone
ANAVAR — 5 to 10 mg. po daily

Oxymetholone
ANADROL-50 — 1 to 5 mg./kg. po daily for anemia

Stanozolol
WINSTROL — 6 mg. po daily

Testolactone
TESLAC — 250 mg. po four times daily for breast carcinoma

bolic steroids' effect on performance results from retrospective efforts trying to compare different analyses using different study designs. Dosage, type, and duration of steroid used, diet, status of training prior to steroid usage, method of strength evaluation, and method of measuring body composition represent only some of the confounding variables. In view of the toxic effects of anabolic steroids, particularly at the larger doses often used by athletes, it is unlikely that ethically or legally endorsed prospective studies will be forthcoming in this country, and the effect of steroids on performance will likely con-

Table 4–2—*Continued*

GENERIC AND BRAND NAMES	CHEMICAL STRUCTURE	RECOMMENDED DOSAGE

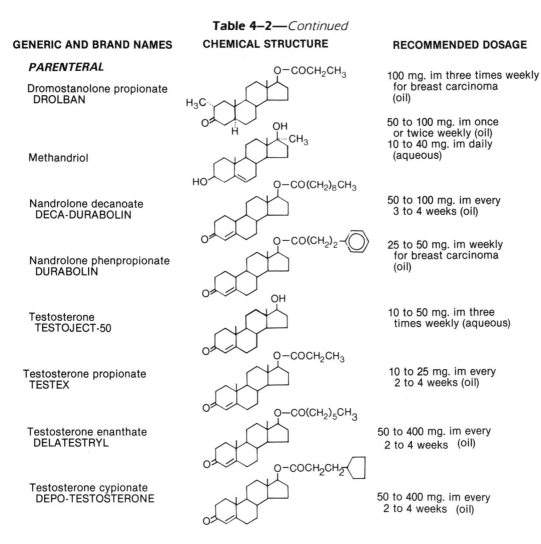

PARENTERAL

Dromostanolone propionate
DROLBAN

100 mg. im three times weekly
for breast carcinoma
(oil)

Methandriol

50 to 100 mg. im once
or twice weekly (oil)
10 to 40 mg. im daily
(aqueous)

Nandrolone decanoate
DECA-DURABOLIN

50 to 100 mg. im every
3 to 4 weeks (oil)

Nandrolone phenpropionate
DURABOLIN

25 to 50 mg. im weekly
for breast carcinoma
(oil)

Testosterone
TESTOJECT-50

10 to 50 mg. im three
times weekly (aqueous)

Testosterone propionate
TESTEX

10 to 25 mg. im every
2 to 4 weeks (oil)

Testosterone enanthate
DELATESTRYL

50 to 400 mg. im every
2 to 4 weeks (oil)

Testosterone cypionate
DEPO-TESTOSTERONE

50 to 400 mg. im every
2 to 4 weeks (oil)

tinue to be a source of controversy and speculation.

If any degree of athletic enhancement is to be attributed to anabolic steroids, a number of explanations are plausible:

1. Increased aggressiveness and motivation;
2. An anticatabolic effect (a reversal of the catabolic effect of glucocorticoids released during periods of stress associated with training);
3. Enhanced utilization of protein resulting in a positive nitrogen balance.

With respect to enhanced protein utilization, in situations other than hypogonadism, any positive nitrogen balance is short lived and probably lasts no more than several months.[3]

In research animals, muscle overload increases anabolic steroid receptor sites.[11] Extrapolating to humans, it is possible that the high level of training required prior to steroid usage in order to detect an increase in strength may reflect an increase in receptor sites in the skeletal muscle. It should be noted, however, that even in hypertrophied muscles, the number of free receptor sites is small.

As previously noted, the standard used for assessing the efficacy of anabolic steroids has been their effect on the ability to increase the maximal weight lifted in a single repetition of a lifting exercise (maximal voluntary isometric contraction). How this benchmark correlates with actual performance in a variety of competitive sports remains highly speculative.

At least some of the increase in weight following anabolic steroid use is from fluid retention secondary to salt retention.[3] In some sports, increased bulk, whether from increased mass or fluid retention, may actually impede performance, particularly where coordinated muscular movement and flexibility are required.

Detailed information regarding the effect of anabolic steroids in women similarly remains speculative and almost completely anecdotal. Strauss and associates[52] reported the results of 10 women athletes who acknowledged their use of anabolic steroids. They all reported a significant increase in muscle size, muscle strength, and performance when they first started using anabolic steroids. Such a response is not surprising since the clinical use of anabolic steroids in women for medical indications suggests that their muscular development can be enhanced, as it can in hypogonad males, both groups having low endogenous testosterone levels. Physiologically, the number of unsaturated anabolic-androgen receptors in the skeletal muscle of female and castrated male animals is higher than in normal male animals.

The use of anabolic steroids in women also induces virilization and an increased sense of aggressiveness. In addition to their illegality in competitive sports, the masculinizing side effects of these hormones often preclude their usage in women to a significant degree.

Few data are available regarding the effects of anabolic steroids on motor coordination and reaction time. Ariel and Saville[53] reported reduced reflex latencies in the patellar reflex components in anabolic steroid users in a study in which subjects served as their own controls for anabolic steroid use versus placebo. The significance of this finding is uncertain and has no obvious correlation to athletic performance.

Fowler and associates[49] noted no significant difference in vertical or long jump ability in subjects taking steroids versus those taking placebos. Both groups trained for 16 weeks under similar conditions. Johnson and co-workers[29] found no significant difference in the time of a mile run when comparing three groups of athletes who trained under similar conditions. One group of athletes received anabolic steroids, one group placebo, and the third group no drugs.

In adolescents, anabolic steroid use promotes an acceleration in skeletal and muscular growth, but premature closure of epiphyseal plates occurs, which in the end may stunt growth.

Neuromuscular and behavioral changes secondary to anabolic steroid use are difficult to tabulate succinctly,[54] as noted in this chapter. Further compounding the issue is the lack of reliable data on dosage of drug taken by the athlete and the mixture of drugs which may be ingested or injected. Some athletes have been reported to supplement anabolic steroids with human growth hormone for additive effects—a treatment strategy which has no good scientific basis in the adult. Others have been reported to add human chorionic gonadotropin in the hopes of preventing oligospermia and decreased sexual drive.[55] Still others have supplemented the drugs with stimulants to prevent the plateau of aggressivity which may occur with chronic usage.[4]

Anabolic steroid use is banned by the National Collegiate Athletic Association (NCAA), the International Olympic Committee (IOC), the National Football League (NFL), and the U.S. Powerlifting Federation. Human chorionic gonadotropin has been added to the list of banned drugs by the IOC.

Case Vignette

A 33-year-old white male decided to stop using anabolic steroids because of marital problems. He first began experimenting with oral anabolic steroids as part of preseason training for high school football, and he increased the frequency and amount of use in college. He had obtained the drugs through the black market, but was uncertain about the dosage of drug used. Once he became a professional football player, he felt obligated to use anabolic steroids, and he did so in a much more compulsive fashion. He felt pressured to use the drugs because he felt that they gave him an edge, not only in allowing him to play more aggressively, but also in preventing injuries.

Typically, he took anabolic steroids in 2- to 3-month cycles. He would ingest 50 to 100 mg per day of stanozolol and would inject

300 to 600 mg per week of nandrolone decanoate. During this period of time, he would intensively train with weights. He claimed that his ability to bench press bulk weights improved considerably during the anabolic steroid cycles, and his overall stamina seemed improved. He also felt incredibly charged, more so than when he had experimented with amphetamines. He noticed not only an increased aggressiveness, but also an increase in irritability and a tremendous sexual drive.

His wife readily recognized when he was on an anabolic steroid cycle. He increased his sexual demands and became physically rougher. His moods fluctuated widely, and insomnia interrupted his nights.

Eventually, after the patient began using anabolic steroids on a more regular basis, his testes shrank in size and his voice pitch rose. Despite these signs of feminism, he was unwilling to stop using the drugs because of a fear that he would be at a considerable disadvantage on the field without them, particularly as he was past his athletic prime and his career was winding down. He finally sought medical help after his wife left him. She no longer could tolerate his unpredictable violent behavior and obsession with anabolic steroid use.

ADVERSE EFFECTS

Legality aside, any potential benefit that might be derived from anabolic steroids in competitive athletics must be measured against their actual or potential side effects[54] (Table 4–3). Athletes often take anabolic steroids for many weeks prior to an event. The so-called stacking of steroids,[17,55,56] that is, combining oral and parenteral anabolic steroids so that the amount of drug used exceeds clinical doses by many fold, further increases the potential for side effects. Much of the data relative to side effects of these hormones probably are understated because they derive from studies of users ingesting the drugs in manufacturer's recommended doses for medical reasons.

Liver function abnormalities have been frequently reported in studies of athletes using oral (17 alpha alkylated) anabolic steroids. Since muscular exertion can cause elevations of SGOT and CPK, better indices of

Table 4–3. ADVERSE EFFECTS OF ANABOLIC STEROIDS

Liver function abnormalities
Peliosis hepatis
Benign and malignant liver tumors
Wilms' tumor
Prostate adenocarcinoma
Hypogonadotropic hypogonadism
Azoospermia
Testicular atrophy
Feminization (enlarged breasts, high-pitched voice)
Decreased high-density lipoprotein
Increased low-density lipoprotein
Hypercholesterolemia
Behavioral changes/psychiatric disorders
Impaired humoral immunity
Acne
Hair loss
Premature epiphyseal closure in prepubescent children

adverse effects on the liver can be obtained by monitoring liver-specific enzymes. Few data are available as to the reversibility of these enzymatic changes. Peliosis hepatis, a rare condition characterized by blood-filled cysts in the liver, has been reported in 23 cases.[7] All were associated with the taking of oral anabolic steroids as treatment for medical illnesses for periods greater than 6 months.

Anabolic steroids have been associated with the development of both liver and kidney tumors.[57,58] One report describes 36 benign and malignant liver tumors in patients who received anabolic steroids for more than 24 months to treat medical illnesses.[7] Another describes hepatocellular carcinoma in an athlete who had taken anabolic steroids intermittently over a 4-year period.[59] Wilms' tumor, a rare kidney malignancy, has been reported in association with anabolic steroid use,[59a,b] and adenocarcinoma of the prostate has been described in another young male athlete who used anabolic steroids.[60] AIDS has been reported in an anabolic steroid user without other risk factors other than sharing used needles for anabolic steroid injections.[61]

Prolonged use of anabolic steroids frequently results in lowering of plasma protein–bound testosterone.[7] Their effects on gonadotropin levels are less predictable,[55] although secondary hypogonadotropic hypogonadism may be observable for at least 16 weeks after the cessation of 3 months of high-dose anabolic steroids.[62] Prolonged use of these hormones also interferes with spermatogenesis and may result in azoospermia and testicular atrophy.[3,7] Paradoxically, anabolic steroids can produce feminizing side effects in males, most notably gynecomastia and a high voice, secondary to increased plasma estradiol—a metabolite of testosterone. Many, if not all, of the above described endocrine changes will reverse themselves if one stops the drug usage for several months.

To avoid testicular atrophy while taking anabolic steroids, some men have taken injections of human chorionic gonadotropin.[55,63] However, it has been demonstrated that continuous gonadotropic stimulation is needed to maintain normal spermatogenesis in athletes using anabolic steroids for prolonged periods of time.[62]

Some athletes inject human chorionic gonadotropin not only to prevent testicular atrophy, but also to stimulate the production of endogenous gonadal testosterone.[63] Not only is the effectiveness of this regimen questionable, but human chorionic gonadotropin itself can cause adverse reactions, including headache, mood swings, depression, and edema.[63]

Large doses of anabolic steroids produce detrimental changes in plasma lipid metabolism, as evidenced by large reductions in high-density lipoprotein cholesterol and increases in low-density lipoprotein cholesterol.[64–66a] In experimental animals, the effects of these changes are not mitigated by the beneficial changes produced by exercise.[67] The long-term side effects of such changes with regard to the development of atherosclerosis, coronary artery disease, and cerebral vascular disease are currently unknown, although a recent case report suggests a causal relationship between anabolic steroid use and acute myocardial infarction in a 22-year-old male weight lifter.[67a]

Humoral immunity may be impaired with anabolic steroid use. Immunoglobulins IgG, IgM, and IgA are significantly lower in anabolic steroid users as compared with controls.[68] The clinical significance of this finding is at present unknown.

Psychiatric side effects of anabolic steroids are rarely mentioned in the literature. In 1980, Annitto and Layman[68a] described a case of an acute schizophrenic episode in a 17-year-old male athlete who had been using illegally obtained anabolic steroids. In 1988, Pope and Katz[69] performed structured interviews of 41 steroid users in an effort to better define the problem of steroid-induced psychiatric changes. Nine subjects (22 percent) displayed manic or depressive symptomatology while taking anabolic steroids, and five (12 percent) had transiently become psychotic. Although this study was retrospective and may not reflect the true incidence of steroid-induced behavioral changes, the psychiatric changes mentioned are of serious concern.

Anabolic steroids obtained from the black market are often unsterile preparations, and frequently are deliberately mislabeled.[70] The potential complications from unknown and impure preparations are, needless to say, enormous.

FINAL NOTE

The abuse of anabolic steroids by athletes to enhance performance presents an especially difficult challenge to sports medicine. Power athletes have long recognized that anabolic steroids have ergogenic properties; these drugs increase bulk and strength and induce aggressiveness, all traits that are desirable in certain sports. Yet many in the medical community remain skeptical. Even leading experts disagree on how to interpret the same studies. However, there appears to be little doubt that strength can be increased by using anabolic steroids in conjunction with a high-protein diet and a vigorous weight-lifting program. Whether actual performance in athletic competition improves remains the subject of debate.

The credibility gap between physician and athlete has spilled over to the question of the adverse effects of anabolic steroids. Many athletes believe the adverse effects are overstated and are used by physicians as a scare tactic. In fact, most of the data have not been derived from the study of athletes but from studies in which anabolic steroids were used in pharmacologic doses to treat medical illnesses. Many of these adverse effects can be anticipated on the basis of hormonal physiology, and some are reversible after the drug is discontinued. Other adverse effects are less well understood, for example, structural changes in the liver and the development of various tumors. Since the doses of anabolic steroids used by athletes may be in excess of 1000 times the normally prescribed doses, it is reasonable to anticipate that the number and severity of adverse effects will significantly exceed those reported with therapeutic doses. However, even if the risk is well established, there are those athletes who feel the potential benefits derived from anabolic steroid use are so compelling that they are willing to use the drug no matter what the consequences.

As noted by Wright[54]: "If the public and government are concerned with equality and fair play as well as with the health of athletes and the future of sports, then comprehensive research studies must be undertaken on national and, if possible, international levels to conclusively determine the efficacy and hazards of the multitude of physical and chemical treatments currently being used or considered by athletes." Although Wright is correct, from a practical perspective it is unlikely that prospective research studies will be approved utilizing the dosages of anabolic steroids currently used by athletes for the purpose of enhancing performance.

Anabolic steroids have become a battleground for the athlete and the drug tester. The athlete, in an effort to avoid detection, has used various combinations of anabolic steroid preparations, rest periods from anabolic steroid use, and drugs that either dilute the urine or block the detection of anabolic steroids in the urine. The drug testers counter with lower detection limits and a better understanding of both anabolic steroid metabolites and possible blocking agents. But what of the athlete who succeeds in escaping the drug testers' urine screen at a particular athletic event? Is year-round testing the answer? What about probable cause testing?

These are but some of the issues that surface in this seemingly endless game. The issue is further clouded by the fact that there are physicians who believe that anabolic steroids speed healing by improving nitrogen balance and that physicians should be permitted to prescribe anabolic steroids—legal drugs that can be obtained with a prescription—for this purpose. Some have suggested that anabolic steroids should be categorized as controlled substances, but this might simply increase the flow of black market drugs into the athletic community.

The two major issues at hand are medical and ethical. We encourage any further studies, such as the retrospective analysis proposed by Wright,[71] that will improve the current understanding of the medical risks of anabolic steroid use. However, even if the risks are found to be relatively small, should attempts by athletes to improve performance through anabolic steroid use be allowed? As columnist George Will[72] notes: "A society's recreation is charged with moral significance. Sport—and a society that takes it seriously—would be debased if it did not strictly forbid things that blur the distinction between the triumph of character and the triumph of chemistry."

REFERENCES

1. Forbes, TR: Crowing hen: early observations on spontaneous sex reversals in birds. Yale J Biol Med 19:955, 1947.
2. Berthold, AA: Transplantation der hoden. Arch Anat Physiol Wiss Med 16:42, 1849.
3. Murad, F and Haynes, RC, Jr: Androgens. In Gilman, AG, et al. (eds): Goodman and Gilman's The Pharmacologic Basis of Therapeutics, 7th ed. Macmillan, New York, 1986, p 1440.
4. Goldman, B: Death in the Locker Room: Steroids, Cocaine & Sports. The Body Press, Tucson, 1987.
5. Ryan, AJ: Anabolic steroids are fool's gold. Fed Proc 40:2682, 1981.
6. Perlmutter, G and Lowenthal, DT: Use of anabolic steroids by athletes. Am Fam Physician 32:208, 1985.
7. Haupt, HA and Rovere, GD: Anabolic steroids: A review of the literature. Am J Sports Med 12:469, 1984.
7a. Johnson, WO and Moore, K: The loser. Sports Illustrated, October 3, 1988, p 20.
8. Wade, NA: Anabolic steroids: Doctors denounce them, but athletes aren't listening. Science 176:1399, 1972.
9. Logan, G: Jets' Cadigan: I'll do anything to succeed. Newsday, March 28, 1988.
9a. Kochakian, CD: Anabolic, Androgenic Steroids. Springer Verlag, New York, 1976.
10. Saartok, T, Dahlbey, E, and Gustafsson, J: Relative binding affinity of anabolic-androgenic steroids: Comparison of the binding to the androgen receptors in skeletal muscle and in prostate, as well as to sex hormone–binding globulin. Endocrinology 114:2100, 1984.
11. Hickson, RC and Kurowski, TG: Anabolic steroids and training. Clin Sports Med 5:461, 1986.
12. Hickson, RC, et al: Skeletal muscle cytosol (3H)methyl trienolone receptor binding and serum androgens: Effects of hypertrophy and hormonal state. J Steroid Biochem 19:1705, 1983.

13. Schiavi, RC, et al: Sex chromosome anomalies, hormones, and aggressivity. Arch Gen Psychiatry 41:93, 1984.
14. Mattsson, A, et al: Plasma testosterone, aggressive behavior, and personality dimensions in young male delinquents. J Am Acad Child Psychiatry 19:476, 1980.
15. Olweus, D, et al: Testosterone, aggression, physical, and personality dimensions in normal adolescent males. Psychosom Med 42:253, 1980.
16. Rose, RM, Holaday, JW, and Bernstein, IS: Plasma testosterone, dominance rank and aggressive behaviour in male Rhesus monkeys. Nature 231:366, 1971.
17. Hollister, LE, Davis, KL, and Davis, BM: Hormones in the treatment of psychiatric disorders. Hosp Pract 10:103, 1975.
18. American Medical Association Department of Drugs, Division of Drugs and Technology: Androgens and Anabolic Steroids. In AMA Drug Evaluations, 6th ed. Philadelphia, WB Saunders, 1986, p 675.
19. Anderson, WA and McKeag, DB: The Substance Use and Abuse Habits of College Student-Athletes. Presented to National Collegiate Athletic Association Council by College of Human Medicine, Michigan State University, June, 1985.
20. Elite Women Athletes Survey. Hazelden Health Promotion Services, January, 1987.
20a. Dezelsky, TL, Toohey, JV, and Shaw, RS: Nonmedical drug use behavior at five United States universities: A 15-year study. Bull Narc 37:49, 1985.
20b. Pope, HG, Katz, DL, and Champoux, R: Anabolic-androgenic steroid use among 1,010 college men. Phys Sportsmed 16(7):75, 1988.
21. Runner's World 22:12, 1987.
22. Strauss, RH: Drug abuse in sports: A three-pronged response. Phys Sportsmed 16(2):47, 1988.
23. Of steroids and sports. Emergency Medicine 20:190, 1988.
24. American College of Sports Medicine, Position Stand: Anabolic Steroids and Athletes, Indianapolis, 1987.
25. Nightingale, SL (From the FDA): Illegal marketing of anabolic steroids to enhance athletic performance charged. JAMA 256:1851, 1986.
26. Cowart, V: Some predict increased steroid use in sports despite drug testing, crackdown on suppliers. JAMA 257:3025, 1987.
27. Anabolic Steroid Abuse. FDA Drug Bulletin. October, 1987.
28. Johnson, LC, et al: Anabolic steroid: Effects on strength, body weight, oxygen uptake and spermatogenesis upon mature males. Med Sci Sports 4:43, 1972.
29. Johnson, LC, et al: Effect of anabolic steroid treatment on endurance. Med Sci Sports 7:287, 1975.
30. Hervey, GR, et al: "Anabolic" effects of methandienone in men undergoing athletic training. Lancet 2:699, 1976.
31. Bowers, RW and Reardon, JP: Effects of methandostenolone (Dianabol) on strength development and aerobic capacity. Med Sci Sports 4:54, 1972.
32. Loughton, SJ and Ruhling, RO: Human strength and endurance responses to anabolic steroid and training. J Sports Med Phys Fitness 17:285, 1977.
33. O'Shea, JP: Anabolic steroid: Effect on competitive swimmers. Nutr Report Int 1:337, 1970.
34. O'Shea, JP and Winkler, W: Biochemical and physical effects of an anabolic steroid in competitive swimmers and weightlifters. Nutr Report Int 2:351, 1970.
35. Stromme, SB, Meen, HD, and Aakvaag, A: Effects of an androgenic-anabolic steroid on strength development and plasma testosterone levels in normal males. Med Sci Sports 6:203, 1974.
36. Win-May, M and Mya-Tu, M: The effect of anabolic steroids on physical fitness. J Sports Med Phys Fitness 15:266, 1975.
37. Fahey, TD and Brown, CH: The effects of an anabolic steroid on the strength, body composition, and endurance of college males when accompanied by a weight training program. Med Sci Sports 5:272, 1973.
38. Ariel, G: The effect of anabolic steroid (methandrostenolone) upon selected physiological parameters. Ath Training 7:190, 1972.
39. Ariel, G: Residual effect of an anabolic steroid upon isotonic muscular force. J Sports Med Phys Fitness 14:103, 1974.
40. Freed, DL, et al: Anabolic steroids in athletics: crossover double-blind trial on weightlifters. Br Med J 2:471, 1975.
41. Hervey, GR, et al: Effects of methandienone on the performance and body composition of men undergoing athletic training. Clin Sci 60:457, 1981.
42. O'Shea, JP: The effects of an anabolic steroid on dynamic strength levels of weightlifters. Nutr Report Int 4:363, 1971.
43. O'Shea, JP: A biochemical evaluation of the effects of stanozolol on adrenal, liver and muscle function in humans. Nutr Report Int 10:3831, 1974.
44. Stamford, BA and Moffatt, R: Anabolic steroid: Effectiveness as an ergogenic aid to experienced weight trainers. J Sports Med 14:191, 1974.
45. Tahmindjis, AJ: The use of anabolic steroids by athletes to increase body weight and strength. Med J Aust 1:991, 1976.
46. Ward, P: The effect of an anabolic steroid on strength and lean body mass. Med Sci Sports 5:277, 1973.
47. Casnser, SW, Jr, Early, RG, and Carlson, BR: Anabolic steroid effects on body composition in normal young men. J Sports Med Phys Fitness 11:98, 1971.
48. Crist, DM, Stackpole, PJ, and Peake, GT: Effects of androgenic-anabolic steroids on neuromuscular power and body composition. J Appl Physiol 54:366, 1983.
49. Fowler, WM, Jr, Gardner, GW, and Egstrom, GH: Effect of an anabolic steroid on physical performance of young men. J Appl Physiol 20:1038, 1965.
50. Golding, LA, Freydinger, JE, and Fishel, SS: Weight, size, and strength—unchanged with steroids. Phys Sportsmed 2:39, 1974.
51. Samuels, LT, Henschel, AF, and Keys, A: Influence of methyl testosterone on muscular work and creatine metabolism in normal young men. J Clin Endocrinol Metab 2:649, 1942.
52. Strauss, RH, et al: Anabolic steroid use and perceived effects in ten weight-trained women athletes. JAMA 253:2871, 1985.

53. Ariel, G and Saville, W: The effect of anabolic steroids on reflex components. Med Sci Sports 4:120, 1972.

54. Wright, JE: Anabolic steroids and athletics. Exer Sport Sci Rev 8:149, 1980.

55. Strauss, RH: Drugs in Sports. In Strauss, RH (ed): Sports Medicine. WB Saunders, Philadelphia, 1984, p 481.

56. Burkett, LN and Falduto, MT: Steroid use by an athlete in a metropolitan area. Phys Sportsmed 12(8):69, 1984.

57. MacDougall, D: Anabolic steroids. Phys Sportsmed 11(9):95, 1983.

58. Johnson, FS: The association of oral androgenic-anabolic steroids and life-threatening disease. Med Sci Sports 7:284, 1975.

59. Overly, WL, et al: Androgens and hepatocellular carcinoma in an athlete (Letter). Ann Intern Med 100:158, 1984.

59a. Pratt, J, et al: Wilms' tumor in an adult associated with androgen abuse. JAMA 237:2322, 1977.

59b. Windsor, RE and Dumitru, D: Anabolic steroid use by athletes. How serious are the health hazards? Postgraduate Medicine 84:37, 1988.

60. Roberts, JT and Essenhigh, DM: Adenocarcinoma of prostate in 40-year-old body-builder. Lancet 2:742, 1984.

61. Sklarek, HM, et al: AIDS in a bodybuilder using anabolic steroid. N Engl J Med 311:1701, 1984.

62. Martikainen, H, et al: Testicular responsiveness to human chorionic gonadotrophin during transient hypogonadotrophic hypogonadism induced by androgenic/anabolic steroids in power athletes. J Steroid Biochem 25:109, 1986.

63. Voy, RO: IOC bans human chorionic gonadotrophin. Sportsmediscope 7:I1, 1988.

64. Webb, Ol, Laskarzewski, PM, and Glueck, CJ: Severe depression of high-density lipoprotein cholesterol levels in weight lifters and body builders by self-administered exogenous testosterone and anabolic-androgenic steroids. Metabolism 33:971, 1984.

65. Costill, DL, Pearson, DR, and Fink, WJ: Anabolic steroid use among athletes: Changes in HDL-C levels. Phys Sportsmed 12(6):113, 1984.

66. Peterson, GE and Fahey, TD: HDL-C in five elite athletes using anabolic-androgenic steroids. Phys Sportsmed 12(6):120, 1984.

66a. Cohen, JC, Noakes, TD, and Benade, AJS: Hypercholesterolemia in male power lifters using anabolic-androgenic steroids. Phys Sportsmed 16(8):49, 1988.

67. Leeds, EM, et al: Effects of exercise and anabolic steroids on total and lipoprotein cholesterol concentrations in male and female rats. Med Sci Sports Exer 18:663, 1986.

67a. McNutt, RA, et al: Acute myocardial infarction in a 22-year-old world class weight lifter using anabolic steroids. Am J Cardiol 62:164, 1988.

68. Duda, M: Study: Steroids lower immunity, lipids. Phys Sportsmed 16(2):56, 1988.

68a. Annitto, WJ and Layman, WA: Anabolic steroids and acute schizophrenic episode. J Clin Psychiatry 41:143, 1980.

69. Pope, HG and Katz, DL: Affective and psychotic symptoms associated with anabolic steroid use. Am J Psychiatry 145:487, 1988.

70. Voy, RO: Steroid users beware! Sportsmediscope 7:I1, 1988.

71. Cowart, VS: Study proposes to examine football players, power lifters for possible long-term sequelae from anabolic steroid use in 1970s competition. JAMA 257:3021, 1987.

72. Will, A: Why the chemistry has to be right. Newsday, October 2, 1988.

Human Growth Hormone

HISTORY

Growth hormone abuse among athletes appears to represent another chapter in the never-ending quest by athletes to gain a competitive edge by turning to pharmaceutics. Prior to 1985, exogenous human growth hormone was obtained from cadaver pituitary extracts, and the supply was quite scarce. The development of Creutzfeldt-Jakob disease in four boys who were treated with cadaver-derived human growth hormone[1] led to the discontinuation of all products derived from the human pituitary. Shortly after pituitary-derived products were banned, genetically engineered human growth hormone for exogenous use became available.

In the United States, two genetically engineered drugs have been approved by the Food and Drug Administration for therapeutic use as exogenous human growth hormone supplements: somatotropin (Humatrope) and somatrem (Protropin). Growth hormone supplementation is officially restricted to the approximately 4000 patients with documented growth hormone deficiency.[2] Distribution of human growth hormone is monitored by the manufacturer, and rigorous screening and postmarketing surveillance procedures have been implemented.[3]

CHEMISTRY AND PHYSIOLOGY

Exogenous human growth hormone mimics the actions of the endogenous hormone. Growth hormone is a polypeptide secreted by the anterior pituitary into the general circulation. Metabolic effects are divided into acute and delayed. Acute effects of growth hormone secretion are insulin-like and include:

1. Increased amino acid uptake and incorporation into protein in muscle and liver
2. Stimulation of glucose uptake in muscle and adipose tissue
3. Antilipolytic effects in adipose tissue

The acute metabolic effects are observed following physiologic doses of growth hormone and cease after three to four hours.[4] Delayed effects are seen after 4 hours and produce the long-term metabolic consequences of chronic growth hormone exposure:

1. Increased mobilization of free fatty acids from adipose tissue secondary to triglyceride lipolysis
2. Increased sensitivity to the lipolytic effects of catecholamines
3. Inhibition of glucose uptake and utilization

Nearly every organ is dependent on growth hormone for proper growth and development.[5] Increased somatic growth appears to be mediated by growth-promoting polypeptides, which in turn are dependent on growth hormone. Somatomedin C and insulin-like growth factor are growth hormone–dependent serum growth factors which stimulate cellular processes (DNA, RNA, protein synthesis) and cause growth of

Table 5–1. FACTORS AFFECTING GROWTH HORMONE SECRETION

Stimulative	Suppressive*
Physiologic	
Sleep	Postprandial hyperglycemia
Exercise	Elevated free fatty acids
Stress (physical or psychological)	
Postprandial hyperaminoacidemia	
Postprandial hypoglycemia (relative)	
Pharmacologic	
Hypoglycemia:	Hormones:
Absolute: insulin or 2-deoxyglucose	Somatostatin
Relative: postglucagon	Somatomedin C (IGF-I)
Hormones:	Growth hormone
Peptides (GRH, ACTH, α-MSH, vasopressin)	Progesterone
Estrogen	Glucocorticoids
Neurotransmitters:	Neurotransmitters:
α-Adrenergic agonists (clonidine)	α-Adrenergic antagonists (phentolamine)
β-Adrenergic antagonists (propranolol)	β-Adrenergic agonists (isoproterenol)
Serotonin precursors (5-hydroxytryptamine)	Serotonergic antagonists (methysergide)
Dopaminergic agonists (L-dopa,	Dopaminergic antagonists (phenothiazines)
apomorphine, bromocriptine)	Cholinergic (muscarinic) antagonists
GABA agonists (muscimol)	(pirenzepine)
Enkephalin analogues	
Pathologic	
Protein depletion and starvation	Obesity
Anorexia nervosa	Hypothyroidism and hyperthyroidism
Chronic renal failure	Acromegaly: dopaminergic agonists
Acromegaly:	
TRH	
GnRH	

*Suppressive effects of some factors can be demonstrated only in the presence of a stimulus.

From Frohman, LA: Diseases of the Anterior Pituitary. In Felig, P, et al (eds): Endocrinology and Metabolism. McGraw-Hill, New York, 1987, p 268, with permission.

skeletal and extraskeletal tissue. Linear bone growth and increased skeletal mass are the most apparent skeletal effects of growth hormone exposure in adolescents.

Although exogenous human growth hormone administration will cause more normal skeletal growth in growth hormone–deficient children, accelerated statural growth will also occur following exogenous growth hormone administration to children who do not have classical growth hormone deficiency.[6-8] However, it is not known if the final height obtained in the latter case will exceed that which would have occurred without exogenous growth hormone administration.

The human pituitary contains 5 to 10 mg growth hormone. Daily production is 0.4 to 1.0 mg per day in adult males and is slightly higher in adolescents and females. Serum levels range from 0.5 to 3.0 μg per liter and are influenced by many factors (Table 5–1). Growth hormone–releasing hormone (GHRH, GRH) and somatostatin are hypothalamic-released polypeptides which exhibit direct excitatory and inhibitory effects, respectively, on pituitary release of growth hormone. In addition to the stimulative factors listed in Table 5–1, ingestion of certain amino acids (arginine aspartase; combination of l-arginine pyrrolidone carboxylate and l-lysine hydrochloride) may transiently cause increased growth hormone secretion.[9]

The influence of exercise on growth hormone secretion and metabolism is not clearcut. In general, high-intensity exercise, either of short or long duration, is associated with an elevated growth hormone level. Women, the elderly, and untrained individuals tend to have higher postexercise levels than trained men.[10] High-intensity exercises lead to increased growth hormone secretion independent of associated emotional stress.[10]

CLINICAL PHARMACOLOGY

The half-life of growth hormone varies from 17 to 45 minutes and is unchanged by exercise, but the biological effects are much longer lasting due to the stimulation of somatomedins. Somatomedins are protein bound and have a half-life of 3 to 4 hours.[5] Growth hormone is extensively metabolized in the liver, and only a small fraction is excreted by the kidney in an immunologically recognizable form.[4]

The optimal dosage of exogenous human growth hormone for the therapeutic treatment of growth hormone deficiency is not known. The recommended dose of somatotropin (Humatrope) is 0.06 mg per kg, three times per week; the recommended dose of somatrem (Protropin) is 0.1 mg per kg three times per week. Both are given as an intramuscular injection. Doses higher than the currently recommended dose may produce further growth increases in adolescents.[11]

Growth hormone assays are often difficult to perform and to interpret,[12] but assays of somatomedin C may provide useful information regarding the amount of exposure to biologically active human growth hormone in an individual.[13]

Clinical Uses

The only indication for exogenous human growth hormone administration is for the treatment of growth hormone deficiency.[2] Possible future uses of the drug include the treatment of osteoporosis, obesity, and trauma.[14]

USE IN SPORTS

No data exist regarding the incidence of human growth hormone use among amateur or professional athletes. However, since the marketing of synthetic human growth hormone in 1985, there has been an alarming increase in the number of inquiries by athletes about the drug.[14] Several aspects of human growth hormone use appear to seduce both the athlete and parents of the young athlete:

1. Because of widespread anabolic steroid testing, many athletes feel that human growth hormone use will give the beneficial effects of anabolic steroids but cannot be detected.

2. The prospect of increased size combined with decreased fat stores is very appealing.

3. Some athletes feel that the advantages of anabolic steroids can be obtained without any of the associated side effects.

4. Parents may feel justified, or obligated, to help their athletically gifted, but short or average-sized child.

Already, instances of athletes using megadose amounts—in the range of 20 times the recommended therapeutic dose—have been reported. Physicians have reported early signs of acromegaly among some athletes who abuse the drug.[14] One physician was indicted for using his license to buy large amounts of human growth hormone and then selling it for nonmedical purposes.[14]

Effects on Performance

Despite the apparent increase in human growth hormone use as an ergogenic aid, no study to date has demonstrated an improvement in physical or physiologic parameters which could potentially be of benefit to the athlete. In view of the toxic effects of growth hormone excess, it is unlikely that ethically or legally endorsed prospective studies will be forthcoming in this country, and the effect of growth-hormone—as with anabolic steroids—on performance will likely continue to be a source of controversy and speculation.

Several animal studies which focus on muscle size and strength following exogenous growth hormone administration may be of relevance to the athlete. Bigland and Jehring[15] noted an increase in quadriceps weight and cross-sectional diameter in rats exposed to high-dose growth hormone for 21 days. However, muscle tension per gram of tissue was decreased in the treated animals. Goldberg and Goodman[16] noted an increase in muscle size in atrophied and hypertrophied rat muscle after growth hormone treatment. In rats with atrophied muscles, Apostolakis and associates[17] demonstrated an increase in both size and strength following growth hormone administration. The general consensus from rat studies is that growth hormone may increase the size and strength of atrophied muscles, but the effects on contractile elements and functional performance in normal muscles are less certain.[9]

The applicability of animal studies to humans is unclear. Although it has been stated that supraphysiologic doses of human growth hormone would be needed for an athletic advantage,[14] clinical experience with adult acromegalics reveals myopathic signs (i.e., muscle weakness) despite increased muscle mass.[4] No improved performance effect has ever been demonstrated from the use of this hormone.

Although no urine test is available for human growth hormone, its use is banned by the United States Olympic Committee, and evidence confirming its use will result in the same punitive action as that for using any banned substance. The National Collegiate Athletic Association also prohibits the use of human, animal, or synthetic growth hormone.

ADVERSE EFFECTS

The safety of exogenous human growth hormone for therapeutic purposes has not been established.[2] Less is known about its use in normal subjects, although adverse effects of endogenous growth hormone hypersecretion are well established (Table 5–2).

Growth hormone excess in children may cause gigantism due to accelerated linear bone growth. In addition, supraphysiologic doses of growth hormone in children may cause the metabolic and systemic side effects of hypersecretion in adults.[18] In adults, growth hormone hypersecretion causes acromegaly. Of particular concern vis-à-vis the athlete, acromegalics typically develop a myopathy, peripheral neuropathy, and cardiac disease, including coronary artery disease and cardiomyopathy. The musculoskeletal and cardiac disease associated with growth

Table 5–2. ADVERSE EFFECTS OF ELEVATED HUMAN GROWTH HORMONE LEVELS

Adults	Children/Adolescents
Soft tissue swelling	Gigantism
Bony hypertrophy/prominence	As per adults
Thickened skin	
Hirsutism	
Fibroma molluscum	
Acanthosis nigricans	
Sebaceous gland hypersecretion	
Increased sweating	
Peripheral neuropathy	
Myopathy	
Visceromegaly:	
salivary glands	
liver	
spleen	
kidney	
heart	
Colonic polyps	
Cardiovascular disease	
Cardiomyopathy	
Hypertension	
Glucose intolerance/diabetes	

hormone excess may be irreversible, even after physiologic growth hormone levels are restored.[4]

An additional concern with exogenous human growth hormone administration is the development of growth hormone antibodies, which could potentially interfere with the activity of endogenous growth hormone.[2]

FINAL NOTE

Human growth hormone represents a particular challenge to the sports community, and the scientific and ethical questions regarding its use may become more urgent if unlimited quantities of the drug become available to the public.[18] The romantic appeal of the drug is obvious, but no usefulness as an ergogenic aid has been established. Clinical experience with acromegalics suggests that, if anything, prolonged exposure to supraphysiologic doses of human growth hormone produces detrimental neuromuscular side effects.

More serious ethical issues arise with its use in children. Not only are children unable to understand the consequences of their actions, but also the abuse of human growth hormone among adolescents carries with it an unknown medical future. Athletes, coaches, trainers, parents, and physicians should realize that no ergogenic effects have been documented following human growth hormone administration, and the potential long-term side effects of the drug are irreversible and may be life-threatening.

REFERENCES

1. Brown, P, et al: Potential epidemic of Creutzfeldt-Jakob disease from human growth hormone therapy. New Engl J Med 313:718, 1985.

2. A new biosynthetic human growth hormone. The Medical Letter 29 (745):73, 1987.
3. Council Report: Drug abuse in athletes. Anabolic steroids and human growth hormone. JAMA 259:1703, 1988.
4. Frohman, LA: Diseases of the Anterior Pituitary. In Felig, P, et al: Endocrinology and Metabolism, 2d edition. McGraw-Hill, New York, 1987, p 247.
5. Murad, F and Haynes, RC: Adenohypophyseal Hormones and Related Substances. In Gilman, AG, et al (eds): Goodman and Gilman's The Pharmacological Basis of Therapeutics, 7th Edition. Macmillan, New York, 1985, p 1362.
6. Van Vliet, G, et al: Growth hormone treatment for short stature. New Engl J Med 309:1016, 1983.
7. Spiliotis, BE, et al: Growth hormone neurosecretory dysfunction. A treatable cause of short stature. JAMA 251:2223, 1984.
8. Rosenfeld, RG, et al: Methionyl human growth hormone and oxandrolone in Turner syndrome: Preliminary results of a prospective randomized trial. J Pediatr 109:936, 1986.
9. Macintyre, JG: Growth hormone and athletes. Sports Medicine 4:129, 1987.
10. Shephard, RJ and Sidney, KH: Effects of physical exercise on plasma growth hormone and cortisol levels in human subjects. Exercise Sports Sci Rev 3:1, 1975.
11. Gerner, JM, et al: Renewed catch-up growth with increased replacement doses of human growth hormone. J Pediatr 110:425, 1987.
12. Legwook, G: Have we learned a lesson about drugs in sports? Phys Sportsmed 12:175, 1985.
13. Kao, PK, Abboud, CF, and Zimmerman, D: Somatomedin C: An index of growth hormone activity. Mayo Clin Proc 61:908, 1986.
14. Cowart, VS: Human growth hormone: The latest ergogenic aid? Phys Sportsmed 16(3):175, 1988.
15. Bigland, B and Jehring, B: Muscle performance in rats, normal, and treated with growth hormone. J Physiol 116:129, 1952.
16. Goldberg, AL and Goodman, HM: Relationship between growth hormone and muscle work in determining muscle size. J Physiol 200:655, 1969.
17. Apostolakis, M, Deligiannis, A, and Madena-Pyrgaki, A: The effects of human growth hormone administration on the fractional status of rat atrophied muscle following immobilization. Physiologist 23 (Suppl):S111, 1980.
18. Underwood, LE: Report of the conference on uses and possible abuses of biosynthetic human growth hormone. New Engl J Med 311:606, 1984.

CHAPTER 6

Amphetamine

HISTORY

Since Piness and associates'[1] 1930 publication on the pressor effects of amphetamines, these drugs have been the subject of much investigation and controversy. In 1935, Prinzmetal and Bloomberg[2] exploited the central stimulant effects of amphetamine to treat narcolepsy. The Germans, who became interested in amphetamines during World War II as a means of delaying the onset of fatigue in troops, demonstrated that the time of running to the point of exhaustion was increased by the use of intramuscular amphetamine.[3,4] Reports appeared of soldiers who had received amphetamines successfully marching long distances despite severe blisters on their feet.[4] Following the war, reports of enhanced endurance in cycling and hand ergometry experiments appeared.[4]

Amphetamine abuse began to occur in the 1940s, became widespread in Japan in the 1950s, and peaked in the United States in the 1960s.[5] Even though the Food and Drug Administration classified amphetamine as a prescription drug in 1938, vast amounts of the drug were diverted into illegal channels in the 1960s.[6] In 1969, over 13 percent of American college students had used amphetamines at least once.[7]

In 1957, in response to reports of amphetamine use to improve athletic performance, the American Medical Association (AMA) condemned such use.[8] However, an ad hoc committee of the AMA, the Committee on Amphetamines and Athletics, working with the National Collegiate Athletic Association and other groups, reported that "the use of these drugs is apparently very small."[8] According to Mandell and associates,[9] professional football players began to use amphet-

75

amines in the 1940s. Their published observations of the extent of amphetamine usage by a National Football League team in 1968 and 1969 were startling and will be discussed later in this chapter.

Throughout the 1960s, amphetamines were readily available and were extensively used for weight control. However, it was increasingly recognized that this was an unsatisfactory approach, in part at least, because of problems with side effects, psychological dependency, and tolerance.

In 1970, amphetamines constituted 14 percent of all psychoactive drugs prescribed by physicians. The Controlled Substances Act of 1970 abruptly changed the availability of amphetamines by imposing severe manufacturing quotas and by establishing strict guidelines for their use. Within 2 years, the production of amphetamines fell to 12 percent of the 1970 levels, and amphetamine abuse declined significantly.[6]

CHEMISTRY AND PHYSIOLOGY

Catecholamines

Amphetamine and the sympathomimetic amines mimic the actions of the endogenous catecholamines epinephrine, norepinephrine, and dopamine. "Catecholamine" refers to a compound that contains a catechol nucleus and an amine group (Fig. 6–1). Catecholamines exert their actions through specific central and peripheral alpha- and beta-adrenergic and dopamine receptors. An understanding of the catecholamine-receptor system is necessary to appreciate the effects

Table 6–1. END ORGAN RESPONSE TO CATECHOLAMINES

Organ	Receptor	Response
Heart	β-1	Increase heart rate and force of contraction
Lung	β-2	Bronchial dilatation
Arterioles	α	Constriction
	β-2	Dilatation
Liver	α, β-2	Glycogenolysis, gluconeogenesis
Skeletal Muscle	β-2	Increase contractility, glycogenolysis
Intestines	α, β-1, β-2	Decrease motility, tone

of amphetamine and the sympathomimetic agents.

In the peripheral nervous system, alpha- and beta-adrenergic receptors are the primary mediators of the effects of amphetamine. Traditionally, alpha receptors are classified as alpha-1 (postsynaptic) and alpha-2 (presynaptic or autoreceptor), and beta receptors are divided into beta-1 and beta-2. The release of endogenous catecholamines normally occurs under conditions of stress or increased physical activity. The diverse biologic effects occur because of the predominance of one or another receptor in a particular organ, and the effect mediated by that receptor. The responses of some peripheral organs to stimulation by catecholamines are summarized in Table 6–1.

In the central nervous system, norepinephrine and dopamine receptors are the primary catecholamines and are similarly classified as postsynaptic (delta-1, alpha-1, beta-1) or as an autoreceptor (delta-2, alpha-2, beta-2). Virtually all of the central nervous system noradrenergic pathways studied to date are efferent pathways of the locus ceruleus. From here, major norepinephrine tracts project to the cerebral cortex, cerebellum, brain stem, and spinal cord (Fig. 6–2). A major function of the locus ceruleus and its projections may be to determine the orientation of the brain to events in the external world or within the internal organs of the body.

The dopamine systems in the brain are more complex. Short and intermediate-length systems exist in the retina and the hy-

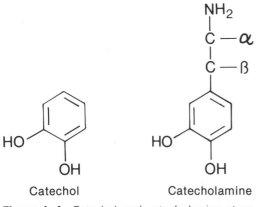

Figure 6–1. Catechol and catecholamine structure.

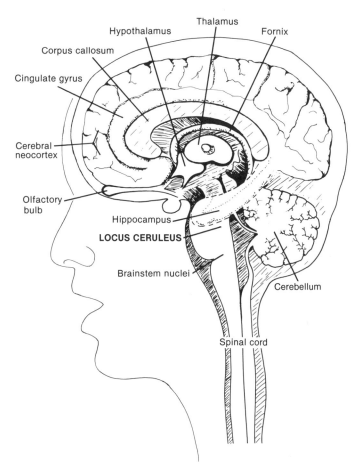

Thalamus
Hypothalamus
Fornix
Corpus callosum
Cingulate gyrus
Cerebral neocortex
Olfactory bulb
Hippocampus
LOCUS CERULEUS
Brainstem nuclei
Cerebellum
Spinal cord

Figure 6–2. Schematic diagram of the projections of the locus ceruleus viewed in the sagittal plane.

pothalamic-pituitary axis, respectively. The more important central nervous system dopamine projections for mediating motor and cognitive/emotional behavior include:

1. Mesocortical/mesolimbic system: ventral tegmental and substantia nigra dopamine cells project to the medial prefrontal, cingulate, and entorhinal cortex plus other limbic regions, including the septum, pyriform cortex, amygdaloid complex, stria terminalis nuclei, lateral septal nuclei, and the olfactory tubercle (Fig. 6–3). This system—the "pleasure brain"—is important in regulating aspects of behavior, including affect and memory, and plays a central role in mediating the effects of amphetamines.

2. Tuberoinfundibular system: arcuate nucleus dopamine cell bodies of the median eminence project to the pituitary. This system is involved in neuroendocrine regulation.

3. Nigrostriatal system: substantia nigra dopamine cells project to the caudate and putamen. This system is involved in important aspects of movement; degeneration of this system causes Parkinson's disease.

Catecholamines are synthesized in the brain, sympathetic nerves, sympathetic ganglia, and chromaffin cells of the adrenal medulla from the amino acid precursor tyrosine (Fig. 6–4). Tyrosine hydroxylase is the rate-limiting enzyme (see pathway 1 in Fig. 6–4). Metabolic transformation of catecholamines occurs primarily via two enzymes: monoamine oxidase (MAO), and catechol-O-methyltransferase (COMT).

Amphetamines

Sympathomimetic drugs share common chemical structures with the chemicals referred to as catecholamines. They both have

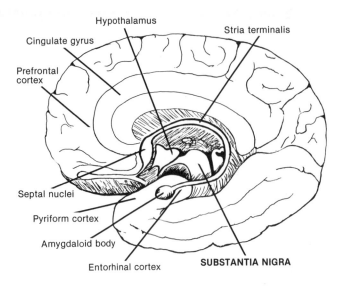

Hypothalamus

Stria terminalis

Cingulate gyrus

Prefrontal cortex

Septal nuclei

Pyriform cortex

Amygdaloid body

Entorhinal cortex   **SUBSTANTIA NIGRA**

Figure 6–3. Schematic diagram illustrating the distribution of the main central neuronal pathways containing dopamine.

beta-phenylethylamine as their parent compound with substitutions made either on the aromatic ring, the alpha or beta carbon atoms, or the amino group. The type and location of these various substitutions will determine the final pharmacologic effect. However, for a sympathomimetic amine to be categorized as a catecholamine, it must have hydroxyl substitutions in the aromatic ring. Amphetamines do not have these hydroxyl substitutions and therefore are not referred to as catecholamines (Fig. 6–5).

Amphetamine was first synthesized in 1887.[10] In addition to its powerful central nervous system effects, amphetamine, like other sympathomimetic drugs, acts on peripheral alpha- and beta-adrenergic receptors. The proposed modes of action of amphetamine on the peripheral and central nervous system include:

1. Displacement of catecholamine, thus causing direct release into the synaptic cleft
2. Partial catecholamine agonist, thus mimicking the action of endogenous catecholamine
3. Inhibition of synaptic catecholamine reuptake, thus increasing the availability of catecholamine at the synaptic cleft
4. Inhibition of monoamine oxidase, thus preventing the metabolic degradation of endogenous catecholamine, thereby increasing its availability[11]

The most prominent peripheral effect of amphetamine is elevation of both systolic and diastolic blood pressure. Heart rate is usually reflexly slowed,[12] and the effects on the intestinal tract are less predictable.

The most prominent behavioral responses following amphetamine ingestion are from the powerful central nervous system stimulating effects. These effects are mediated through both the norepinephrine and dopamine projection systems and are secondary to partial agonist properties as well as an increased availability of endogenous norepinephrine and dopamine. Many of the stimulating effects of amphetamine can be blocked through α-methyltyrosine, an inhibitor of the rate-limiting catecholamine enzyme, tyrosine hydroxylase (see pathway 1 of Fig. 6–4), thus limiting available endogenous catecholamine.

The main psychic effects of amphetamine include wakefulness, alertness, decreased sense of fatigue, elevation of mood, increased initiative and self-confidence, an increase in motor and speech activity, and a decreased appetite.

Amphetamine is a potent reinforcer in that animals and humans will have a drive or urge to self-administer the drug under a variety of conditions.[13] The reinforcing effects are attenuated by dopamine antagonists. The mesocortical/mesolimbic dopamine projections—the "pleasure brain"—are important in mediating this reinforcing behavior. The circuitry of the "pleasure brain" is self re-exciting, thereby intensifying the reward.

Amphetamine use in animals also can

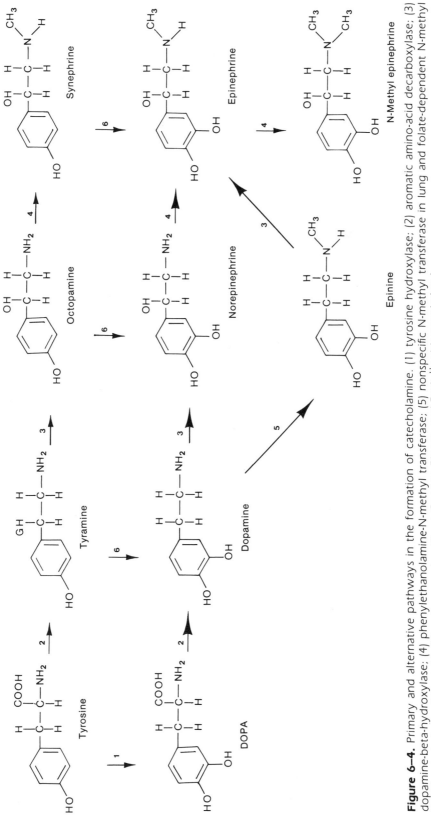
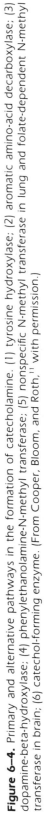

Figure 6–4. Primary and alternative pathways in the formation of catecholamine. (1) tyrosine hydroxylase; (2) aromatic amino-acid decarboxylase; (3) dopamine-beta-hydroxylase; (4) phenylethanolamine-N-methyl transferase; (5) nonspecific N-methyl transferase in lung and folate-dependent N-methyl transferase in brain; (6) catechol-forming enzyme. (From Cooper, Bloom, and Roth,[11] with permission.)

CHEMICAL STRUCTURES AND MAIN CLINICAL USES OF IMPORTANT SYMPATHOMIMETIC DRUGS†

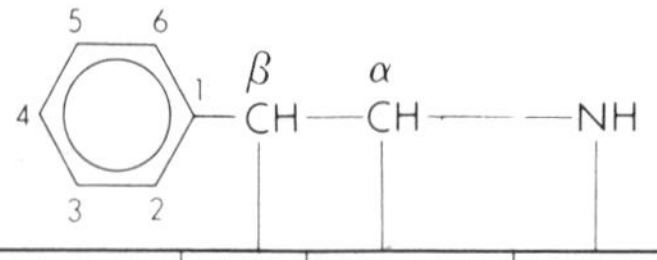

Prototypical formula: benzene ring (positions 5, 6, 4, 1, 3, 2) — $CH(\beta)$ — $CH(\alpha)$ — NH

	Ring	β	α	NH—	α Receptor A N P V	β Receptor B C U	CNS,0
Phenylethylamine		H	H	H			
Epinephrine	3-OH,4-OH	OH	H	CH_3	A. P,V	B,C	
Norepinephrine	3-OH,4-OH	OH	H	H	P		
Dopamine	3-OH,4-OH	H	H	H	P		
Dobutamine	3-OH,4-OH	H	H	1 *		C	
Ethylnorepinephrine	3-OH,4-OH	OH	CH_2CH_3	H		B	
Isoproterenol	3-OH,4-OH	OH	H	$CH(CH_3)_2$		B,C	
Isoetharine	3-OH,4-OH	OH	CH_2CH_3	$CH(CH_3)_2$		B	
Metaproterenol	3-OH,5-OH	OH	H	$CH(CH_3)_2$		B	
Terbutaline	3-OH,5-OH	OH	H	$C(CH_3)_3$		B, U	
Metaraminol	3-OH	OH	CH_3	H	P		
Phenylephrine	3-OH	OH	H	CH_3	N,P		
Tyramine	4-OH	H	H	H			
Hydroxyamphetamine	4-OH	H	CH_3	H			
Ritodrine	4-OH	OH	CH_3	2 *		U	
Prenalterol	4-OH	OH ‡	H	-$CH(CH_3)_2$		C	
Methoxamine	2-OCH_3,5-OCH_3	OH	CH_3	H	P		
Albuterol	3-CH_2OH,4-OH	OH	H	$C(CH_3)_3$		B, U	
Amphetamine		H	CH_3	H			CNS,0
Methamphetamine		H	CH_3	CH_3			CNS,0
Benzphetamine		H	CH_3	3 *			0
Ephedrine		OH	CH_3	CH_3	N,P	B,C	
Phenylpropanolamine		OH	CH_3	H	N		0
Mephentermine		H	4 *	CH_3	N,P		
Phentermine		H	4 *	H			0
Fenfluramine	3-CF_3	H	CH_3	C_2H_5			0
Propylhexedrine	5 *	H	CH_3	CH_3	N		0
Diethylpropion		6 *					0
Phenmetrazine		7 *					0
Phendimetrazine		8 *					0

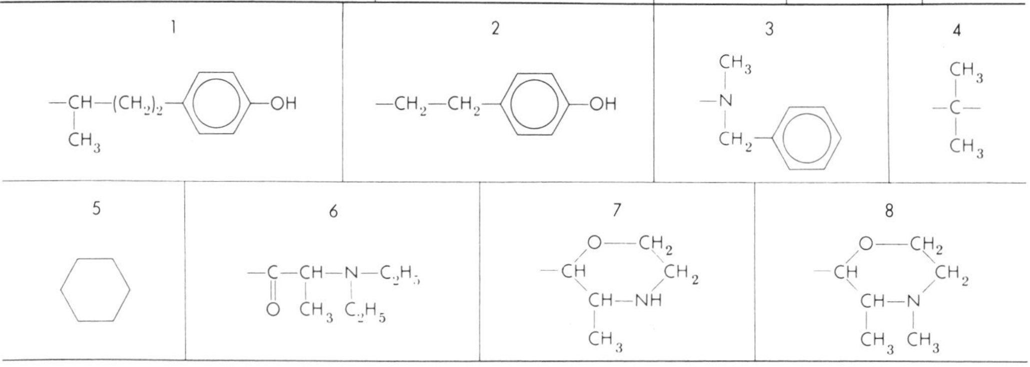

Substituent structures:

1. —CH—$(CH_2)_2$—[ring]—OH ; CH_3
2. —CH_2—CH_2—[ring]—OH
3. —N< (CH_3 above; CH_2—[ring] below)
4. —C— (CH_3, CH_3, CH_3)
5. [cyclohexane ring]
6. —C—CH—N—C_2H_5 (O ; CH_3 C_2H_5)
7. O—CH_2 / —CH CH_2 / CH—NH / CH_3
8. O—CH_2 / —CH CH_2 / CH—N / CH_3 CH_3

α Activity
A = Allergic reactions (includes β action)
N = Nasal decongestion
P = Pressor (may include β action)
V = Other local vasoconstriction
    (e.g., in local anesthesia)

β Activity
B = Bronchodilator
C = Cardiac
U = Uterus

CNS = Central nervous system
0 = Anorectic

* Numbers bearing an asterisk refer to the substituents numbered in the bottom rows of the table; substituent 3 replaces the N atom, substituent 5 replaces the phenyl ring, and 6, 7, and 8 are attached directly to the phenyl ring, replacing the ethylamine side chain.

† The α and β in the prototypical formula refer to positions of the C atoms in the ethylamine side chain.

‡ Prenalterol has —OCH_2— between the aromatic ring and the carbon atom designated as β in the prototypical formula.

Figure 6–5. Chemical structures and main clinical uses of important sympathomimetic drugs. (From Weiner,[12] with permission.)

Table 6–2. NOMENCLATURE FOR AMPHETAMINES

Generic Name	Trade Name	Street Name
Amphetamine	Benzedrine	Ups, bennies, greenies
Dextroamphetamine	Dexedrine	Dexies, copilots, oranges, greenies
Dextroamphetamine + Amphetamine	Biphetamine	Footballs
Methamphetamine		Speed, crystal

cause repetitive, stereotyped motor activity, which can include repetitive gnawing, picking, or other compulsive motor activities. This effect is probably mediated through nigrostriatal dopamine projections.[12,14] The increase in locomotor activity following amphetamine administration may be mediated through both norepinephrine and dopamine projections.[11,12]

An interesting phenomenon of tolerance and sensitivity occurs after repetitive amphetamine use. Tolerance to the mood-enhancing properties occurs after prolonged or repetitive dosing,[13] but tolerance for the drive to continue taking the drug does not occur. On the other hand, increased sensitivity to the stereotyped behavior and locomotor effects occurs after repeated doses.[13] This may lead to a pattern of continued increases in the dosage of amphetamine in an attempt to achieve the mood-enhancing effects, which in turn may cause progressive compulsive and stereotyped behavior. In addition, prolonged amphetamine use at high doses may lead to serious adverse effects of the drug (see Adverse Effects).

Of interest is that experienced drug users cannot differentiate amphetamine from cocaine in a controlled clinical setting.[15]

CLINICAL PHARMACOLOGY

Benzedrine is the racemic mixture of the *d* and *l* isomers of amphetamine, and is available in 5- and 10-milligram tablets. Dextroamphetamine (Dexedrine) is the *d* isomer of amphetamine and likewise is available in 5- and 10-milligram tablets, as well as 15-milligram slow-release form. With respect to CNS excitatory effects, the *d* isomer is three to four times more potent than the *l* isomer.[12]

Amphetamines are rapidly absorbed, with blood levels peaking in 1 to 2 hours. The clinical effects can appear within half an hour and can last in excess of 3 hours. The plasma half-life is about 2 hours. Most amphetamine is excreted unchanged in the urine. Since it is a noncatecholamine sympathomimetic, amphetamine is not metabolized by catechol-O-methyltransferase. It is also not metabolized by monoamine oxidase. As a weak base, the renal clearance of amphetamines can be increased by acidification of the urine, and it can be decreased by alkalinization of the urine, thereby prolonging its effects.

Some nomenclature for illicit amphetamines is shown in Table 6–2. In addition to the amphetamines, some noncatecholamine central nervous system stimulants (Table 6–3) may produce effects similar to the amphetamines.

Clinical Uses

The indications for the legitimate use of amphetamines have become increasingly narrow: childhood hyperkinetic syndrome (minimal brain dysfunction); attention-deficit disorder; narcolepsy (no longer a first-line drug); an adjunct in chronic pain patients taking opiates; for certain central nervous

Table 6–3. NON-CATECHOLAMINE CENTRAL NERVOUS SYSTEM STIMULANTS

Strychnine
Picrotoxin
Pentylenetetrazol
Doxapram
Nikethamide
Methylphenidate (Ritalin)
Pemoline (Cylert)

system diseases to overcome somnolence. Of the noncatecholamine stimulants listed in Table 6–3, only methylphenidate (Ritalin) and pemoline (Cylert) are used therapeutically.

USE IN SPORTS

Amphetamines delay the point of fatigue during sustained intense exercise.[10] Their most dramatic effects occur when performance has been reduced by fatigue and the lack of sleep, a principle widely exploited by students and truck drivers alike.

Amphetamines' potential effects on performance, concentration, and weight control led to athletes experimenting with their use. In the 1984 Michigan State drug study of college athletes,[16] 8 percent of the 2039 respondents reported having used amphetamines in the prior 12 months; 61 percent of users did so for social or personal reasons, 37 percent to enhance performance. In the 1986 Elite Women Athletes Survey, 6 and 3 percent of respondents used amphetamines before or during competition, respectively.[17]

Mandell and associates[9] reported dramatic amphetamine use by professional football players, although their report has been disputed by National Football League officials. From purchase data alone in 1968 and 1969, a mean of 60 to 70 tablets of amphetamines per man per game were used. Mandell and associates[9] further reported that interviews conducted between 1972 and 1975 with 87 players representing 11 NFL teams revealed that "⅔ of the players used amphetamines at least sometimes; more than half used them regularly." The dosage used tended to parallel the positions played. The range for wide receivers was 5 to 15 mg per game; quarterbacks ingested 10 to 15 mg per game; linebackers, 10 to 60 mg per game; and defensive linemen 30 to 150 mg per game. Dosages in the range of 50 to 200 mg are used by "speed freaks" and have been associated with both paranoid and manic behavior.

Although no firm data are available for professional baseball, many anecdotes exist about players ingesting "greenies" during a game both to improve performance and to relieve boredom. Bill Madlock, third baseman for the Los Angeles Dodgers, stated that amphetamines used to be handed out in the clubhouse.[18] Such reports are not surprising, given the long season and mental fatigue which can accompany baseball playing conditions.

Eating disorders have been increasingly recognized as a problem in certain competitive activities. These include gymnastics, ballet, wrestling,[3] thoroughbred racing,[3] and perhaps women's tennis. These sports tend to have certain features in common. They are individual sports, they are entered into at a high level during the teenage years, and weight control is important. In this regard, reports of substance abuse and in particular amphetamine abuse to control weight are not surprising,[19,20] especially since amphetamine was originally used as an appetite suppressant.

Effects on Performance

Until 1959, there were scant data on the effect of amphetamines on athletic performance in general, as well as on sport-specific performance. In an effort to address this controversial question, the AMA commissioned two studies,[21,22] one of which was performed by Smith and Beecher at Harvard.[21] Their paper, "Amphetamine and Athletic Performance," is a classic on the effects of drugs on athletic performance. Subjects consisted of highly trained runners, swimmers, and throwers. Amphetamines in doses of 14 mg per 70 kg improved the performance of the majority (75 percent) of athletes in all three classes. The maximum performance increase was in the throwers (3 to 4 percent), followed by the runners (approximately 1.5 percent). The swimmers showed varying degrees of improvement ranging from 0.59 to 1.16 percent. Although the increments of improvement were small, such differences can be the difference between winning and losing at the world-class level. The analysis of data must be tempered by two factors. First, these sports required essentially maximal effort activities, and second, factors that are operative in other sports, such as eye-hand coordination, judgment, timing, stance stability, and hand-arm steadiness, were not addressed.

Various studies[23–28] have addressed some of these latter factors, but they have shortcomings which include the use of a limited number of subjects, crude design, single-dose levels, testing at only one period following drug administration, and failure to establish baseline performance levels. Despite these shortcomings, it is noteworthy that enhancement of fine motor coordination and thinking skills, factors which are operative in many sports, have been demonstrated. For example, in a nonfatigued condition, low-dose amphetamine (5 to 15 mg per 70 kg) can improve performance in tasks requiring prolonged attention,[23] especially if rapid motor responses are required.[24] By contrast, delayed auditory feedback, a test of mental performance not requiring prolonged attention, appears to be unaffected by amphetamine usage.[25] This data suggest that tasks requiring prolonged attention may be favorably affected by amphetamine, a phenomenon which is certainly exploitable by the athlete under certain conditions.

Although it is widely believed that amphetamine causes jitteriness and anxiety, symptoms that should interfere with fine motor coordination, direct study contradicts the assumption. Hand-arm steadiness, resting tremor, and tasks of precision-hole steadiness do not differ significantly when comparing subjects treated with amphetamines versus placebo.[24,26] Stability of stance is not significantly different in varying doses of amphetamine (5 to 15 mg per 70 kg) versus placebo, and is even improved significantly over placebo if the subjects close their eyes.[25] In sleep-deprived subjects, significant improvement in tracking performance tasks involving eye-hand coordination skills may occur with amphetamine usage.[28]

Studies of effects of amphetamine on bulk strength yield conflicting results. With regard to endurance, that is, time to exhaustion, Chandler and Blair have shown that anaerobic capacity and time to exhaustion increase following amphetamine ingestion, even though no discernible change in $\dot{V}O_2$max occurs. A significant increase in lactate production occurs in association with the increased endurance, which suggests that amphetamine does not prevent fatigue from a physiologic standpoint, but masks the symptoms of fatigue, thereby allowing prolonged endurance.[29] However, conflicting data regarding amphetamine use and endurance exist. For example, Williams and Thompson observed no beneficial effect of varying doses of amphetamine upon time to exhaustion. They studied 12 college students, using time

to exhaustion on a bicycle ergometer as the end point. Each student received either placebo or d-amphetamine in varying doses of 5 mg per kg, 10 mg per kg, or 15 mg per kg, 2 hours prior to exercise. No discernible effect was noted among the four groups.[29a] Other authors have reported similar results.[29b–29d]

Animal experiments may help to explain why endurance may increase following amphetamine ingestion. Mice increase their swimming capacity with methamphetamine usage, and the change correlates with more efficient glucose utilization, increased lipolysis, and increased availability of nonesterified fatty acids.[30] In rats, despite conditions of extreme stress, amphetamines restore exploratory behavior to a degree that correlates with a prevention of brain norepinephrine reduction.[31]

In a pilot study comparing amphetamine (Dexedrine 10 mg) to placebo in poststroke victims undergoing rehabilitation, amphetamine-treated patients appeared to achieve significantly greater increments in motor performance scores.[32] It is unclear if this improvement is secondary to enhancement of catecholamine effects which modulate recovery after brain injury or from other effects of amphetamine on the nervous system. It is also unclear what implications such a study has for normal athletes wishing to enhance motor performance.

In sum, the available evidence suggests that amphetamine use can enhance skills which play a key role in athletic performance, including speed, power, endurance, concentration, and fine motor coordination. In addition, some athletes may use amphetamines regardless of any actual benefit, believing it will provide a competitive edge.[33] It may be true that certain doses of amphetamine are more useful for specific athletic endeavors, that is, sport-specific or position-specific dosing, as the data provided by Mandell and colleagues suggest. Unfortunately, firm data regarding amphetamine use and doses in various sports are unavailable.

Case Vignette

A 24-year-old male baseball player reached a plateau in his career, which was less successful than he had expected. He found it difficult to become "psyched up" for games, and he often lost his concentration after the first few innings. A teammate recommended that he try some "greenies."

The greenies were supplied by the teammate the following game, and were probably Dexedrine, 10 mg. The player took the pill just before the game started, and at about the time of the second inning he noted a tremendous surge in energy. He felt faster, stronger, and better able to concentrate on the details of the game. His performance that game was quite good. Fearing addiction, he took the greenies for only major games or during long road trips during the remainder of the season.

The following year, however, he had more difficulty concentrating and remaining energetic during games. He began taking greenies before most games, and he enjoyed a rather successful first half of the season. Typically a low-key individual, he acquired the nickname "chatter-box" because of his marked verbalization following games. On several occasions, he had to drink several beers following games in order to calm down from the pregame amphetamine use.

During the latter part of the season, his playing skills again seemed to plateau, and he began to double the amount of amphetamine prior to games. At this point, his playing skills deteriorated further. He often missed routine ground balls. On one occasion, he was intensely digging his spikes into the ground in a repetitive fashion, and he made no attempt to field a routine grounder. On other occasions, he started fights with opposing players for minor incidents. He be-

came withdrawn, even from friends, and sometimes exhibited paranoid behavior. At the recommendation of a friend, he eventually sought medical treatment for amphetamine dependence.

ADVERSE EFFECTS

Any potential benefits of amphetamines must be weighed against their known side effects, particularly under the conditions of competition, and especially in high doses (Table 6–4). Side effects listed as acute may occur at any time, even after an individual has been using the drug for a prolonged period of time.

Common acute behavioral side effects of amphetamines result from the central nervous system excitatory effects. Restlessness, dizziness, tremor, irritability, and insomnia can all result from amphetamine ingestion, and occur more commonly in higher doses.[12] More severe behavioral changes may occur, including confusion, assaultiveness, delirium, paranoia, and hallucinations.[3,12,34,35] These effects may occur acutely or following long-term use. Convulsions, coma, and death may follow severe central nervous system stimulation from amphetamine use.[36]

Chronic amphetamine use may cause other central nervous system–related side effects. Dyskinesias, both chorea and athetosis, particularly of the facial and masticatory muscles, have been described.[10] Compulsive and stereotypic repetitive behavior may occur.[10] A paranoid delusional state indistin-

Table 6–4. SIDE EFFECTS OF AMPHETAMINES

Acute, Mild	Acute, Severe	Chronic
Restlessness	Confusion	Addiction
Dizziness	Assaultiveness	Weight loss
Tremor	Delirium	Psychosis
Irritability	Paranoia	Paranoid delusions
Insomnia	Hallucinations	Dyskinesias
Euphoria	Convulsions	Compulsive/stereotypic/repetitive
Uncontrolled movements	Cerebral hemorrhage	behavior
Headache	Angina/myocardial infarction	Vasculitis
Palpitations	Hypertension	Neuropathy
Anorexia	Circulatory collapse	
Nausea		
Vomiting		

guishable from schizophrenia has been noted.[13]

Systemic side effects include hypertension, angina, and life-threatening cardiac arrhythmias.[12,37] Vomiting, abdominal pain, weight loss, and excessive diaphoresis may occur immediately after amphetamine ingestion.[12]

Necrotizing vasculitis indistinguishable from periarteritis nodosa can occur with long-term oral as well as intravenous use.[38,39] The vasculitis may also result in mononeuritis multiplex.[40] Reports indicate that intracerebral hemorrhage can occur with doses as low as 20 mg of amphetamine, in both chronic and first-time users.[27] Subarachnoid hemorrhage has similarly been reported following amphetamine use.[41,42] As discussed earlier, central hyperexcitability can cause seizures, particularly in persons taking higher doses of amphetamines.[36]

Amphetamines may produce irreversible dopaminergic neuronal degeneration distinct from the vascular changes. Following amphetamine administration, massive synaptic accumulation and subsequent auto-oxidation of dopamine produces a selective dopaminergic neurotoxin, 6-hydroxydopamine.[43] Neuronal degeneration and subsequent irreversible reductions in the central concentrations of dopamine occur, although the long-term behavioral sequelae are unknown.

Abrupt withdrawal of amphetamines may produce chronic fatigue, lethargy, somnolence, and depression.[12,19] Toxic effects of amphetamines vary widely and may occur idiosyncratically with doses as low as 2 mg or with tolerance doses as high as 500 mg. The strongly positive reinforcing effects of amphetamine may lead to a pattern of continued use and dependency, which may further potentiate any of the above-mentioned adverse effects.

FINAL NOTE

Amphetamines, unlike anabolic steroids, are taken just prior to an athletic event and have no long-term role in neuromuscular training. Also unlike anabolic steroids, amphetamine abuse is more likely to occur by athletes under a variety of circumstances. A baseball player may use these drugs to improve concentration and alertness. A football lineman may take massive doses to increase aggressiveness and prolong endurance. A sprinter may use amphetamine to increase energy and speed before a race.

Amphetamines share many central nervous system effects with cocaine. Whereas amphetamines (relatively long-acting drugs) are used primarily as performance enhancers, cocaine (a relatively short-acting drug) is more often used by athletes for recreational purposes. Most drug testing protocols call for the testing of cocaine because it is an illicit recreational drug, while amphetamines are tested for as performance-enhancing agents. Testing for performance enhancement appears justified because of the fairly convincing evidence of amphetamine ergogenicity.

In addition to drug testing, educational programs for the athlete should emphasize that amphetamines are dangerous, both psychologically and physically. The positive reinforcing effects lead to a high abuse potential, which in turn increases the risk of physical and psychological damage with each subsequent ingestion.

REFERENCES

1. Piness, G, Miller, H and Alles, GA: Clinical observations on phenylaminoethanol sulphate. JAMA 94:790, 1930.
2. Prinzmetal, M and Bloomberg, W: The use of benzedrine for the treatment of narcolepsy. JAMA 105:2051, 1935.
3. Strauss, RH: Drugs in sports. In Strauss, RH (ed): Sports Medicine. WB Saunders, Philadelphia, 1984, p 481.
4. Laties, VG and Weiss, B: The amphetamine margin in sports. Fed Proc 40:2689, 1981.
5. Brill, H and Girose, T: Semin Psychiatry 1:179, 1969.
6. Lake, CR and Quirk, RS: CNS stimulants and the look-alike drugs. Psychiatr Clin North Am 7:689, 1984.
7. Iverson, LI, Iverson, SD and Snyder, SH (eds): Handbook of Psychopharmacology, Vol II. Plenum Press, New York, 1978, p 99.
8. Ryan, AJ: Use of amphetamines in athletics. JAMA 170:562, 1959.
9. Mandell, AJ, Stewart, KD and Russo, PV: The Sunday syndrome: From kinetics to altered consciousness. Fed Proc 40:2693, 1981.
10. Langston, JW and Langston, EB: Neurological consequences of drug abuse. In Asbury, AK, McKhann, GM and McDonald, WI (eds): Diseases of the Nervous System: Clinical Neurobiology. WB Saunders, Philadelphia, 1986, p 1333.
11. Cooper, JR, Bloom, FE and Roth, RH: The Biochemical Basis of Neuropharmacology, ed 5. Oxford University Press, New York, 1986.
12. Weiner, N: Norepinephrine, Epinephrine and the Sympathomimetic Amines. In Gilman, AG et al

(eds): Goodman and Gilman's The Pharmacological Basis of Therapeutics, ed 7. Macmillan, New York, 1985, p 145.

13. Fischman, MW: Cocaine and the Amphetamines. In Meltzer, HY (ed): Psychopharmacology: The Third Generation of Progress. Raven Press, New York, 1987, p 1543.

14. Ando, K and Johanson, C: Sensitivity changes to dopaminergic agents in fine motor control of rhesus monkeys after repeated methamphetamine administration. Pharm Biochem Behav 22:737, 1985.

15. Fischman, MW, et al: Cardiovascular and subjective effects of intravenous cocaine administration in humans. Arch Gen Psychiatry 33:983, 1976.

16. Anderson, WA and McKeag, DB: The substance use and abuse habits of college student athletes. Research paper no. 2: General findings. Presented to NCAA Executive Committee Drug Education Committee by College of Human Medicine, Michigan State University, June, 1985.

17. Elite Women Athletes Survey. Hazelden Health Promotion Services, Minneapolis, January, 1987.

18. Anderson, D: Madlock sees no hard drug discipline. The New York Times, February 23, 1986.

19. American Medical Association Department of Drugs, Division of Drugs and Technology: Agents used in obesity. In AMA Drug Evaluations, ed. 6. WB Saunders, Philadelphia, 1986, pp 927–936.

20. Jonas, JM and Gold, MS: Cocaine abuse and eating disorders (letter). Lancet 1:390–391, 1986.

21. Smith, GM and Beecher, HK: Amphetamine sulfate and athletic performance: 1. Objective effects. JAMA 170:542–557, 1959.

22. Karpovich, PV: Effect of amphetamine sulfate on athletic performance. JAMA 170:558–561, 1959.

23. Blum, B and Stern, M: A comparative evaluation of the action of depressant and stimulant drugs on human performance. Psychopharm 6:173–177, 1964.

24. Domino, E and Albers, J, et al: Effects of d-amphetamine on quantitative measures of motor performance. Clin Pharmacol Ther 13:251–257, 1972.

25. Evans, M, Martz, R, et al: Effects of dextroamphetamine on psychomotor skills. Clin Pharmacol Ther 19:777–781, 1976.

26. Lovingood, B, Blyth, C, et al: Effects of d-amphetamine sulfate, caffeine and high temperature on human performance. Res Quart 38:64–71, 1965.

27. Harrington, H, Heller, H, et al: Intracerebral hemorrhage and oral amphetamine. Arch Neuro 40:503–507, 1983.

28. Belleville, J and Dorey, F: Effect of nefopam on visual tracking. Clin Pharmacol Ther 26:457–463, 1979.

29. Chandler, J and Blair, S: The effect of amphetamines on selected physiological components related to athletic success. Med Sci Sports Exer 12:65–69, 1980.

29a. Williams, MH and Thompson, J: Effect of variant dosages of amphetamine upon endurance. Res Quart 44:417, 1973.

29b. Golding, L and Barnard, J: The effect of d-amphetamine sulfate on physical performance. J Sports Med Phys Fitness 3:221, 1963.

29c. Karpovich, P: Effect of amphetamine sulfate on athletic performance. JAMA 170:558, 1959.

29d. Foltz, E, et al: The influence of amphetamine (Benzedrine) sulfate and caffeine on the performance of rapidly exhausting work by untrained subjects. J Lab Clin Med 28:601, 1943.

30. Estler, C and Gabrys, M: Swimming capacity of mice after prolonged treatment with psychomotor stimulants. Psychopharm 60:173–176, 1979.

31. Stone, E: Swim-stress-induced inactivity: Relation to body temperature and brain norepinephrine, and effects of d-amphetamine. Psychosom Med 32:32–51, 1970.

32. Crisostomo, EA, Duncan, PW, Probst, M, et al: Evidence that amphetamine with physical therapy promotes recovery of motor function in stroke patients. Ann Neurol 23:94, 1988.

33. McArdle, WD, Katch, FI and Katch, VL: Exercise Physiology—Energy, Nutrition and Human Performance. Lea and Febiger, Philadelphia, 1981, p 308.

34. Kulberg, A: Substance abuse: Clinical identification and management. Ped Clin North Am 33:325, 1986.

35. Richter, RW: Drug abuse. In Rowland, LP (ed): Merritt's Textbook of Neurology, ed 7. Lea and Febiger, Philadelphia, pp 730–735, 1984.

36. Schuster, C and Fischman, M: Amphetamine toxicity: Behavioural and neuropathological indexes. Fed Proc 34:1845–1851, 1975.

37. Guyton, AG: The autonomic nervous system: The adrenal medulla. In Textbook of Medical Physiology, ed 7. WB Saunders, Philadelphia, 1986.

38. Citron, B, Halpern, M, et al: Necrotizing angiitis associated with drug abuse. N Engl J Med 2873:1003–1011, 1970.

39. Bostwick, D: Amphetamine induced cerebral vasculitis. Hum Path 12:1031–1033, 1981.

40. Stafford, CR, et al: Mononeuropathy multiplex as a complication of amphetamine angiitis. Neurology 25:570, 1975.

41. Chynn, KY: Acute subarachnoid hemorrhage. JAMA 233:55–56, 1975.

42. Caplan, LR, Hier, DB and Banks, G: Current concepts of cerebrovascular disease—stroke: Stroke and drug abuse. Stroke 13:869, 1982.

43. Gawin, FH and Willinwood, EH: Cocaine and other stimulants; actions, abuse, and treatment. New Engl J Med 318: 1173, 1988.

CHAPTER 7

Cocaine

HISTORY

Among abused drugs, cocaine provides the most romantic and subtly dangerous of stories.[1-5] The coca bush was and continues to be indigenous to the Peruvian Andes. During the pre-Inca period, coca leaf chewing was widespread and uncontrolled among the Indians of that area. The Inca religion incorporated coca leaf chewing into its rituals of the priesthood and nobility, as it was believed to be a gift of the Manco Cepac,[5] the son of the Sun God. The nobility, recognizing its favorable effect on endurance, even permitted soldiers and workers on imperial projects to use the substance on select occasions. Gradually, control over cocaine usage eroded, and by the time of Pizarro's Spanish conquest of Peru in the 1530s, abuse of the drug had became uncontrolled and widespread.

By 1550, cocaine found its way into the Old World and 15 years later, the Spanish physician Monardes published the first scientific treatise on coca.[4] For 3 centuries, interest in cocaine in Europe remained limited to its botanical and scientific properties. During the mid-1800s, however, the German chemist Friedrich Gaedcke isolated cocaine from the coca leaf.[3] Shortly thereafter, Niemann characterized the substance chemically[3] and Mantegazza published his work on its physiology.[4]

A little more than a century ago, in 1883, the German army physician Ashenbrandt gave cocaine to Bavarian troops in an effort to delay the onset of fatigue.[5] A year later Freud embraced cocaine as an answer to his depression.[1,4,5] "I took for the first time 0.05 gm of cocaine. . . . A few minutes later, I experienced a sudden exhilaration and a feel-

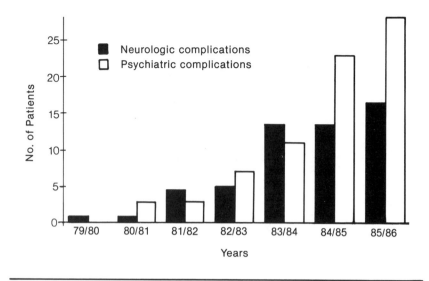

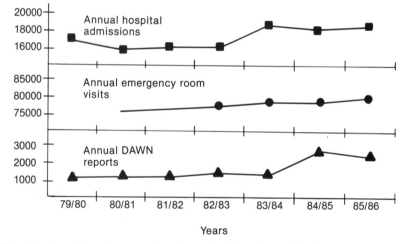

Figure 7–1. *Top,* Number of cocaine-associated neurologic and psychiatric complications identified between July 1979 and June 1986. *Bottom,* Number of annual hospital admissions, emergency room visits, and DAWN reports for the San Francisco General Hospital during the same time period (emergency room visits prior to July 1982 are approximated). (From Lowenstein et al,[17] with permission.)

ing of ease.[1]" His review, "On Coca," fermented heightened interest in the drug.[3] In fact, some have speculated that Freud wrote his great works under the influence of cocaine.[5] An ardent proponent, Freud recommended using cocaine for a diversity of purposes including as a stimulant, an aphrodisiac, and a treatment for alcohol and morphine addiction.[1,3–5] Both Freud in Europe and Halsted, the great American surgeon, recognized the anesthetic potential of cocaine.[2–6] Koller, with Freud's assistance, operated on Freud's father's glaucomatous eyes using cocaine anesthesia,[4] while Halstead, who developed a severe cocaine habit, performed the first nerve block by applying cocaine to the peripheral nerve.[1,3–6] Soon cocaine, in one form or another, became the panacea for a potpourri of ailments ranging from cancer to hemorrhoids.[1,4] It is even reported that Robert Louis Stevenson wrote "The Strange Case of Dr. Jekyll and Mr.

Hyde" in less than a week while receiving cocaine as part of his treatment for tuberculosis.[4,5]

By the end of the 19th century, numerous tonics, powders, and patent medicines included cocaine,[1,2,6] and the drug soon became a part of the beverage industry. Angelo Mariani, the Corsican chemist, incorporated the coca leaf into the widely acclaimed Mariani wine.[1,2,4,5] By 1886, John Smythe Pemberton, in Atlanta, developed what was to become an American tradition, Coca Cola.[1,3-5] Initially, Coca Cola's formula included water, syrup, coca leaf, and kola berry extract. Not until 20 years later did the Coca Cola Company agree to use decocainized leaves in its formulation.[1,4]

In 1906, the Federal Pure Food and Drug Act[1,2,4] regulated the distribution of narcotics and cocaine for the first time. The Harrison Act of 1914[2,4] put additional restrictions on opiates and cocaine. By 1930, interest in cocaine waned dramatically, only to re-emerge in the 1960s.[4] The Controlled Substances Act of 1970[2,4] placed cocaine in Category II, indicating that it had a legitimate medical use but possessed a high potential for abuse and inducing dependency. Its usage escalated greatly,[8] so that by 1974, 5.4 million Americans reported using cocaine at least once, and by 1982 the number had risen to 21.6 million.[9] As its usage increased, the age of its users fell.[10] A 1986 federal report of a 3-year national survey indicated that 5.8 million people used cocaine at least monthly, representing a 38 percent increase in 3 years.[11] Though there was a 2 percent decrease in 18- to 25-year-old individuals using cocaine in that 3-year period, there was an increase in usage in both the 12 to 17 and the 26 and over age groups.[11] By 1987, 17.3 percent of high school seniors had tried cocaine.[12]

By 1986, the development of crack (which is pure cocaine; see below) placed a new, dangerous dimension on the problem of cocaine abuse.[13-16] Deaths associated with this highly addictive and dangerous agent underscored the magnitude of the cocaine problem in the United States.[7] According to the National Institute on Drug Abuse's DAWN system, a 91 percent increase in cocaine-related deaths occurred in the United States between 1980 and 1983, eliminating the perception that cocaine was a "safe" drug.[17] Illustrating this point, Lowenstein and colleagues report a substantial increase in the number of neurologic and psychiatric complications from cocaine use as reflected by admissions and emergency room visits to San Francisco hospitals between 1979 and 1986[18] (Fig. 7–1).

Possibly, cocaine use is beginning to decline. In its 13th annual drug survey, the University of Michigan's Institute of Social Research recently reported the first substantial decline in cocaine use among high school and college students and young adults.[12] The decreased use appears to represent a change in demand rather than supply since, if anything, cocaine is perceived as more available, purer, and less expensive than it had been previously. Nevertheless, many young cocaine users remain: 1 in every 6 high school seniors admits to trying cocaine and 1 in 18 has tried crack. Nearly 40 percent of adults in their late 20s have tried cocaine.[12]

CHEMISTRY AND PHYSIOLOGY

Cocaine is an ecgonine alkaloid obtained from the leaf of the coca plant, *Erythroxylon coca* and related species[19] (Fig. 7–2). Acid and solvent extraction of such leaves produces a variety of alkaloids, the hydrolysis of which yields ecgonine, an amino alcohol base. Methanol/benzoic acid esterification produces the product, cocaine hydrochloride (benzoyl/methylecgonine hydrochloride)[4] (Fig. 7–3). So-called free-based cocaine (benzoyl methylecgonine) is produced by the extraction of cocaine hydrochloride by a base, such as buffered ammonia, and a solvent, usually ether.[4,20] "Crack," which like free-based cocaine is essentially pure cocaine, is made by preparing an aqueous solution of

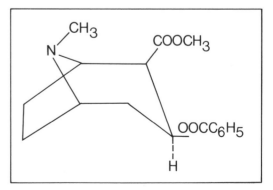

Figure 7–2. Structure of cocaine.

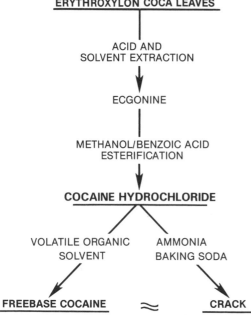

ERYTHROXYLON COCA LEAVES

ACID AND
SOLVENT EXTRACTION

ECGONINE

METHANOL/BENZOIC ACID
ESTERIFICATION

COCAINE HYDROCHLORIDE

VOLATILE ORGANIC   AMMONIA
SOLVENT   BAKING SODA

FREEBASE COCAINE   ≈   **CRACK**

Figure 7–3. Preparation of freebase cocaine and crack.

cocaine hydrochloride and adding ammonia, with or without sodium bicarbonate, to alkalinize the solution and precipitate the cocaine in its alkaloid form.[13] The production of crack, as contrasted to the production of free-based cocaine powder, does not require the use of the volatile solvent, ether.[16] Whereas free-based cocaine and crack are readily volatilized into smoke when heated, cocaine hydrochloride powder decomposes with heating.[16]

Cocaine is primarily metabolized to benzoylecgonine and ecgonine methyl ester, both of which are excreted in the urine.[21] Less than 20 percent of cocaine is excreted unchanged by the kidney.[5] Cholinesterases are important in the metabolism of cocaine. They are present in the plasma, liver, and brain. Cholinesterase activity varies among individuals. Those with hereditary cholinesterase deficiency may have fatal reactions to small doses of cocaine.[6,21]

Cocaine exerts complex physiologic effects on the brain and shares similarities in this respect with amphetamine.[22] Both increase concentrations of dopaminergic and noradrenergic transmitters at the neuronal synapse; whereas amphetamine augments release and blocks reuptake, cocaine works primarily by blocking reuptake (Fig. 7–4). Following cocaine ingestion, individuals typically show a decrease in fatigue and an increase in activity and talkativeness and have a general sense of euphoria and well-being.[23] Cocaine, like amphetamine, produces enhancement in a number of scales of the Profile of Mood States, including friendliness, arousal, elation, vigor, and positive mood state.[23] The mood elevation and overall behavioral enhancement is similar to amphetamine and accounts for the seductiveness of the drug. The potent reinforcing action of cocaine accounts for its frequent repetitive dosing among users.

Current evidence suggests that much of cocaine's effect is mediated through the reward or reinforcing circuitry of the "pleasure brain"—mesocortical (medial prefrontal, cingulate, and entorhinal cortex) and mesolimbic (septum, olfactory tubercle, nucleus accumbens, amygdaloid complex, and pyriform cortex) dopamine tracts (see Fig. 6–3). This reward system appears to originate from the lateral hypothalamus—the center of nonthinking reflexes—which in turn projects via the median forebrain bundle to the ventral tegmental area, where linkage with dopamine tracts occurs.[22,24] In essence, the reward and reinforcing circuitry of the "pleasure brain" involves much of the limbic system—an area of the brain known to subserve emotions, sexual drive, autonomic function, and memory. This circuitry is self-re-exciting and intensifies the reward. It is the pharmacologic manipulation of the "pleasure brain" that explains neurochemically the compulsivity, preoccupation, craving, and relapse behavior so often seen in cocaine users.[25]

The potent reinforcing effects of the drug may have roots in specific binding sites in the brain.[26] Although cocaine binds to several brain sites, the drug's addictive properties appear to be mediated by a binding site on the dopamine transporter, which normally functions to remove dopamine from the synaptic cleft. Other neurotransmitters, including serotonin and norepinephrine, appear to have little influence on the self-administration effects of cocaine.[26]

It is not surprising that a dysphoria follows cocaine-induced psychic stimulation (euphoria) with its concomitant synaptic cleft dopamine excess. At least in part, the dys-

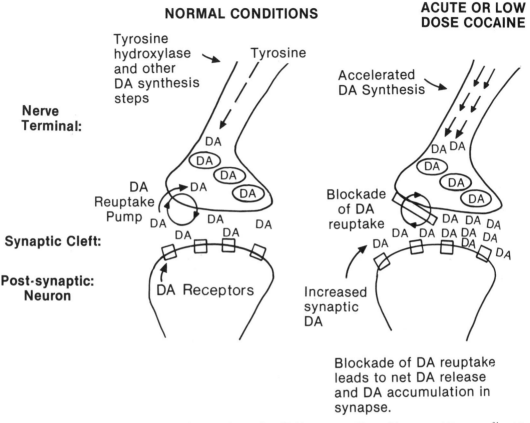

NORMAL CONDITIONS

ACUTE OR LOW DOSE COCAINE

Tyrosine hydroxylase and other DA synthesis steps

Tyrosine

Accelerated DA Synthesis

Nerve Terminal:

DA Reuptake Pump

Blockade of DA reuptake

Synaptic Cleft:

Post-synaptic: Neuron

DA Receptors

Increased synaptic DA

Blockade of DA reuptake leads to net DA release and DA accumulation in synapse.

Figure 7–4. Effects of low-dose cocaine on dopamine (DA) neurons. (From Nunes and Rosecan,[24] with permission.)

phoria can be attributed to a depletion of presynaptic dopamine consequent to a reuptake blockade (Fig. 7–5).

Another proposed CNS mechanism for the dysphoria and craving that follows cocaine abuse relates to the development of receptor site supersensitivity (see Fig. 7–5). The efficacy of desipramine in decreasing postcocaine depressive symptoms supports this concept. Investigators postulate that the tricyclic antidepressants, including desipramine, produce receptor site subsensitivity, thereby offsetting cocaine-induced supersensitivity.[27,28]

With increasing doses of cocaine, subcortical and brain stem centers are affected, producing tremors and convulsive movements.[20] Spinal cord reflexes are increased, perhaps as a result of a depression of inhibitory neurons, and eventually tonic-clonic convulsions appear. Lower brain stem stimulation initially increases the respiratory rate but

eventually stimulation gives way to medullary depression and potentially death from respiratory failure.

Following repetitive dosing of cocaine, sensitization occurs, resulting in enhancement of stereotyped behavior and locomotor stimulant effects. Even though tolerance to the subjective effects of the drug occur, the reinforcing properties are little affected.[23] These properties of sensitization and tolerance, coupled with the continued reinforcing properties of cocaine, account in large part for its potential lethal toxicity. In animal studies, this point is well documented. The mortality rate for rats given unlimited access to cocaine is 90 percent, whereas only 36 percent of rats given unlimited access to heroin will die.[29] In another study, rhesus monkeys were given a choice between cocaine and food pellets and chose almost exclusively cocaine, leading to weight loss and marked behavioral impairment, including

CHRONIC OR HIGH DOSE COCAINE

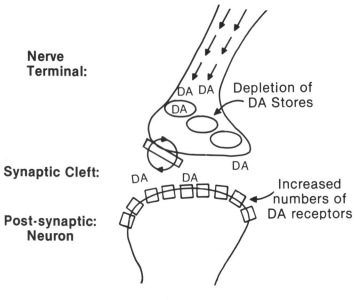

Nerve Terminal:

DA DA
DA
Depletion of DA Stores
DA

Synaptic Cleft:

DA DA
Increased numbers of DA receptors

Post-synaptic: Neuron

DA synthesis cannot keep pace with DA release. DA depletion and DA receptor supersensitivity result.

Figure 7–5. Effects of chronic or high-dose cocaine on dopamine (DA) neurons. (From Nunes and Rosecan,[24] with permission.)

excessive grooming, scratching, facial grimacing, and stereotyped movements of the head.[30] Similarly, human subjects will consistently choose intravenous cocaine over placebo when given the choice in an experimental setting.[31]

From a neurophysiologic perspective, cocaine's effects may not be limited to the sympathomimetic system. For example, cocaine has been shown to slow the conversion of tryptophan to serotonin and to diminish acetylcholine uptake, and it may involve endorphin mechanisms.[22]

Cocaine potentiates the peripheral response of sympathetically innervated organs to norepinephrine, sympathetic nerve stimulation, and, to a lesser degree, epinephrine. Such sympathetic neurons may have either excitatory or inhibitory functions. Here, too, the mechanism of action probably relates to the prevention of the reuptake of catecholamines in the synapse, thereby sensitizing neurons to sympathomimetic amines.[32]

Very high doses of cocaine can produce dramatic increases in the body temperature, partly from central nervous system stimulation producing shaking chills or convulsions and partly by interfering with heat loss by peripheral vasoconstriction.[20]

Aside from Freud's 1884 studies (see Table 7–2), no evidence supports the notion of increased muscular strength while under the influence of cocaine.[20] Such feelings probably reflect grandiosity of thought and blunted feelings of fatigue.

The local anesthetic effect of cocaine relates to its ability to interfere with nerve conduction.[20] Cocaine increases both the systolic and diastolic blood pressures, as well as the heart rate in a dose-response fashion.[20,31,33,34]

CLINICAL PHARMACOLOGY

The effects of cocaine relate to both the dose and the route of administration (Table 7–1). Although uncommonly used in this

Table 7–1. ROUTE OF
ADMINISTRATION AND PEAK
SUBJECTIVE EFFECTS OF
COCAINE

Route of Administration	Peak Subjective Effect	Return to Baseline
Oral	minutes to 1 hour	>1 hour
Nasal (snorting)	5–15 minutes	1 hour
Intravenous	30 seconds to minutes	30 minutes
Inhalation (free-base, crack)	8 seconds to 1 minute	minutes

fashion nowadays, cocaine can be absorbed by the oral route.[22] Chewing the coca leaf permits absorption through the oral mucous membranes. The swallowed portion is subject to first-pass metabolism by the liver.[22] The Incas chew the coca leaf mixed with an alkaline powder, which increases the plasma concentration of cocaine by as much as tenfold.[3,4] The effects of chewed cocaine tend to be subtle and enduring, with resultant mood elevation, mild stimulation, reduced appetite, and increased physical stamina. Though relatively unpopular in the United States, oral dosing may produce peak subjective effects that are not greatly different than those of the intranasal route.[22]

Most cocaine taken in the United States is through nasal inhalation, "snorting."[5] Following such inhalation, the blood concentration rapidly increases for 20 minutes, peaks at 60 minutes, and then gradually returns to baseline. Measurable levels can be found up to 3 hours after administration.[22] The widespread preference of users for the intranasal route, however, suggests that this route may increase brain cocaine levels faster than measured venous blood levels.[22] The greater the nasal vascularity, the greater the absorption. In support of this notion is the observation that following intranasal cocaine, peak physiologic and subjective effects occur in 5 to 15 minutes and return to baseline within an hour.[34] Absorption of cocaine via continued

intranasal use is somewhat self-limiting because of local vasoconstriction.[35]

With intravenous cocaine, the rate of injection seems to be almost as important in determining the subjective and physiologic effects as are the absolute blood levels. Following the intravenous injection of cocaine, specific effects may begin within 30 seconds and wear off within 30 minutes.[22]

The inhalation of the vaporized cocaine base (both "freebasing" and "crack") may give an even more intense "rush" of sensation than does intravenous cocaine. The vascular bed of the lungs can quickly absorb large quantities of the drug, and subsequent massive delivery of the drug to the brain occurs in about 8 seconds, contrasted with at least 16 seconds and a less sharp peak from arm to brain (intravenous injection). The shorter the time to reach the brain, the less time for degradation by circulating cholinesterases. Craving for repeated dosages occurs most frequently after the inhalation of vaporized cocaine (crack or free-based) because of efforts to abort the intense dysphoria that routinely follows the initial intense euphoria.[16,22,34]

Cocaine users often discover that the euphoria can become intensified with higher doses. With increasing intoxication, the user focuses less on external pleasurable experiences and more on intense euphoric internal sensations, leading to social withdrawal and a disregard for personal habits.[36] The rapid decline in the effect of drug, coupled with the memory of intense euphoria, may lead to binges in which the drug is taken as frequently as every 10 minutes in an effort to re-create the pleasurable experience and to prevent the development of an intense dysphoria.[36]

The pharmacology of cocaine abuse is complicated by the fact that most cocaine is adulterated by various substances, including: (1) stimulants such as caffeine, phenylpropanolamine, and even strychnine; (2) local anesthetics such as procaine and lidocaine; (3) hallucinogens such as LSD and PCP; (4) depressants such as diazepam; (5) inert substances such as talc and various sugars; and (6) miscellaneous substances such as quinine and sodium bicarbonate.[16,30]

Illicit cocaine goes by a variety of street names, including snow, dama blanca, flake, gold dust, C girl, Charlie, candy girl, nose candy, lady, green gold, coke, and toot.[11,16,30] A similar jargon covers dosages: the terms "hit," "snort," "line," and "dose" are used interchangeably. A "spoon" is equivalent to a half gram.[5] Typically a line of cocaine is 3 to 5 cm long, each containing 25 mg.[19] However, the amount of cocaine in a given dose can vary from 0 to 200 mg. Vials of crack generally contain 1 to 3 "rocks," each weighing approximately 100 mg.[16]

Clinical Uses

Cocaine, usually in combination with epinephrine, is widely used as a topical anesthetic for nasal surgical procedures in the United States, the estimate being that the drug is applied in more than half of the 370,000 such operations performed annually.[6] Cocaine is not legitimately prepared for either internal use or injection in the United States.

USE IN SPORTS

In 1986, the cocaine-related deaths of Len Bias and Don Rogers provided a major impetus to drug testing in sports and catalyzed an increased awareness of the potential morbidity and mortality of cocaine abuse among athletes and nonathletes alike. Satisfactory epidemiological data, however, of cocaine use patterns and associated medical complications among amateur and professional athletes remain largely nonexistent.

In 1984, before the escalation in cocaine abuse, the Michigan State University College of Human Medicine attempted to quantitate cocaine usage in NCAA athletics.[37] Of 2,039 athletes responding in Division I, II, and III colleges, 17 percent admitted to using cocaine in the prior 12 months and 13 percent were still taking the drug at the time of the survey. In the 1986 Elite Women Athletes Survey, 7 percent of respondents reported using cocaine; 3 and 2 percent of Olympic-caliber women athletes reported using cocaine before or during competition, respectively.[38]

A 1986 survey of the National Football League Players' Association revealed that half of the respondents felt that cocaine was the number one drug of abuse in the NFL.[39] Anecdotal information suggested that ath-

letes used cocaine primarily for social reasons rather than to enhance athletic performance.

Effects on Performance

Unlike amphetamine, systematic studies regarding potential ergogenic effects are not available for cocaine. Remarkably, the most detailed study of relevance to the athlete was done by Freud in 1884 (Table 7–2). Freud found that muscle strength, as measured by a dynamometer, as well as reaction time, improved within minutes of intranasal cocaine use, and this effect persisted for over 3 hours.[40]

Aside from potential effect on endurance and creating a sense of enhanced mental prowess, no evidence other than Freud's earlier data suggests that cocaine enhances athletic performance in a sustained fashion. If the analogy with amphetamine holds true, however, theoretically it is possible that, at certain points on the dose-response curve, cocaine may well be ergogenic in ways similar to amphetamine. At properly titrated low doses, the heightened arousal and increased alertness initially appear to be essentially free of negative consequences.[36]

Theoretical considerations aside, most observers have reported athletic deterioration among cocaine users. Tim Raines, an outfielder for the Montreal Expos, discussed his involvement with cocaine. "It certainly hurt my performance. I struck out a lot more; my vision was lessened. A lot of times I'd go up to the plate and the ball was right down the middle and I'd jump back, thinking it was at my head. The umpire would call it a strike and I'd start arguing. . . . When you're on drugs, you don't feel you're doing anything wrong."[41] Lonnie Smith of the Kansas City Royals noted: "I think it slowed me down, not just running but my mental thinking. . . . I started to lose interest in things. . . . Whitey thought I was having problems but not drugs. . . . No one wants to believe a guy is doing bad because of drug problems. But the more I did it, the worse I felt. My need kept getting greater and I couldn't fight that need."[41] Gold has observed an impairment of eye-hand coordination. He notes: "Hitters have a hard time making contact with the ball. Pitchers lose something off their fastball and their curve and lose concentration. Bas-

Table 7–2. FREUD'S EXPERIMENTS WITH COCAINE

Time	Pressures	Max.	Average	Remarks
Experiment of November 9, 1884. Dynamometer for two hands.				
8:00	66-65-60	66	63.6	fasting
10:00	67-55-50	67	57.3	after morning rounds
10:22	67-63-56	67	62	after breakfast
10:30	65-58-67	67	63.6	—
10:33			0.10 cocaïnum muriaticum*	
10:45	82-75-69	82	75.3	first ruptus
10:55	76-69-64	76	69.6	tired
11:20	78-71-77	78	75.3	euphoria
12:30	72-66-74	74	70.6	before lunch
12:55	77-73-67	77	72.6	—
1:35	75-66-74	75	71.6	after lunch
1:50	76-71-61	76	69.3	—
3:35	65-58-62	65	61.6	euphoria over
Experiment of November 10, 1884. (Same apparatus.)				
8:00	60	60	60	tired
10:00	73-63-67	73	67.6	after rounds
—		thereupon, a small indeterminate quantity of cocaine		
10:20	76-70-76	76	74	cheerful
10:30	73-70-68	73	70.3	—
11:35	72-72-74	74	72.6	—
12:50	74-73-63	74	70	—
2:20	70-68-69	70	69	—
4:00	76-74-75	76	75	normal condition
6:00	67-64-58	67	63	after strenuous work
8:30	76-64-67	74	68.3	somewhat tired
—		thereupon, 0.10 cocaïnum muriaticum†		
8:43	80-73-74	80	75.6	ruptus
8:58	79-76-71	79	75.3	—
9:18	77-72-67	77	72	buoyant feeling

Time	Reaction Times	Max.	Min.	Av.	Remarks
Experiment of November 26, 1884.					
7:10	15½-21½-19-21-18½-24-24	24	15½	20.5	motor energy, 36−, tired
	about 7:30, 0.10g cocaïn. mur.				
7:38	17-21½-16-21-17-16	21½	16	18	motor energy, 39+
8:05	17-17-18-17	18	17	17.2	a little more cocaine
8:15	13½-11-16-15-16-12	16	11	13.9	euphoria
10:30	15½-14½-15-13½-17½	17½	14½	15.2	remaining good feeling motor energy, 37.5
Experiment of December 4, 1884. Well-being. No cocaine.					
8:15	13½-13-14½-13½	14½	13	13.6	motor energy, 38–39k
8:30	15-14-14-19-15½-15½	19	14	15.5	during 4th reaction a disturbing sound
8:45	11½-13½-14½-12½-16½	16½	12½	13.7	—
9:00	12½-13-13-15½-14-18½	18½	12½	14.2	motor energy, 38

*Freud did not state the measurement here but it was almost certainly grams, as later specified in his experiment of November 26, 1884. Ed.

†Once again, Freud did not state the measurement here but it was almost certainly grams. Ed.

(From Freud, S: Cocaine Papers [edited by R. Byck], Stonehill Publishing, New York, 1974, with permission).

ketball players lose their shooting touch and become confused during rapidly changing game situations, and football players have difficulty following the game plan."[42] Czechowicz of the National Institute on Drug Abuse has noted that coaches consistently report that an early clue to cocaine abuse is a distortion of a sense of time—athletes show up either early or late to practice. Practices may be missed altogether, and fights with teammates are not uncommon.[42]

All in all, the data for cocaine and its effects on parameters of athletic performance are incomplete, and it is unlikely that well-controlled prospective studies will be forthcoming.

Case Vignette

A 20-year-old college basketball player was about to begin his final season after having played a reasonably good season during his junior year. Typically an upbeat person on the court, off the court he had mood swings which often included mild depressive symptoms. He enjoyed socializing, and during the offseason prior to his senior year, he experimented with intranasal cocaine for the first time. He snorted about 4 lines, and he remembers having felt exhilarated that evening. His memories of the evening were so pleasant that he snorted cocaine on several other occasions.

Initially, he snorted cocaine only with friends, and he limited his amount to no more than 6 lines per evening. Three months after having started using cocaine, he purchased his first gram. When the drug was available in his own room, he could not resist the temptation of using it. For the first time, he snorted cocaine while alone.

Once the basketball season began, he vowed to no longer use the drug. However, after his team's first victory, several friends invited him over for some postgame snorting. Although initially reluctant, he spent the entire evening snorting cocaine and used approximately 2 grams over 8 hours.

Postgame partying began to occur more frequently, and the individual was now using cocaine 2 to 3 times per week. In order to support his habit, he began selling the drug on campus. On two occasions, he arrived late for practice due to oversleeping,

and he was severely reprimanded. The night following his second late practice, he again snorted cocaine and stayed up most of the night. The next morning he awoke on time for practice, but he was exhausted. He tried 2 lines of cocaine and immediately felt energetic, and he enjoyed a rather good practice session.

The cycle of late-night partying and prepractice or pregame cocaine use became routine. In addition, he often drank heavily after using cocaine in order to help himself fall asleep. As he became more and more dependent on cocaine, his social and private life centered around selling, buying, and using the drug. He became distant from friends, his grades suffered, and he was often irritable with teammates. During games, however, he usually played well, and he never used more than 2 to 3 lines of cocaine prior to a given game, although at times he snorted an additional 1 to 2 lines during halftime.

He completed the season rather uneventfully, not having played up to preseason expectations. His postseason use of cocaine escalated, and he became more withdrawn and at times paranoid. Following a 3-day binge of intranasal cocaine use, he suffered a generalized tonic-clonic seizure and was treated at a local hospital. A confession of cocaine abuse led to his transfer to a rehabilitation institute for detoxification.

ADVERSE EFFECTS

The risks of cocaine abuse to the athlete are not inconsequential (Table 7–3). The incidence of sudden death has increased with the increased use of cocaine and particularly with the use of crack.[13,43-47] Competitive athletics further increase the potential of cocaine's powerful adverse cardiovascular stimulating effects, namely, life-threatening cardiac arrhythmias and myocardial infarction.[48-57] Myocardial infarction in young cocaine abusers has been reported in the absence of structural coronary artery disease.[45,50,52,58-61] Recent experimental work demonstrates that the adrenergic nervous system can cause coronary artery vasoconstriction,[62] suggesting this as a mechanism in which cocaine can be lethal to the young athlete.[44] Dilated cardiomyopathy has been

Table 7–3. COMPLICATIONS OF
COCAINE USE

Cardiac
Ventricular arrhythmia
Sudden death
Angina pectoris
Myocardial infarction
Myocarditis
Neuropsychiatric
Cerebrovascular
Cerebral infarction
Cerebral hemorrhage
Subarachnoid hemorrhage
Cerebral vasculitis
Transient ischemic attacks
Addiction
Seizures
Tourette's exacerbation
Headache
Visual scotoma/blindness
Optic neuropathy
Behavioral
Insomnia
Euphoria/dysphoria
Confusion
Assaultiveness
Delirium
Paranoia
Hallucinations
Psychosis
Repetitive behavior
Anorexia
Ob/Gyn
Abruptio placentae
Spontaneous abortion
Congenital malformations of fetus
Placental transfer to infant and secondary
acute toxicity
Breast milk transfer to infant and secondary
acute toxicity
Other Medical
Sexual dysfunction
Liver toxicity
Osteolytic sinusitis
Pneumomediastinum
Aortic dissection
Gastrointestinal ischemia
Necrosis/perforation of nasal septum
Loss of smell
Hyperthermia/tachycardia

noted in two chronic cocaine abusers—a 42-year-old male and a 28-year-old female—one of whom had normal coronary arteries.[61]

Intracerebral and subarachnoid hemorrhages have been reported shortly after cocaine abuse. In most instances, there had been an underlying vascular anomaly, either an aneurysm or an arteriovenous malformation,[52,63–67] although spontaneous hemorrhage without a structural predisposition has been reported.[66] Cerebral ischemia and infarction may occur, either as a complication of vasculitis or from acute vasospasm.[64,65,68–71]

Convulsions following cocaine have been reported as far back as 1922,[72,73] and the drug has been used to induce temporal lobe epilepsy in animals.[74] The epileptogenic mechanism is not presently known, although the acute sympathomimetic effects of the drug may play an important role.[73,75] Even repeated small doses of the drug have been shown to produce seizures, the so-called kindling effect.[8,74] Various other neurologic complications may occur following cocaine abuse, including exacerbations of Tourette's syndrome, visual scotoma and blindness, optic neuropathy, and headache.[18,71,76,77]

Acute and chronic behavioral changes are similar to those observed with amphetamine abuse and may include insomnia, euphoria and dysphoria, confusion, assaultiveness, delirium, paranoia, hallucinations, psychosis, repetitive behavior, and anorexia.[19,23,71]

Various other medical, gynecological, and obstetrical complications are outlined in Table 7–3. Systemic medical complications seem to occur as a result of some combination of acute hypertension, tachycardia, and peripheral vasospasm.[71] Of concern are reports of acute cocaine toxicity in infants resulting in one case from transfer through breast milk[78] and in another from placental transfer just prior to birth.[79]

The strongly positive reinforcing effects of cocaine lead to a pattern of continued use and drug addiction, which may further potentiate any of the above-mentioned adverse effects.

FINAL NOTE

The ergogenic abuse potential for cocaine theoretically might be similar to amphetamine. However, not only does cocaine's short duration of action make it impractical as an ergogenic aid, but its route of administration and associated intense euphoric effect appear to seduce individuals into more serious recreational abuse patterns than those seen with amphetamine. One rarely hears of athletes binging on amphetamine during the off-season, and current national surveys indicate that cocaine abuse is a much more serious threat to both athletes and nonathletes.

The euphoria following cocaine use is in some ways similar to the intense euphoria following an outstanding athletic performance; both are in part mediated through the "pleasure brain." The individual feels energetic, exhilarated, and hyperalert. Is the athlete, then, more susceptible than the nonathlete to cocaine abuse in an effort to replicate this feeling? No evidence supports such a conclusion. One fact, however, is clear: The abuse potential of cocaine is compelling. The seductive nature of the drug coupled with its potent behavioral reinforcing actions make cocaine a dangerously addictive substance.

The deaths of world-class athletes from cocaine have heightened public awareness to the problem of cocaine abuse in the athletic community, and they have brought the problem of cocaine abuse by the population at large into focus. The problem of cocaine abuse by the athlete and nonathlete lends itself to no simplistic solutions. However, any effort to impact on this problem first requires an understanding of the abuse and addiction potential of this drug. Accordingly, if education is to be relied on as a deterrent, then education must be predicated on facts and not fiction born of ignorance.

Similarly, an understanding of the extent of the problem in both professional and amateur sports must be based on fact derived from sound epidemiology and not from hearsay and anecdote. Drug testing plays an important role not only in providing epidemiologic data but also in encouraging an ongoing dialogue among members of the sports community on how best to address the dangerously seductive nature of cocaine.

REFERENCES

1. Gomez, L: Cocaine—America's 100 years of euphoria and despair. Life Magazine, May, 1984.
2. Stone, N, Fromme, M and Kagan, D: Cocaine—Se-duction and Solution. Clarkson N Potter, Inc., New York, 1984.
3. Van Dyke, C and Byck R: Cocaine. Scientific Amer 246:128, 1982.
4. Kunkel, DB: Cocaine then and now. Part I. Its history, medical botany and use. Emerg Med, June 15, 1986, p 125.
5. Haddad, LM: Cocaine abuse: background, clinical presentation, and emergency treatment. Int Med for Specialist 7:67, 1986.
6. Fairbanks, DNF and Fairbanks, GR: Cocaine uses and abuses. Primary ENT 2:2, 1986.
7. Thomal, E: America's crusade. What is behind the latest war on drugs. Time, Sept 15, 1986, p 60.
8. Barron, J: Use of cocaine, but not other drugs, seen rising. The New York Times, Sept 29, 1986.
9. Adams, EH and Kozel, NJ: Cocaine use in America: Introduction and overview. In Kozel, NJ and Adams, EH (eds): Cocaine Use in America: Epidemiologic and Clinical Perspectives. NIDA Research Monograph 61. Rockville, Maryland, 1985, p 1.
10. Morganthau, T, et al: Kids and cocaine. Newsweek, March 17, 1986, p 58.
11. Brinkley, J: Drug use held mostly stable or better. The New York Times, Oct 10, 1986.
12. Johnston, L and Bachman, J: The Monitoring the Future Study. Institute for Social Research, The University of Michigan, 1987.
13. "Crack." The Medical Letter 28:69, 1986.
14. Rust, M: Very addictive, appealing to youth, crack poses major health worries. Am Med News, Sept 12, 1986.
15. Kerr, P: Extra-potent cocaine: Use rising sharply among teen-agers. The New York Times, March 20, 1986.
16. Washton, AM, Gold, MS and Pottash, AC: "Crack"—early report of a new drug epidemic. Postgrad Med 80:52, 1986.
17. Pollin, W: The danger of cocaine (editorial). JAMA 254:98, 1985.
18. Lowenstein, DH, et al: Acute neurologic and psychiatric complications associated with cocaine abuse. Am J Med 83:841, 1987.
19. Jaffe, JH: Drug Addiction and Drug Abuse. In Gilman, AG, et al (eds): Goodman and Gilman's The Pharmacological Basis of Therapeutics, ed 7. Macmillan, New York, 1985, p 532.
20. Ritchie, JM and Greene, NM: Local Anesthetics. In Gilman, AG, et al (eds): Goodman and Gilman's The Pharmacological Basis of Therapeutics, ed 7. Macmillan, New York, 1985, p 302.
21. Wise, RA: Neural Mechanisms of the Reinforcing Action of Cocaine. In Grabowski, J (ed): Pharmacology, Effects, and Treatment of Abuse. NIDA Research Monograph 50, NIDA, Rockville, Maryland, 1984, p 15.
22. Jones, RT: The pharmacology of cocaine. In Grabowski, J (ed): Pharmacology, Effects, and Treatment of Abuse. NIDA Research Monograph 50. NIDA, Rockville, Maryland, 1984, p 34.
23. Fischman, MW: Cocaine and the amphetamines. In Meltzer, H (ed): Psychopharmacology: The Third Generation of Progress. Raven Press, New York, 1987, p 1543.
24. Nunes, EV and Rosecan, JS: Human neurobiology of cocaine. In Spitz, HI and Rosecan, JS (eds): Co-

caine Abuse: New Directions in Treatment and Research. Brunner/Mazel, New York, 1987, p 48.

25. Miller, WS, Dackis, CA and Gold, MS: The relationship of addiction, tolerance, and dependence to alcohol and drugs: A neurochemical approach. J Substance Abuse Treatment 4:197, 1987.

26. Ritz, ML, et al: Cocaine receptors on dopamine transporters are related to self-administration of cocaine. Science 237:1219, 1987.

27. Giannini, AJ, et al: Treatment of depression in chronic cocaine and phencyclidine abuse with desipramine. J Clin Pharmacol 26:211, 1986.

28. Gawin, FH and Kleber, HD: Cocaine abuse treatment. Arch Gen Psychiatry 41:903, 1984.

29. Bozarth, M and Wise, R: Toxicity associated with long-term intravenous heroin and cocaine self-administration in the rat. JAMA 254:81, 1985.

30. Aigner, TG and Balster, RL: Choice behavior in rhesus monkeys: Cocaine versus food. Science 201:534, 1978.

31. Fischman, MW and Schuster, CR: Cocaine self-administration in human. Fed Proc 41:241, 1982.

32. Collins, GB: Clues to cocaine dependency. Diagnosis, 1985, p 57.

33. Fischman, MW, et al: Cardiovascular and subjective effects of intravenous cocaine administration in humans. Arch Gen Psychiatry 33:983, 1976.

34. Resnick, RB and Resnick, EB: Cocaine abuse and its treatment. Psychiatr Clin North Am 7:713, 1984.

35. Kulberg, A: Substance abuse: Clinical identification and management. Med Clin North Am 33:325, 1986.

36. Gawin, FH and Ellinwood, EH: Cocaine and other stimulants; actions, abuse and treatment. N Engl J Med 318:1173, 1988.

37. Anderson, WA and McKeag, DB: The Substance Use and Abuse Habits of College Student Athletes. Research Paper No. 2: General Findings. Presented to NCAA Executive Committee Drug Education Committee by College of Human Medicine, Michigan State University, June 1985.

38. Elite Women Athletes Survey. Hazelden Health Promotion Services, Minneapolis, January, 1987.

39. The Washington Post, November 26, 1986.

40. Freud, S: On the general effect of cocaine. In Byck, R (ed): Cocaine Papers. Stonehill Publishing, New York, 1974, p 111.

41. Chass, M: Cocaine disrupts baseball from field to front office. New York Times, August 20, 1985, p 1.

42. Kirkman, D: Experts: Coke even hurts best athletes. Newsday, April 24, 1986.

43. Duda, M: Cocaine deaths may increase drug tests. Phys Sportsmed 14(8):37, 1986.

44. Weiss, RJ: Recurrent myocardial infarction caused by cocaine abuse. Am Heart J 111:793, 1986.

45. Ring, ME and Butman, SM: Cocaine and premature myocardial infarction. Drug Therapy, September 1986, p 117.

46. Drug deaths revive test issue. Newsday, July 1, 1986.

47. Cocaine use can affect heart. The New York Times, June 26, 1986.

48. Benchimol, A and Bartall, H: Accelerated ventricular rhythm and cocaine abuse. Ann Intern Med 88:519, 1978.

49. Simpson, RW and Edwards, WD: Pathogenesis of cocaine-induced ischemic heart disease. Arch Pathol Lab Med 110:479, 1986.

50. Isner, JM, et al: Acute cardiac events temporally related to cocaine abuse. N Engl J Med 315:1438, 1986.

51. Coleman, E, Ross, T. Naughton, JL: Myocardial ischemia and infarction related to recreational cocaine use. West J Med 315:1438, 1986.

52. Cregler, L and Mark, H: Cardiovascular dangers of cocaine abuse. Am J Cardiol 57:1185, 1986.

53. Gould, L and Gopalaswamy, C: Cocaine-induced myocardial infarction. NY State J Med 85:660, 1985.

54. Kossowsky, W and Lyon, A: Cocaine and acute myocardial infarction—a probable connection. Chest 86:729, 1984.

55. Nanji, A and Filipenko, J: Asystole and ventricular fibrillation associated with cocaine intoxication. Chest 85:132, 1984.

56. Boag, F and Havard, C: Cardiac arrhythmia and myocardial ischemia related to cocaine and alcohol consumption. Postgrad Med J 61:997, 1985.

57. Pasternack, P, et al: Cocaine-induced angina pectoris and acute myocardial infarction in patients younger than 40 years. Am J Cardiol 55:847, 1985.

58. Rollinger, IM, et al: Cocaine-induced myocardial infarction. Can Med Assoc J 135:45, 1986.

59. Howard, R, et al: Acute myocardial infarction following cocaine abuse in a woman with normal coronary arteries. JAMA 254:95, 1985.

60. Mathias, DW: Cocaine-associated myocardial ischemia—review of clinical and angiographic findings. Am J Med 81:675, 1986.

61. Wiener, RS, Lockhart, JT and Schwartz, RG: Dilated cardiomyopathy and cocaine abuse. Am J Med 81:699, 1986.

62. Buffington, CW and Feigl, EO; Adrenergic coronary vasoconstriction in the presence of coronary stenosis in the dog. Cir Res 48:416, 1981.

63. Lichtenfeld, P and Rubin, D: Subarachnoid hemorrhage precipitated by cocaine snorting. Arch Neurol 41:223, 1984.

64. Caplan, L and Hier, D: Current concepts of cerebrovascular disease—stroke: Stroke and drug abuse. Stroke 13:869, 1982.

65. Levine, SR and Welch, KMA: Cocaine and stroke. Stroke 22:25, 1987.

66. Wojak, JL and Flamm, ES: Intracranial hemorrhage and cocaine use. Stroke 18:712, 1987.

67. Tuchman, AJ, et al: Intracranial hemorrhage after cocaine abuse. JAMA 257:1175, 1987.

68. Brust, J and Richter, R: Stroke associated with cocaine abuse. NY State J Med 77:1473, 1977.

69. Kaye, BR and Fainstat, M: Cerebral vasculitis associated with cocaine abuse. JAMA 258:2104, 1987.

70. Golbe, LI and Merkin, MD: Cerebral interaction in a user of free-base cocaine ("crack"). Neurology 36:1602, 1986.

71. Cregler, LI and Mark, H: Medical complications of cocaine abuse. New Engl J Med 315:1495, 1986.

72. Pulay, E: Cocaine poisoning. JAMA 78:1855, 1922.

73. Myers, J and Earnest, M: Generalized seizures and cocaine abuse. Neurology 34:675, 1984.

74. Eidelberg, E, et al: An experimental model of temporal lobe epilepsy: Studies of the convulsant properties of cocaine. In Glaser, GH (ed): EEG and Behavior. Basic Books, New York, 1963, p 272.

75. Jonsson, S, et al: Acute cocaine poisoning: Importance of treating seizure and acidosis. Am J Med 75:1061, 1983.

76. Mesulam, MM: Cocaine and Tourette's syndrome. New Engl J Med 315:398, 1986.

77. Newman, NM, et al: Bilateral optic neuropathy and osteolytic sinusitis: Complications of cocaine abuse. JAMA 259:72, 1988.

78. Cocaine found in breast milk of nursing mother who used drugs. Am Med News, 1/8/88, p 42.

79. Chasnoff, J, et al: Perinatal cerebral infarction and maternal cocaine use. J Pediatr 108:456, 1986.

CHAPTER 8

Phenylpropanolamine, Ephedrine, and the "Look-Alikes"

HISTORY

Phenylpropanolamine and ephedrine are prototypic sympathomimetic amines commonly called "look-alikes"—drugs usually combined with caffeine which may mimic the actions of amphetamines. These central nervous system stimulants are available over-the-counter without a prescription. Their emergence as potential drugs of abuse dates back to the early 1970s, coincident with the controls placed on amphetamines by the Controlled Substances Act of 1970. To circumvent the intent of this act, psychoactive drugs were formulated and marketed as amphetamine look-alikes. These look-alikes were referred to by such names as black beauties, white crosses, Christmas trees, greens, and clears.[1] The most common formulation was that of caffeine, ephedrine, and phenylpropanolamine.[2]

The problem of amphetamine look-alikes grew to sufficient proportions to warrant Congressional hearings in the early 1980s.[2] Ironically, the look-alikes fell between jurisdictional cracks. The Drug Enforcement Agency had no authority to regulate these licit over-the-counter drugs. The Food and Drug Administration similarly had limited jurisdiction. By 1982, phenylpropanolamine was conservatively estimated to be the fifth most widely used drug in the United States.[3] That same year, the Food and Drug Administration circumvented jurisdictional constraints by banning the sale of the triple combination of phenylpropanolamine, caffeine, and ephedrine until an investigational new drug license for such a combination could be obtained.[4] A game of cat and mouse ensued between the pharmaceutical industry and the Food and Drug Administration. The industry removed one of the three stimulants. In turn, the Food and Drug Administration, in 1983, mandated that a new license be obtained for drugs combining phenylpropanolamine and caffeine.[2] Since 1986,[5] no combinations of phenylpropanolamine with either caffeine or ephedrine have been listed in the *Physician's Desk Reference*. However, given the ubiquitous nature of caffeine, ephedrine, and phenylpropanolamine, practical concerns regarding the interplay of these drugs persist.

CHEMISTRY AND PHYSIOLOGY

Phenylpropanolamine and ephedrine are structurally similar to amphetamine (see Fig. 6–5). Phenylpropanolamine differs only by the presence of a single hydroxyl group on the beta carbon; ephedrine additionally has a methyl substitution on the terminal amino group. The substitution of the hydroxyl group on the beta carbon decreases lipid solubility, thereby decreasing penetration into the brain and central stimulatory effects.[6]

Phenylpropanolamine and ephedrine exert their effect indirectly on the sympathetic nervous system by displacing norepinephrine and other monoamine transmitters from storage sites.[2] This indirect sympathetic activity is enhanced by intraneuronal monoamine oxidase resistance because of the presence of the methyl group on the alpha carbon.[6] Additionally, direct effects on both alpha and beta receptors exist.[2] The principal effects of phenylpropanolamine and ephedrine are associated with alpha-adrenergic activity.[3]

Phenylpropanolamine and ephedrine exhibit significantly less potency than *d*-amphetamine with respect to increases in locomotor activity, stereotyped behavior, and reduction in food intake.[7] In the experimental animal, even with extremely high doses of phenylpropanolamine, there appears to be significantly less depletion of central monoamines than with amphetamines, and the depletion appears limited to the frontal cortex.[7]

Woolverton[7] concluded from behavioral

studies of the rhesus monkey that phenylpropanolamine should have only limited amphetamine-like subjective effects and even then at doses significantly higher than is required for its anorectic properties. Further, he concluded from self-administration data that phenylpropanolamine should not have amphetamine-like dependence potential. However, this may be a dose-dependent phenomenon, as evidenced by Martin and associates,[8] who reported similar physiologic and subjective responses in subjects exposed to 75 and 150 mg per 70 kg ephedrine versus 15 and 30 mg per 70 kg amphetamine. The latter study suggests that at high enough doses, sufficient blood-brain barrier penetration of drug occurs to allow the similarity with amphetamines in central nervous system effects.

Peripheral effects of phenylpropanolamine and ephedrine are similar to other sympathomimetic drugs and include elevated blood pressure, increased pulse rate, and bronchodilatation.

Psychic effects are usually mild at normally prescribed doses, but larger doses, as with amphetamines, may result in euphoria and increased alertness.[8] Like amphetamine, large doses of ephedrine may cause overstimulation of the central nervous system with subsequent psychosis, hallucinations, and complusive, stereotypic drug-seeking behavior.[9,10]

CLINICAL PHARMACOLOGY

Phenylpropanolamine is available as 18.75 and 25 mg tablets, and 75 mg time-release capsules. Ephedrine is available as the l-isomer in 25 and 50 mg capsules. Both are usually formulated with other drugs such as antihistamines, and they occur in numerous over-the-counter common cold remedies.

The clinical effects of the look-alikes appear as early as 30 minutes after ingestion and last up to 3 hours.[11] Time-release capsules can produce a clinical effect for 12 to 16 hours. Therapeutic doses of phenylpropanolamine are associated with plasma levels of 60 to 200 ng per ml, but toxic plasma concentrations have not been estalished.[3]

Phenylpropanolamine and ephedrine are rapidly absorbed, producing peak blood levels in 1 to 2 hours,[11] although the kinetics are different in the sustained-release form. Most is excreted unchanged in the urine, though some is metabolized by the liver.[11] The plasma half-life is 2 to 3 hours. As non-catecholamine sympathomimetics (no hydroxyl groups on the third and fourth positions of the benzene ring—see Fig. 6–5), phenylpropanolamine and ephedrine, like amphetamines, are not metabolized by catechol-O-methyltransferase. The presence of methyl groups in the alpha position of phenylpropanolamine, ephedrine, and amphetamines blocks oxidation by monoamine oxidase (MAO), thereby prolonging the duration of action.[6,11]

Clinical Uses

Phenylpropanolamine and ephedrine are widely available as over-the-counter cold remedies. Phenylpropanolamine is a common ingredient in diet pills; ephedrine is commonly used in the treatment of asthma, hay fever, sinusitis, allergic rhinitis, urticaria, and other allergic disorders.

USE IN SPORTS

No epidemiologic data regarding the use of look-alikes among athletes have been reported. Although other sympathomimetic amines have similar mechanisms of action, phenylpropanolamine and ephedrine are thought to be the most commonly abused of the look-alikes. The most dramatic story of look-alike "abuse" in sports occurred during the 1972 Olympic Games. Rick DeMont, an American swimmer with asthma, was disqualified for taking medication containing ephedrine.[12]

Effects on Performance

Sidney and Lefcoe[12] performed the only prospective study to examine the possible ergogenicity of the look-alikes. Twenty-one males, age 19 to 30 years, were given either ephedrine, 24 mg, or placebo, in a double-blind modified crossover design. Subjects were studied on 3 separate occasions during a 3-week period. The following variables were assessed:

1. Strength
2. Endurance and power
3. Lung function, $\dot{V}O_2$max

4. Reaction time
5. Hand-eye coordination
6. Anaerobic capacity and speed
7. Cardiorespiratory endurance
8. Response to maximal and submaximal effort
9. Perceived exertion
10. Speed of recovery from effort

Physiologic changes following ephedrine administration relative to placebo included widening of resting pulse pressure, minor increases in exercise heart rate, and slowing of the rate of recovery following muscular effort. Despite these physiologic changes, ephedrine had no effect on the physical performance variables studied, and no subjective effects of improved performance were noted by the subjects.

Sidney and Lefcoe's data are useful because a clinically prescribed dose of ephedrine is examined. Aside from anecdotal evidence and the data by Martin and associates,[8] no study has convincingly demonstrated enhanced athletic performance following large doses of ephedrine, phenylpropanolamine, or the look-alikes. However, these drugs are on the National Collegiate Athletic Association and International Olympic Committee banned list of drugs (Table 8–1) because of the concern that they may be easily abused as ergogenic aids.

The significance of phenylpropanolamine and ephedrine use in sports is severalfold. First, they may be available as amphetamine look-alike formulations. Consequently, any athlete who might be suspect for taking amphetamines should be suspect for abusing phenylpropanolamine or ephedrine, either

Table 8–1. SYMPATHOMIMETIC AMINES BANNED BY THE NCAA AND IOC

Chlorprenaline
Ephedrine
Etafedreine
Isoetharine
Isoprenaline
Methoxyphenamine
Methylephedrine
Phenylpropanolamine
AND RELATED COMPOUNDS

knowingly or unwittingly. Second, the medical complications attendant to the abuse of phenylpropanolamine and ephedrine, especially when used in combination with some other drugs, should be familiar to sports medicine physicians.

Case Vignette

A 20-year-old female tennis player sought medical help at the urging of a close friend. She had lost 40 pounds and was becoming somewhat bizarre.

Always somewhat overweight as a child, she began dieting in her teenage years, but usually without effect. When she began playing tennis more seriously, she found that a major limiting factor in her performance was her weight, which interfered with her desired mobility. At age 17, she began using diet pills and initially lost 15 pounds, but within months the anorectic effect of the pills waned and she regained her weight.

A friend had recommended taking "white crosses," and she obtained a constant supply of the pills. Not only did she again start to lose weight, but she felt energetic and alert after taking the drug. Initially she took one pill each morning, but after several months she began increasing the daily dose. On several occasions she took the pill prior to working out, and she felt better able to concentrate and anticipate her opponent's shots.

One year after beginning white cross use, she generally felt better about her physical appearance and seemed more confident about herself. She continued to take several white cross pills per day, and soon she developed a compulsive ritual: one each morning; one before each meal; one before each practice session or match; one in the evening if she were to socialize; one or two as needed if she felt particularly fatigued.

For the 2 months prior to medical evaluation, she took 6 to 10 pills daily, rarely ate, and became socially isolated. She often paced alone back and forth between matches and was easily irritated by others. She lost several friends, and occasionally became suspicious that others were plotting to ruin her career. She finally listened to her one remaining friend and sought medical help. An analysis of the white cross pills revealed a combination of caffeine, phenylpropanolamine and ephedrine.

ADVERSE EFFECTS

Table 8–2 lists the adverse effects of phenylpropanolamine and ephedrine. Although most of the serious adverse effects of the look-alikes have been noted in patients using combination drugs usually containing caffeine,[2,3,13,14] they also have been noted with phenylpropanolamine or ephedrine alone.

Excessive quantities of the look-alikes have been associated with a variety of neurologic and psychologic sequelae, although less commonly than with amphetamines.[14] Paranoid ideation has been noted in association with homicidal behavior.[15] Excessive doses have been found to produce anxiety and agitation.[3] Restlessness, headaches, dizziness, and confusion have been reported,[14] in addition to mania, hallucinations, and seizures.[3,13–16]

Stroke and transient ischemic attacks have been noted following the ingestion of phenylpropanolamine in association with other stimulants.[3,17] Several cases of cerebral vasculitis and intracerebral hemorrhage secondary to ephedrine and phenylpropanolamine—used either alone or in combination with caffeine—have been reported.[18–25] The vasculitis is indistinguishable from that of amphetamine abuse and presumably is similarly mediated.

Table 8–2. ADVERSE EFFECTS OF THE LOOK-ALIKES

Acute, Mild	Acute, Severe
Nervousness	Agitation
Irritability	Confusion
Insomnia	Paranoia
Anorexia	Mania
Dizziness	Hallucinations
Headaches	Stroke/TIA
Tachycardia	Cerebral vasculitis
Palpitations	Cerebral hemorrhage
Mild hypertension	Severe hypertension
	Myocardial ischemia
	Ventricular arrhythmia
	Rhabdomyolysis

Another hazardous property of the look-alikes is the development of acute hypertension. Phenylpropanolamine has a low therapeutic index and can produce potentially life-threatening hypertension at doses of 85 mg, only three times the standard over-the-counter dose.[3] In some patients, a considerable blood pressure rise may occur with doses as low as 25 mg.[26] Horowitz and associates[27] prospectively studied the effects of phenylpropanolamine in 34 young normotensive subjects. They found that 85 mg produced a mean diastolic blood pressure increase of 24 mm Hg; in four subjects, the diastolic pressure increased to over 115 mm Hg, and in one to 142 mm Hg. Similarly, Lake and colleagues[27a] noted a significant increase in both the systolic and diastolic blood pressures after subjects ingested either 150 mg sustained-release phenylpropanolamine (twice the recommended dose) or 75 mg sustained-release phenylpropanolamine in combination with 400 mg caffeine. Individuals on MAO inhibitors are at particular risk of a hypertensive crisis.[3,14]

As noted by Lee and associates,[28] phenylpropanolamine may also cause significant hypertension when used in association with nonsteroidal anti-inflammatory drugs. They described a 27-year-old female who developed severe hypertension following the ingestion of phenylpropanolamine and indomethacin. Indomethacin reduces prostaglandin synthesis. Prostaglandins control the negative feedback loop that regulates the release of catecholamines at sympathetic nerve endings. Thus, the phenylpropanolamine-augmented release of catecholamines at sympathetic nerve endings is left unopposed. Furthermore, the synthesis of vasodilator prostaglandins, such as prostacyclin, within the vessel wall will be suppressed. The end result is an unopposed indirect effect of phenylpropanolamine on sympathetic nerves and an unopposed direct effect on small arterioles.[14,27,28] Any drug that is a prostaglandin inhibitor, such as aspirin and the nonsteroidal anti-inflammatory agents, could act similarly.

The hypertensive effects of the look-alikes, especially in combination with caffeine or nonsteroidal anti-inflammatory drugs, are particularly disturbing vis-à-vis the athlete. Athletes frequently take over-the-counter drugs, and weight-conscious athletes such as gymnasts may rely on phenylpropanolamine for its anorectic properties. Since the use of nonsteroidal anti-inflammatory drugs and caffeine is so high among athletes, they may be particularly vulnerable if they simultaneously take other look-alike drugs, either knowingly or unknowingly. Additional adverse reactions of the look-alikes are myocardial injury,[29] ventricular arrhythmias,[29,30] and rhabdomyolysis in association with acute renal failure.[31]

The widespread availability of phenylpropanolamine and ephedrine in both prescription and over-the-counter preparations represents a particular point of vulnerability for the athlete, both from a drug testing perspective and a medical standpoint.

FINAL NOTE

Amateur athletes are tremendously burdened with a long list of banned substances, and they must be especially careful before taking any over-the-counter medication for everyday ailments. One may well ask if such an approach is appropriate. For example, if an athlete does have a common cold, International Olympic Committee guidelines suggest that he or she may take an antihistamine rather than using a decongestant for symptomatic relief. Antihistamines not only cause drowsiness in most individuals—which might further impair performance—but they also, at best, provide only partial symptomatic relief in the treatment of the common cold.

Perhaps the original intent of abolishing all sympathomimetic amines from amateur athletic competition was correct, but the current system of banning all substances, regardless of the dose taken or the concentration of the drug in the urine, makes little sense. Is it reasonable to preclude the use of medications appropriately prescribed by medical doctors in accordance with standards of good medical practice, particularly in the absence of evidence of enhanced athletic performance at therapeutic doses of these drugs? Shouldn't the pharmacologic principles of dose-response be addressed? Such a step has been taken with caffeine and should be taken with phenylpropanolamine, ephedrine, and related compounds used in the symptomatic treatment of common ailments suffered by all.

REFERENCES

1. Morgan, JP: Phenylpropanolamine. A Critical Analysis of Reported Adverse Reactions and Overdosage. Jack K. Burgess, Inc., New Jersey, 1986.
2. Lake, CR and Quirk, RS: CNS stimulants and the look-alike drugs. Psychiatr Clin North Am 7:689, 1984.
3. Pentel, P: Toxicity of over-the-counter stimulants. JAMA 252:1898, 1984.
4. Wesson, DR: Substance abuse. JAMA 252:2286, 1984.
5. Physician's Desk Reference 1986. Medical Economics Company, Oradell, NJ.
6. Weiner, N: Norepinephrine, Epinephrine and the Sympathomimetic Amines. In Gilman, AG, et al (eds): Goodman and Gilman's The Pharmacological Basis of Therapeutics, ed 7, Macmillan, New York, 1985, p 145.
7. Woolverton, WL, et al: Behavioural and neurochemical evaluation of phenylpropanolamine. J Pharmacol Exp Therap 237:926, 1986.
8. Martin, WR, et al: Physiologic, subjective, and behavioral effects of amphetamine, methamphetamine, ephedrine, phenmetrazine, and methylphenidate in man. Clin Pharmacol Ther 12:245, 1971.
9. Herridge, CF and Brook, MF: Ephedrine psychosis. Br Med J 2:160, 1968.
10. Prokop, H: Halluzinose bei ephedrinsucht (Hallucinosis in ephedrine addiction). Nervenarzt 39:71, 1942.
11. Kulberg, A: Substance abuse: Clinical identification and management. Med Clin North Am 33:325, 1986.
12. Sidney, KH and Lefcoe, WM: The effects of ephedrine on the physiological and psychological responses to submaximal and maximal exercises in man. Med Sci Sports 9:95, 1977.
13. Phenylpropanolamine over the counter. Lancet 1:839, 1982.
14. Bernstein, E and Diskant, BM: Phenylpropanolamine: A potentially hazardous drug. Ann Emerg Med 11:311, 1982.
15. Cornelius, JR, et al: Paranoia, homicidal behaviour and seizures associated with phenylpropanolamine. Am J Psychiatry 141:120, 1984.
16. Mueller, SM and Solow, EB: Seizures associated with a new combination "pick-me-up" pill. Ann Neurol 11:322, 1982.
17. Johnson, DA, et al: Stroke and phenylpropanolamine use (Letter). Lancet 2:970, 1983.
18. Wooter, MR, Khangure, MS and Murphy, MJ: Intracerebral hemorrhage and vasculitis related to ephedrine abuse. Ann Neurol 13:337, 1983.
19. Maher, LM: Postpartum intracranial hemorrhage and phenylpropanolamine use. Neurology 37:399, 1987.
20. King, J: Hypertension and cerebral haemorrhage after trimolets ingestion (Letter). Med J Aust 2:258, 1979.
21. Fallis, RJ and Fisher, M: Cerebral vasculitis and hemorrhage associated with phenylpropanolamine. Neurology 35:405, 1985.
22. Kikta, DG, Devereaux, MW and Chandar, K: Intracranial hemorrhages due to phenylpropanolamine. Stroke 16:510, 1985.
23. Stoessl, AJ, Young, GB and Feasby, TE: Intracerebral haemorrhage and angiographic beading following ingestion of catecholaminergics. Stroke 16:734, 1985.
24. Mueller, SM, Muller, J and Asdell, SM: Cerebral hemorrhage associated with phenylpropanolamine in combination with caffeine. Stroke 15:119, 1984.
25. Kase, CS, et al: Intracerebral hemorrhage and phenylpropanolamine use. Neurology 37:399, 1987.
26. Drug found harmful in some cases: Warning labels urged. Am Med News February 5, 1988, p 36.
27. Horowitz, JD, et al: Hypertensive response induced by phenylpropanolamine in anorectic and decongestant preparations. Lancet 1:60, 1980.
27a. Lake, CR, et al: A double dose of phenylpropanolamine causes transient hypertension. Am J Med 85:339, 1988.
28. Lee, KY, et al: Severe hypertension after ingestion of an appetite suppressant (phenylpropanolamine) with indomethacin. Lancet 1:1110, 1979.
29. Pentel, PR, Mikell, FL and Zavoral, JH: Myocardial injury after phenylpropanolamine ingestion. Br Heart J 47:51, 1982.
30. Peterson, RB: Phenylpropanolamine-induced arrhythmias (Letter). JAMA 223:324, 1973.
31. Swenson, RD, Golper, TA and Bennet, WM: Acute renal failure and rhabdomyolysis after ingestion of phenylpropanolamine-containing diet pills. JAMA 248:1216, 1982.

Caffeine

HISTORY

Man's earliest involvement with caffeine and related substances may date back to paleolithic times.[1,2] To capture its stimulant properties, the raw fruit of the coffee plant, *Coffea arabica*, was used to prepare very strong caffeinated beverages. With time, the raw fruit was replaced by the roasted coffee bean.[3] The Turks monopolized coffee cultivation until the seventeenth century. From Turkey it found its way to Europe by way of Venice. Thereafter, assertions appeared in France that coffee cured smallpox, gout, and scurvy, while the English claimed it cured venereal disease, indigestion, and the common cold.[3]

In Colonial America, tea, introduced into the Western world by China, was the principal source of caffeine until the Boston Tea Party of 1773.[3] Subsequently, coffee became the major source of caffeine in North America.

Concerns regarding caffeine's potential adverse health effects are not new. In the sixteenth century, the sale of coffee in Egypt was forbidden and coffee stores were burned. Because some Muslim sects believed caffeine-containing beverages to be intoxicating, it was prohibited by the Koran. In the United States, concern was voiced at the turn of the twentieth century that coffee addiction was in a class with morphine and alcohol addiction.[3] In recent years increasing concern has been voiced regarding the adverse effects of caffeine on health.[4] Nonetheless, caffeine remains the most widely consumed drug in Europe and America.[4]

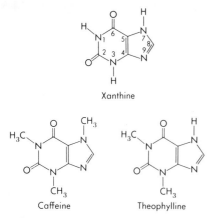

Figure 9–1. Structures of xanthine, caffeine, and theophylline.

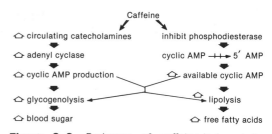

Figure 9–2. Pathway of caffeine-induced increased glycogenolysis and lipolysis.

CHEMISTRY AND PHYSIOLOGY

Caffeine originates naturally in 63 species of plants.[5] Caffeine, theophylline, and theobromine are all methylated xanthines[1] (Fig. 9–1). Xanthine per se is a dioxypurine, and it is structurally related to uric acid. Caffeine is 1,3,7-trimethylxanthine; theophylline is 1,3-dimethylxanthine; and theobromine is 3,7-dimethylxanthine. The methylation of position 1 accounts for the central nervous system stimulation, the methylation of position 3 is predominantly responsible for the diuretic effect, and the methylation of the 7 position correlates with cardiac stimulation.[5] Caffeine is complexed to compounds such as sodium benzoate to increase its solubility.

Caffeine exerts its effects through at least three proposed mechanisms of action at the cellular level:

1. Translocation of intracellular calcium
2. Increase in available cyclic AMP
3. Competitive antagonism of adenosine receptors[1,6,7]

In vitro studies have suggested that caffeine increases the permeability of the sarcoplasmic reticulum to calcium, thereby increasing the amount of intracellular calcium available for muscular contraction.[1,7] Caffeine increases cellular cyclic AMP by two mechanisms (Fig. 9–2). First, by raising circulating catecholamine levels, it increases adenyl cyclase activity with consequently greater production of cyclic AMP.[7] Second, caffeine inhibits phosphodiesterase, the en-

zyme that catalyzes the conversion of cyclic AMP to 5'-AMP.[1,7] The resulting increased cyclic AMP, in turn, gives rise to increased glycogenolysis (increased blood sugar) in caffeine-naive subjects[4] and to increased lipolysis (increased free fatty acids) in all subjects.[4,7] Free fatty acids, in particular, may allow greater energy production and work output in endurance exercise.[7–9]

The main psychic effects following caffeine ingestion include increased alertness, clearer thinking, shortened reaction time, and increased capacity for attention-requiring tasks; these generally occur in doses of 85 to 250 mg.[1] Nervousness, restlessness, and insomnia commonly occur with increasing doses and may occur at a low dose in naive or sensitive individuals. Toxic central nervous system stimulatory effects include delirium and seizures and generally occur in doses over one gram. Lethal doses appear to be over five grams.[1]

A number of mechanisms explain the central nervous system stimulant effects of caffeine:

1. Via competitive antagonism, caffeine blocks adenosine receptors; the resulting blockade of the known sedative effects of adenosine leads to central nervous system stimulation[1,7,10,11]
2. Sensitization of central catecholamine postsynaptic receptors, particularly those for dopamine
3. Possible alteration of acetylcholine and serotonin turnover and receptor functions[5]

Coffee contains opiate receptor antagonist activity independent of caffeine and other xanthines,[12] but the physiologic significance of this is at present unknown.

The cardiovascular effects of caffeine differ between caffeine-tolerant and caffeine-naive individuals. Whereas the caffeine-naive individual may experience altered hemodynamics (pressor response and increase in heart rate), the chronic ingestion of caffeine has little or no effect on blood pressure, heart rate, or plasma catecholamine or renin levels.[3,11] Sensitive individuals experience cardiac arrhythmias with high levels of caffeine.[1,11]

Caffeine has a diuretic effect and causes relaxation of smooth muscles, notably bronchial dilatation. Ingestion of caffeine has been reported to improve the capacity for skeletal muscle work.[1]

CLINICAL PHARMACOLOGY

Caffeine is readily absorbed following ingestion. Blood levels begin to rise in 15 minutes, and peak concentrations are reached in 60 minutes.[1,7] The half-life has been variously reported to be 2 to 10 hours.[1,5,7] This doubles during the latter stages of pregnancy and with the chronic use of oral contraceptive steroids.[1]

Concentrations of caffeine in various formulations are shown in Table 9–1.

Caffeine is primarily degraded via hepatic metabolism, with the resultant single methyl group xanthines and methyluric acids then eliminated in the urine. From 0.5 percent to 3.5 percent of ingested caffeine is excreted unchanged in the urine.[1,6]

Clinical Uses

Caffeine has been incorporated into a number of over-the-counter analgesic preparations. It may be useful topically in atopic dermatitis, and systemically it may play a role in the treatment of neonatal apnea.

USE IN SPORTS

Caffeine has long been consumed by athletes in the belief that it will enhance performance.[6,11,13,14] However, an analysis of the available data suggests that a distinction must be made between caffeine's effect on high-intensity, short-duration activities and its effect on endurance activities.[2,7]

Effects on Performance

Caffeine's direct enhancing effect on skeletal muscle has been demonstrated by in situ low-frequency electrical stimulation.[15] This effect, which is primarily mediated through changes in intracellular calcium transport, can be observed in both fatigued and rested muscle. However, with high-frequency electrical stimulation, akin to maximum voluntary contraction, caffeine had no enhancing effect on either fatigued or rested muscle. These observations and others have suggested that caffeine has no significant enhancing effect on high-intensity, short-term work.[7]

Reports on caffeine's effect on the oxygen transport system ($\dot{V}O_2$max) are inconsistent and no firm conclusions can be drawn.[7,9] With respect to metabolic rates, caffeine is known to increase the basal metabolic rate of both caffeine-tolerant and caffeine-naive individuals.[1,16] However, it has been demonstrated that endurance-trained athletes have a blunted response to the thermogenic actions of caffeine.[16]

Table 9–1. CONCENTRATION OF CAFFEINE IN VARIOUS FORMULATIONS

Substance	Milligrams of Caffeine
Food and Beverages	
Coffee (6 oz. cup)	
Brewed	100–150
Instant	65–100
Decaffeinated	3
Tea	
Regular	30–75
Herbal	0
Sodas (12 oz.)	
Colas	32–65
Cocoa (6 oz. cup)	5–50
Chocolates (1 oz.)	
Milk	6
Bittersweet	20
Medications (Per Tablet)	
Cafergot	100
Fiorinal	40
Darvon Compound	32
Vivarin	200
No Doz	100
Excedrin, Extra-Strength	65
Dexatrim	0
Anacin	32
Midol	32

Contrary to caffeine's entirely equivocal effect on short-term, high-intensity work, evidence for its enhancing effects on endurance performance is somewhat stronger, although not absolutely conclusive.[7,8,11,17-22] Observed increased work production (improved times) and the delay in the onset of fatigue have been at least partly attributable to the sparing of muscle glycogen. This, in turn, has been attributed to caffeine's lipolytic effect whereby free fatty acids become an alternate substrate for aerobic metabolism. An alternative explanation is direct neuronal stimulation. The endurance-enhancing effect of caffeine has been demonstrated with doses of 250 mg taken 1 hour prior to the endurance exercise with an additional 250 mg in divided doses taken immediately prior to the exercise and subsequently at 15-minute intervals during the exercise.[8,17,18]

Other studies, however, have not demonstrated enhanced endurance following caffeine ingestion. Perkins and Williams[19] found no significant difference in time of pedaling to exhaustion following caffeine doses up to 10 mg/kg. Similar results were demonstrated by the Essig and Powers groups in separate studies.[18,20]

Although increased lipolysis and subsequent decreased glucose utilization are the purported mechanisms of action of increased endurance with caffeine use,[7-9,23] this claim has been challenged.[21,22] Knapik and associates[21] found no significant change in lipid oxidation or inhibition of carbohydrate use following caffeine intake. Casal and Leon[22] noted no change in the respiratory ratio despite an increased plasma concentration of free fatty acids, suggesting that the use of free fatty acids was unaffected. Nutritional status at the time of study may in part account for these observed differences.[24]

Contradictory data abound with respect to caffeine's effect on other measures of performance that are important in athletic competition. Poorly substantiated reports of less drowsiness, increased vigilance, reduced fatigue, and an increased capacity for sustained intellectual work have all contributed to the widespread use of caffeine.[7,25-28] Mental tasks which require prolonged concentration are reported by some to be significantly improved after caffeine ingestion.[29,30] Others, however, have reported no objective improvement in tests of alertness, psychomotor

performance, and cognition following caffeine ingestion,[31-34] although experimental subjects did report subjective feelings of increased alertness and physical activity.[31] In those subjects who did feel more alert or active, there was a tendency to report feelings of nervousness.[30]

Coordination and other fine motor skills which are important in some aspects of athletic performance are neither clearly enhanced nor diminished following caffeine ingestion. Standing steadiness (body sway) has been shown to be adversely affected by 300 mg of caffeine per 70 kg of body weight,[35] and unsteady hand movements have been noted at caffeine doses of only 150 mg.[36] Other investigators report that 100 to 500 mg of caffeine produce no significant change in performance when measuring hand-arm steadiness, simple reaction time to visual stimulation, and precision-coordination tasks.[29,37] Similarly, tests of manual dexterity reportedly failed to show significant decrements after 300 mg of caffeine per 70 kg of body weight.[35] Koller and associates[38] demonstrated that caffeine only infrequently induces tremor in normal people, and it does not exacerbate pathologic tremor.

The uncertainty as to the ergogenic effects of caffeine on athletic performance has caused the International Olympic Committee (IOC) to vary its standards at different times. In 1972, the IOC removed caffeine from its list of doping agents.[7] More recently, the use of high doses of caffeine has been banned, the assumption being that a dose-response curve exists for the ergogenic effects of the drug. Conservatively, it has been suggested that urinary caffeine levels of 10 μg per ml could be indicative of caffeine ingestion aimed at enhancing athletic performance.[6] Currently, greater than 12 μg per ml of caffeine in the urine is defined as doping by the IOC.[39] The NCAA urine limit for caffeine doping is 15 μg per ml.[40] It is estimated that 2 cups of coffee will yield urine levels of 3 to 6 μg per ml.

Case Vignette _____

A 32-year-old woman was brought to the emergency room with complaints of light-headedness and palpitations. She had no prior medical problems, normally drank 1 to 2 cups of coffee daily, and was a well-trained middle-distance runner. One hour prior to a 10-kilometer race, she drank 5 cups of espresso in the hopes of improving her race time. Thirty minutes later, she developed lightheadedness and palpitations, and she became presyncopal.

Evaluation in the emergency room was notable for a resting pulse of 180 per minute, blood pressure of 90/70, and an otherwise unremarkable general medical and neurological exam, including no discernible cardiac murmur or click. Electrocardiogram revealed a supraventricular tachycardia. The patient was treated conservatively and returned to her baseline in 2 hours. She has since abstained from coffee.

ADVERSE EFFECTS

Numerous adverse health effects have been attributed to the use of caffeine (Table 9–2). In analyzing these reports, a distinction should be made between the adverse health effects of chronic caffeine intake versus acute caffeine usage as it might occur in attempts to enhance athletic performance.

Nervousness, irritability, and insomnia result from the central nervous system stimulant effects and may occur in different individuals at varying doses.[1] High doses of caffeine have been associated with delirium, seizures, coma, and death.[1,41–43]

Transient hypertension usually occurs in caffeine-naive individuals immediately after ingestion[1]; a subgroup of patients with a baseline higher systemic vascular resistance or positive family history of hypertension may be at an increased risk of blood pressures greater than 230/100 following caffeine intake.[44] Various ventricular and supraventricular arrhythmias have been described in association with caffeine and may be secondary to changes in the refractory period.[45,46]

Numerous studies have addressed the issue of caffeine and associated ischemic heart disease,[4,47–52] although a consensus is lacking. Curatolo and Robertson[4] state that such a discrepancy justifies the conclusion "that coffee intake is not a risk factor for this disease." The difficulty lies in separating coffee per se as a risk factor since many heavy coffee users have other risk factors for cardiovascular disease. Serum cholesterol is elevated as a result of caffeine consumption.[47,48]

The issue of teratogenicity, carcinogenicity, and fibrocystic breast disease is excellently reviewed by Curatolo and Robertson.[4] The available evidence suggests that no such link exists. Some individuals develop diarrhea and gastrointestinal discomfort following caffeine ingestion, although an association with peptic ulcer disease is less clearcut.[4]

FINAL NOTE

Caffeine, like cocaine and amphetamines, is primarily a central nervous system stimulant. Also like the amphetamines, its ergogenicity is a function of its dose-response curve. In this regard, it is interesting that caffeine is the only stimulant treated in a dose-response manner in drug testing protocols by the IOC and NCAA. It is not the mere presence of the drug in the urine that is the basis

Table 9–2. ADVERSE EFFECTS OF CAFFEINE

Acute, Mild	Acute, Severe	Chronic
Nervousness	Peptic ulcer	Increased serum cholesterol
Irritability	Delirium	? Increased ischemic heart disease
Insomnia	Seizures	? Increased teratogenicity
Sinus tachycardia	Coma	? Increased carcinogenesis
Hypertension	Arrhythmia	? Increased fibrocystic breast disease
Gastrointestinal distress	Supraventricular	
	Ventricular	
	Death	

for disqualification; a threshold level of 12 and 15 μg per ml is required before sanctions are imposed by the IOC and NCAA, respectively.

Undoubtedly, the imposition of a quantitative standard for caffeine as contrasted with an "all or none" standard for cocaine and amphetamines reflects both the ubiquity and legality of caffeine in society. Although conflicting data make it difficult to know precisely how urine concentrations of a drug correlate with ergogenicity, we agree fully that such an approach should be increasingly used in drug testing protocols, especially for widely available over-the-counter drugs such as ephedrine and phenylpropanolamine.

REFERENCES

1. Rall, TW: Central nervous stimulants—the methylxanthines. In Gilman, AG, et al (eds): Goodman and Gilman's the Pharmacological Basis of Therapeutics, ed 7. Macmillan, New York, 1985, p 589.
2. Slavin, JL and Joensen, DJ: Caffeine and sports performance. Phys Sportsmed 13(5):191, 1985.
3. Goulart, FS: The Caffeine Book—A User's and Abuser's Guide. Dodd Mead and Co., New York, 1984.
4. Curatolo, PW and Robertson, D: The health consequences of caffeine. Ann Intern Med 98:641, 1983.
5. Greden, JF: Caffeine and tobacco dependence. In Kaplan, HI and Sadock, BJ (eds): Comprehensive Textbook of Psychiatry, IV, ed 4. Williams & Wilkins, Baltimore, 1985, p 1026.
6. Delbeke, FT and Debackere, M: Caffeine: Use and abuse in sports. Int J Sports Med 5:179, 1984.
7. Powers, SK and Dodd, S: Caffeine and endurance performance. Sports Med 2:165, 1985.
8. Ivy, JL, et al: Influence of caffeine and carbohydrate feedings on endurance performance. Med Sci Sports 11:6, 1979.
9. Toner, MM, Kirkendall, DT and Delio, DJ: Metabolic and cardiovascular responses to exercise with caffeine. Ergonomics 25:1175, 1982.
10. Daly, JW, Bruns, RF and Snyder, SH: Adenosine receptors in the central nervous system: Relationship to the central actions of methylxanthines. Life Sci 28:2083, 1981.
11. Eichner, ER: The caffeine controversy: Effects on endurance and cholesterol. Phys Sportsmed 14(12):124, 1986.
12. Boublik, JH, et al: Coffee contains potent opiate receptor binding activity. Nature 301:246, 1983.
13. Rogers, CC: Cyclists try caffeine suppositories. Phys Sportsmed 13:38, 1985.
14. Butts, NK and Crowell, D: Effect of caffeine ingestion on cardiorespiratory endurance in men and women. Res Q Exerc Sport 56(4):301, 1985.
15. Lopes, M, et al: Effect of caffeine on skeletal muscle function before and after fatigue. J App Physio 54:1303, 1983.
16. Poehlman, ET, et al: Influence of caffeine on the resting metabolic rate of exercise-trained and inactive subjects. Med Sci Sports Exer 17:689, 1985.
17. Costill, DL, Dalsky, GP and Fink, WJ: Effects of caffeine ingestion on metabolism and exercise performance. Med Sci Sports 10:155, 1978.
18. Essig, D, Costill, DL and Van Handel, PJ: Effects of caffeine ingestion on utilization of muscle glycogen and lipid during leg ergometer cycling. Int J Sports Med 1:86, 1980.
19. Perkins, R and Williams, MH: Effects of caffeine upon maximal muscular endurance of females. Med Sci Sports 7:221, 1975.
20. Powers, SK, et al: Effects of caffeine ingestion on metabolism and performance during graded exercise. Eur J Appl Physiol 50(3):301, 1983.
21. Knapik, JJ, et al: Influence of caffeine on serum substrate changes during running in trained and untrained individuals. In Knuttgen, HG, Vogel, JA and Poortans, J (eds): Biochemistry of Exercise. Human Kinetics Publishers, Inc., Champaign, IL, 1983, p 514.
22. Casal, DC and Leon, AS: Failure of caffeine to affect substrate utilization during prolonged running. Med Sci Sports Exer 17:174, 1985.
23. Erickson, MA, Schwearzkopf, RJ and McKenzie, RR: Effects of caffeine, fructose, and glucose ingestion on muscle glycogen utilization during exercise. Med Sci Sports Exer 19:579, 1987.
24. Weir, J, et al: A high carbohydrate diet negates the metabolic effects of caffeine during exercise. Med Sci Sports Exer 19:100, 1987.
25. Elkins, RN, et al: Acute effects of caffeine in normal prepubertal boys. Am J Psychiatry 138:178, 1981.
26. Cheney, RH: Comparative effect of caffeine per se and a caffeine beverage (coffee) upon the reaction time in normal young adults. J Pharmacol Exp Therap 53:304, 1935.
27. Horst, K and Jenkins, WL: The effect of caffeine, coffee, and decaffeinated coffee upon blood pressure, pulse rate and simple reaction time of men of various ages. J Pharmacol Exp Therap 53:385, 1935.
28. Rapoport, JL, et al: Behavioral and cognitive effects of caffeine in boys and adult males. J Nerv Ment Dis 169:726, 1981.
29. Blum, B and Stern, M: A comparative evaluation of the action of depressant and stimulant drugs on human performance. Psychopharm 6:173, 1964.
30. Holliday, A and Devery, W: Effects of drugs on the performance of a task by fatigued subjects. Clin Pharmacol Ther 3:5, 1982.
31. Goldstein, A, Kaizer, S and Warren, R: Psychotropic effects of caffeine in man. II. Alertness, psychomotor coordination, and mood. J Pharmacol Exp Therap 150:146, 1965.
32. Dureman, EI: Differential patterning of behavioral effects from three types of stimulant drugs. Clin Pharmacol Ther 3:29, 1961.
33. Goldstein, A, Kaizer, S and Warren, R: Psychotropic effects of caffeine in man. I. Individual differences in sensitivity to caffeine induced wakefulness. J Pharmacol Exp Ther 149:156, 1965.
34. Clubley, M, et al: Effects of caffeine and cyclizine alone and in combination in human performance, subjective effects, and EEG activity. Br J Clin Pharmacol 7:157, 1979.
35. Franks, HM, et al: The effect of caffeine on human

performance alone and in combination with ethanol. Psychopharm 45:177, 1975.

36. Gilliland, K and Bullock, W: Caffeine: A potential drug of abuse. Adv Alc Subst Abuse 3:53, 1984.

37. Lovingood, B, et al: Effects of d-amphetamine sulfate, caffeine and high temperature on human performance. Res Quart 38:64, 1965.

38. Koller, W, Lone, S and Herbster, L: Caffeine and tremor. Neurology 37:169, 1987.

39. U.S. Olympic Committee, Division of Sports Medicine and Science: Drug Education & Control Policy, 1988.

40. The 1988–89 NCAA Drug Testing Program Mission, Kansas, NCAA Publishing, 1988.

41. Stillner, V, et al: Caffeine-induced delirium during prolonged competitive stress. Am J Psychiatry 135:855, 1978.

42. Jokela, S and Vartianen, A: Caffeine poisoning. Acta Pharmacol Toxicol 15:331, 1959.

43. Alsott, RL, Miller, AJ and Forney, RB: Report of a human fatality due to caffeine. J Forensic Sci 18:135, 1973.

44. Wilson, MF, et al: Caffeine exaggerates hypertensive response to maximal exercise in normal young men at risk for hypertension. Circulation 76(S):0043, 1987.

45. Prineas, RJ, et al: Coffee, tea and VPB. J Chronic Dis 33:67, 1980.

46. Dobmeyer, DJ: The arrhythmogenic effects of caffeine in human beings. N Engl J Med 308:814, 1983.

47. Walker, WJ and Gregoratos, G: Myocardial infarction in young men. Am J Cardiol 19:339, 1967.

48. Hennekens, CH, et al: Coffee drinking and death due to coronary heart disease. N Engl J Med 294:633, 1976.

49. Rosenberg, L, et al: Coffee drinking and myocardial infarction in young women. Am J Epidemiol 111:675, 1980.

50. Dawber, TR, Kannel, WB and Gordon, T: Coffee and cardiovascular disease: Observations from the Framingham study. N Engl J Med 291:871, 1974.

51. Wilhelmsen, L, et al: Coffee consumption and coronary heart disease in middle-aged Swedish men. Acta Med Scand 201:547, 1977.

52. Pearson, TA: Heavy coffee drinkers risk heart trouble. Hopkins Med News 10:21, 1986.

CHAPTER 10

Barbiturates and Benzodiazepines

HISTORY

Chloral hydrate is perhaps the oldest hypnotic, having been introduced in 1869.[1] The capacity of bromides to depress the central nervous system was recognized in the mid-1800s, when Locock used them to treat epilepsy. The sedative capacity of bromide was sufficiently popular that a single London hospital used several tons annually.[2] Due to the toxic effect of bromide, the barbiturates replaced it as a sedative. Though barbituric acid was first prepared in 1864, it was not until 1903 that the first hypnotic barbiturate, barbital (Veronal) was introduced into clinical medicine.[3] In 1912 phenobarbital made its appearance, and since then over 2500 different barbiturates have been developed, though currently only about 12 are still used.

A number of nonbarbiturate hypnotics replaced most of the barbiturates on the erroneous assumption that these agents would not cause physical or psychic dependence.[1] These, in turn, were largely replaced by the benzodiazepines.

Compounds of the benzodiazepine type were initially synthesized in 1933,[4] but it was not until 1961 that they were introduced into clinical medicine.[5] The first benzodiazepine of clinical significance was chlordiazepoxide (Librium). Since then, more than 3000 benzodiazepines have been synthesized, and more than 25 are in clinical use around the world.[5]

Although originally believed to be effective alternatives to the barbiturates as sedatives and anxiolytic agents, serious public health concerns have been raised about the benzodiazepines. The use of these compounds as anxiolytics steadily increased through 1975, at which time 100 million new prescriptions were filled annually. Since 1981, new benzodiazepine prescriptions have leveled off to approximately 65 million per year.[6]

Twenty-five percent of patients who use benzodiazepines exceed the dose prescribed, use them for nonmedical reasons, or receive them from a nonmedical source.[7] Household survey data indicate that 11 to 13 percent of the United States adult population have taken an anxiolytic at least once in the past year, and approximately 2.5 percent have used anxiolytic agents on a daily basis for at least 4 months.[8] In 1987, 9.6 percent of high school seniors used nonprescription sedatives or tranquilizers at least once.[9] Nonmedical use of benzodiazepines doubled between 1980 and 1985.[10] Such startling statistics led to a 1988 New York State Department of Health recommendation that all benzodiazepines must be prescribed on official triplicate prescription forms, although its implementation has been delayed by court challenge.

CHEMISTRY AND PHYSIOLOGY

Barbiturates

The parent compound, barbituric acid, is 2,4,6-trioxohexahydropyrimidine (Fig. 10–1). Barbituric acid does not have central depressant activity, but this property is conferred by the presence of an alkyl or aryl group at position 5.[5] Barbiturates depress the activity of all excitable central nervous system activity, in particular the reticular activating and vestibular systems.[5,11-13] In all regions of the brain, barbiturates appear preferentially to suppress polysynaptic responses.[5,14] Although no specific barbiturate receptor site has been identified, the precise

molecular requirements for the depressant action suggest that specific receptor mechanisms may play an important role.[15]

Barbiturates appear to exert their central inhibitory effects in two ways:

1. Facilitate the effects of gamma-aminobutyric acid (GABA)—an inhibitory neurotransmitter—by opening chloride ion channels and thereby hyperpolarizing neuronal membranes[16]
2. Cortical suppression unrelated to GABA inhibition[5,16]

The main behavioral effects of barbiturates are sleepiness and decreased anxiety. Due to the general cortical suppressant effect of the barbiturates, the anxiolytic actions are usually associated with sedation.[5] Euphoria and occasionally paradoxical excitement may occur following barbiturate ingestion. Clouding of consciousness and decreased memory are common, especially following large doses.[3]

In animal studies, barbiturates are self-administered, suggesting a reinforcing effect of the drug.[17] Similarly, pentobarbital in humans has been demonstrated to possess a strong reinforcing effect, accounting for its abuse liability.[6] Physical dependence occurs following repeated use of barbiturates, and abrupt discontinuation of the drug may produce withdrawal reactions similar to alcohol withdrawal (see Chapter 11).[18]

In the peripheral nervous system, barbiturates depress autonomic ganglia transmission. In low doses, skeletal neuromuscular responses are augmented, but in high doses, barbiturates reduce the sensitivity of the postsynaptic membrane to the depolarizing effect of acetylcholine.[3] The general clinical effect is muscular relaxation.

Benzodiazepines

The term "benzodiazepine" refers to the 5-aryl-1,4-benzodiazepines.[5] Substitutions in this basic structure have accounted for the many compounds in this family of drugs (Fig. 10–2). Specific benzodiazepine receptors were discovered in 1977.[19,20] Autoradiographic techniques allowed the identification of brain regions that are targets for the benzodiazepines, many of which involve the "pleasure brain" (the mesocortical/mesolimbic system) as well as the substantia nigra,

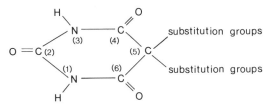

Figure 10–1. General structural formula of barbiturates.

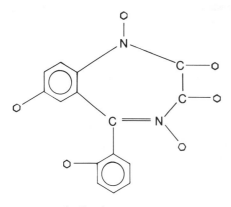

O = substitution groups

Figure 10–2. *General structural formula of benzodiazepines.*

the superior colliculus and the lateral lemniscus.[21] The identification of benzodiazepine receptors in the brain suggests a neuroanatomic-pharmacologic circuitry that mediates fear and anxiety responses.

Benzodiazepine receptors are coupled with gamma-aminobutyric acid (GABA) receptors at the molecular level. Evidence suggests that the benzodiazepines facilitate the synaptic actions of the inhibitory neurotransmitter GABA.[22] GABA is known to inhibit neuronal excitability by activating membrane chloride conductance. Benzodiazepines alone produce little effect on membrane chloride conductance, but in the presence of GABA markedly potentiate GABA-mediated responses.[23] Such selectivity distinguishes benzodiazepines from the barbiturates, which can directly activate chloride conductance to produce neuronal inhibition, thereby accounting in part for the greater toxicity of the barbiturates.[23]

Benzodiazepines act primarily as anxiolytic agents, although sedation and other barbiturate-like effects may occur through the activation of benzodiazepine-GABA pathways. Additionally, benzodiazepines release suppressed behaviors by regulating the firing of neurons which impact on inhibitions related to fear and punishment.[24] For example, a thirsty rat that is shocked when attempting to drink will avoid drinking. Under the influence of benzodiazepines, the rat will be better able to resist the shocks and will continue to drink.[23]

In general, the behavioral reinforcing effects of the benzodiazepines are less than for

the barbiturates. However, differences exist among the various types of benzodiazepines. Lorazepam (Ativan) and diazepam (Valium) produce greater reinforcing and euphoric subjective effects than oxazepam (Serax) and chlordiazepoxide (Librium), and this correlates with a greater abuse potential for lorazepam and diazepam.[23]

Tolerance to the behavioral effects of benzodiazepines develops following repeated use at therapeutic levels, thus resulting in an escalation of dosages. Abrupt discontinuation may cause a distinct withdrawal reaction indicative of the development of physical dependence. Withdrawal symptoms include agitation, depression, panic, delirium, tremors, muscle twitches, and frank convulsions.[25–29] Withdrawal severity and latency to onset appear to be related to the rate of elimination of the metabolically active drug; rapidly eliminated drugs tend to produce more intense withdrawal with a shorter latency from the time of drug discontinuation.[17] (See Table 10–2.)

CLINICAL PHARMACOLOGY

Barbiturates

Lipid solubility is a key determinant of the pharmacokinetics of the barbiturates.[16] Barbiturates with a high degree of lipid solubility are associated with shorter latencies, shorter durations of action, and greater degrees of hypnotic potencies.[5] Traditionally, barbiturates have been divided into four groups based on their duration of action: long-acting, intermediate-acting, short-acting, and ultra-short-acting[1] (Table 10–1). Barbiturates are readily absorbed orally. Those with a high degree of lipid solubility are primarily eliminated via metabolic breakdown products, and those which are more water soluble are predominantly excreted unchanged in the urine. It is important to note that none of the oral barbiturates available in the United States has a sufficiently short half-life to ensure complete elimination in 24 hours.[5] Consequently, accumulation will result from repetitive dosing.

Benzodiazepines

In recent years numerous benzodiazepines have been developed with differences in their pharmacodynamic spectra and phar-

Table 10–1. PHARMACOLOGY OF BARBITURATES

Drug	Trade Name	Street Name	Onset of Action	Half-Life	Average Oral Adult Daily Dose
Long-acting			60 min	80–120 hr	
Mephobarbital	Mebaral				96–400 mg
Metharbital	Gemonil				100–300 mg
Phenobarbital	Luminal	Purple hearts			30–120 mg
Intermediate-acting			45–60 min	8–42 hr	
Amobarbital	Amytal	Goof balls; downs; blue heavens			30–150 mg
Aprobarbital	Alurate				120 mg
Butabarbital	Butisol				45–120 mg
Talbutal	Lotusate				60–180 mg
Amobarbital/ Secobarbital	Tuinal	Tooies; rainbows; Christmas trees			50–200 mg
Short-acting			10–15 min	15–48 hr	
Pentobarbital	Nembutal	Yellow jackets			60–80 mg
Secobarbital	Seconal	Reds; red devils; red birds			90–200 mg
Ultra-short-acting					
Thiopental	Pentothal		10–20 sec	3 min	intravenous only

macokinetic properties. Although some benzodiazepines are marketed for insomnia and others for anxiety, any benzodiazepine can be used for either purpose,[30] and no sound scientific evidence validates the notion that one or another is primarily an anxiolytic or hypnotic drug. Differences among the benzodiazepines relate to the time of onset, in-tensity, and duration of action (Table 10–2). They are all lipid soluble and are essentially completely absorbed after oral administration.

Peak plasma concentrations of benzodiazepines are achieved in 30 minutes to 8 hours, depending on the specific drug. The benzodiazepines are extensively metabolized

Table 10–2. PHARMACOLOGY OF BENZODIAZEPINES

Drug	Trade Name	Onset of Action	Half-life	Active Metabolite(s) Half-life	Average Oral Adult Daily Dose
Long-acting					
Chlordiazepoxide	Librium	15–45 min	5–30 hr	5–200 hr	15–40 mg
Chlorazepate	Tranxene	30–60 min		5–200 hr	15–60 mg
Diazepam	Valium	15–45 min	20–70 hr	5–200 hr	4–40 mg
Flurazepam	Dalmane	15–45 min	2–3 hr	2–200 hr	15–30 mg
Halazepam	Paxipam	15–45 min	14 hr	30–200 hr	60–160 mg
Prazepam	Centrax	30–120 min		5–200 hr	20–60 mg
Intermediate-acting					
Alprazolam	Xanax	15–45 min	12–15 hr	12–15 hr	0.75–1.5 mg
Clonazepam	Klonopin	30–60 min	20–44 hr	none	1–4 mg
Short-acting					
Lorazepam	Ativan	15–45 min	10–20 hr	none	2–3 mg
Oxazepam	Serax	45–90 min	5–15 hr	none	30–60 mg
Temazepam	Restoril	25 min	9–12 hr	none	15–30 mg
Triazolam	Halcion	15–30 min	2–3 hr	none	0.25–0.5 mg

in the liver, and the total duration of action of an individual drug is often determined by the half-life of the biologically active metabolite (see Table 10–2).

Clinical Uses

The benzodiazepines have largely replaced the barbiturates as a class of sedative-hypnotics because of their greater specificity and safety. In addition to their use as anxiolytics, the benzodiazepines are used as muscle relaxants, anticonvulsants, and in conjunction with anesthesia. The barbiturates still play an important role in the management of seizure disorders, and they are useful diagnostically in certain psychiatric disorders.[31]

USE IN SPORTS

As with alcohol, barbiturates and benzodiazepines are not generally perceived as ergogenic drugs. However, in the 1984 Michigan State Study of college athletes,[32] 2 percent of responders used barbiturates and/or tranquilizers during the previous year: 28 percent for sports-related injuries, and 8 percent for performance enhancement. The nature of the hoped-for performance enhancement was not detailed. In the 1986 Elite Women Athletes Survey, 12 percent of professional athletes polled had used sedatives during the prior 12 months, and 3 percent of Olympic athletes had used these drugs during the similar time period.[33]

Effects on Performance

Some studies of relevance to the athlete indicate that barbiturates and benzodiazepines may be beneficial under limited circumstances. Both are useful in the control of tremor. Barbiturates have been extensively studied in this regard, and are an effective alternative to, and in some cases are superior to, propanolol in the treatment of essential tremor.[34–39] Similarly, benzodiazepines are effective in reducing tremor amplitude[39,40] and are particularly useful for individuals requiring only intermittent therapy,[40] which is the scenario for the athlete wishing to steady his hand for a particular event.

In one subgroup of athletes studied by Smith and Beecher,[41] weight throwers demonstrated significant improvement in maximum and mean distance achieved when given secobarbital, 50 mg per 70 kg, as opposed to when given a placebo. Maximum distance improved 2.44 percent, and mean distance improved 2.9 percent. This subgroup represented but one of many groups studied in the experiment and may therefore explain the above finding as statistically not valid. This is referred to as Type I error, meaning that chance alone may account for an apparently significant result if enough variables are simultaneously studied. However, the observation may have some validity. For example, Ritchie[42] has noted that the total amount of work accomplished by an individual under the influence of alcohol may increase secondary to a lessened appreciation of fatigue. Barbiturate use may be an analogous situation, and theoretically may confer "euphoric powers."[41,43]

Aside from the above mentioned benefit obtained in reducing tremor and perhaps in improving mood, other important aspects of performance of relevance to the athlete are impaired following barbiturate or benzodiazepine use. For example, Smith and Beecher[41] demonstrated significant performance impairment in swimmers who took secobarbital, 100 mg per 70 kg.

Other investigators have demonstrated a significant impairment in the psychomotor skills listed below following barbiturate intake:

1. Reaction time
2. Cognitive function and attention (digital subtraction and serial addition)
3. Visual tracking skills[44–47]

Visual tracking is especially impaired during movements which involve angular acceleration, probably secondary to inhibition of visual fixation, suppression of optikinetic nystagmus, and interference with smooth tracking.[14,48–50]

The literature on the effects of benzodiazepines on psychomotor performance is inconsistent and conflicting, at least in part because of individual drug sensitivity, dosing, tolerance, variables measured, and specific benzodiazepines used. For example, some have reported a significant deterioration in the following psychomotor tasks of relevance to the athlete:

1. Maximal rate at which subjects can finger tap[51–56]

2. Tracking skills: subjects indirectly manipulate an object with a joystick device[57−66]

3. Choice reaction time: subjects respond differentially and as quickly as possible to two stimuli presented in random order[59,67−72]

4. Sorting: subjects must sort objects according to some rule[73−75]

5. Divided attention: subjects monitor two stimuli simultaneously and respond differentially[72,76]

6. Reaction time: subjects press a key as quickly as possible in response to a stimulus[58,66,67,77−81]

On the other hand, others have reported tolerance to these detrimental effects. For example, following at least 6 days of repeated dosing, several authors have noted no decrement in psychomotor performance in normal subjects,[51,57,65,82] although tracking skills may remain impaired following daily doses of diazepam, 10 to 90 mg per day.[72,83,84]

In anxious patients, the acute effects of benzodiazepines on measures of psychomotor performance are not appreciably different from normal subjects.[85]

In insomniacs, some investigators have demonstrated deterioration in psychomotor skills the morning following bedtime benzodiazepine use,[86,87] whereas others have shown no change.[87,88] The deterioration observed appears to be related to total dose and duration of action of the drug.[87] Similarly, impairment of performance may be present for many hours after barbiturate ingestion. Airplane pilots tested for proficiency in simulated air missions were impaired for up to 22 hours after taking 200 mg of secobarbital.[89] Following repeated nighttime doses of benzodiazepines, however, most studies demonstrate no detrimental effect in performance skills the following morning.[85]

With the exception of the subgroup of weight throwers in Smith and Beecher's study,[41] no significant beneficial effect on strength or endurance following administration of barbiturates or benzodiazepines has been demonstrated.

Athletes may be susceptible to sedative-hypnotic drug abuse if they seek these drugs' potential calming effect in anticipation of the stress of athletic competition. Additionally, athletes using stimulants may use sedative-hypnotics to counteract the stimulants. For reasons which are not clear, the combination of amphetamines and barbiturates produces

mood elevations in excess of the effect of either drug alone.[90]

Other than the study by Smith and Beecher, the direct applicability to the athlete of the above mentioned detrimental and tolerance effects of sedatives and hypnotics has not been clearly demonstrated.

Case Vignette

A 24-year-old male tennis player sought professional help for benzodiazepine dependency. At the time of evaluation, he was taking 40 to 60 mg diazepam (Valium) per day and 60 mg flurazepam (Dalmane) at bedtime.

The patient always had difficulty falling asleep. During his college years, he frequently drank beer or took over-the-counter sedatives prior to sleeping, especially during examination weeks. On a few occasions he tried triazolam (Halcion), 0.25 mg, and he fell asleep easily and without hangover side effects.

After college, against his family's wishes, he turned down a business career in order to play the tennis circuit. The first 2 years were quite stressful because of financial difficulty and only moderate success in the satellite circuit. He became increasingly anxious and developed severe insomnia. He again obtained some triazolam and initially responded well to the nighttime hypnotic effects. After 2 to 3 months, he was taking triazolam daily and frequently awoke 3 to 4 hours after falling asleep. He began to double and sometimes triple his daily dose but still often awoke in the middle of the night.

A friend recommended trying flurazepam, and he easily obtained a 1-month supply. The first few weeks after beginning flurazepam, 30 mg, he slept much better. Soon, however, he awoke feeling somewhat drowsy and felt less alert during the day. Although initially the fatigue interfered with his daily activities, he soon became tolerant to the sedative effects and noticed that he generally felt calmer during the day.

Approximately 4 months after beginning flurazepam, his nighttime dose was 60 mg, and he often felt anxious and somewhat irritable in the afternoon. Again a friend had some pharmacologic advice, and he began to take diazepam, 5 mg, for his daytime anxiety. The anxiolytic effects of diazepam were not associated with any perceived adverse sedative effects, and within months the daily dose escalated to 40 to 60 mg. When the patient's supply of benzodiazepines diminished, he began seeing different physicians who were willing to give him a 2- to 3-week supply of diazepam and flurazepam. When one physician became suspicious and confronted him, the patient agreed to seek professional help for his benzodiazepine dependency.

ADVERSE EFFECTS

Side effects of barbiturates and benzodiazepines are listed in Table 10–3. Acute side effects such as drowsiness, ataxia, blurred vision, and decreased attention span may occur, especially in drug-naive individuals or with rapid dose escalation. Impaired memory is especially prominent in the elderly[30] following benzodiazepine use. Euphoria sometimes occurs and may be related to rapid absorption, which may explain, in part, the widespread abuse of diazepam.[30]

Cumulative sedation may result with those drugs that have a long duration of action. In this regard, many of the benzodiazepines have metabolites which are biologically active for days (see Table 10–2). Physiologic drug dependence may occur, and tolerance usually develops, leading to an escalation of dosage.[25–29]

Rebound anxiety and insomnia may result from abrupt discontinuation of sedatives and hypnotics.[30] Similarly, withdrawal symptoms and signs following abrupt drug discontinuation may develop; therefore, gradual tapering to achieve abstinence is recommended.[26]

Respiratory depression and coma occur more frequently following large doses of barbiturates, but both benzodiazepines and barbiturates in large enough doses may cause profound central nervous system and respiratory depression, coma, and even death. Benzodiazepines are the drugs most commonly used in suicide attempts.[91]

FINAL NOTE

Anecdotal evidence suggests that, in general, benzodiazepines and barbiturates are not abused as ergogenic aids, although in sporting events where hand steadiness is important, such as riflery and archery, the ergogenic abuse potential is high. It makes sense, then, that drug testing for barbiturates and benzodiazepines to prevent erogenic drug use should be limited to such sports. The results from the subgroup of weight throwers in Smith and Beecher's study,[41] however, is intriguing, and a follow-up study to address this particular issue is warranted.

Whether or not athletes are more susceptible to sedative and hypnotic abuse outside of direct training time and competition is not known. Athletes are at least as susceptible as the population at large, and for this reason more epidemiologic data regarding barbiturate and benzodiazepine use among athletes should be obtained and coupled with educational programs warning of the abuse potential of these drugs.

Table 10–3. SIDE EFFECTS OF BARBITURATES AND BENZODIAZEPINES

Sedation
Blurred vision
Decreased attention
Impaired gait/balance
Impaired memory
Euphoria
Rebound insomnia
Dependence
Tolerance
Clinical withdrawal
Respiratory depression
Stupor/coma

REFERENCES

1. Davis, JM: Minor tranquilizers, sedatives and hypnotics. In Kaplan, HI and Sadock, BJ (eds): Comprehensive Textbook of Psychiatry/IV, ed 4. Williams & Wilkins, Baltimore, 1985, p 1537.
2. Sharpless, SK: Hypnotics and sedatives. II. miscellaneous agents. In Goodman, LS and Gilman, A (eds). The Pharmacological Basis of Therapeutics, ed 4. Macmillan, New York, 1970, p 121.
3. Sharpless, SK: Hypnotics and sedatives: I. The barbiturates. In Goodman, LS and Gilman, A (eds): The Pharmacological Basis of Therapeutics, ed 4. Macmillan, New York, 1970, p 98.
4. Jarvik, ME: Drugs used in the treatment of psychiatric disorders. In Goodman, LS and Gilman, A (eds): The Pharmacological Basis of Therapeutics, ed 4. Macmillan, New York, 1970, p 339.

5. Harvey, SC: Hypnotics and sedatives. In Gilman, AG, et al (eds): Goodman and Gilman's The Pharmacological Basis of Therapeutics, ed 7. Macmillan, New York, 1985, p 339.

6. Griffiths, RR and Sannerud, CA: Abuse of and dependence on benzodiazepines and other anxiolytic/sedative drugs. In Meltzer, Hy (ed): Psychopharmacology: The Third Generation. Raven Press, New York, 1987, p 1535.

7. Frank, B: Testimony before the New York Public Health Council, November 14, 1986.

8. Mellinger, GD, Balter, MB and Uhlenhuth, EH: Prevalence and correlates of the long-term regular use of anxiolytics. JAMA 251:375, 1984.

9. Johnston, L and Bachman, J: The Monitoring the Future Study. Institute for Social Research. The University of Michigan, Ann Arbor, 1988.

10. National Institute on Drug Abuse. 1985 National Household Survey on Drug Abuse. DHHS Pub No (ADM) 87-1539, 1987.

11. Rashbass, C and Russell, G: Action of barbiturate drug (amylbarbitone sodium) on the vestibulo-ocular reflex. Brain 84:329, 1961.

12. Cucchiara, R and Michenfelder, J: The effect of interruption of the reticular activating system in metabolism in canine cerebral hemispheres before and after thiopental. Anesthesiology 39:3, 1973.

13. Killam, E: Drug action on the brain-stem reticular formation. Pharmacol Rev 14:175, 1962.

14. Weakly, J: Effect of barbiturates on "quantal" synaptic transmission in spinal motorneurones. J Physiol Lond 204:63, 1969.

15. Nicoll, R: Selective actions of barbiturates on synaptic transmission. In Lipton, MA, DiMascio, A and Killam, KF (eds): Psychopharmacology: A Generation of Progress. Raven Press, New York, 1978, p 1337.

16. American Medical Association Department of Drugs, Division of Drugs and Technology: Drugs used for anxiety and sleep disorders. In AMA Drug Evaluations, ed 6. WB Saunders, Philadelphia, 1986, p 81.

17. Griffiths, RR, et al: Relative abuse liability of triazolam: Experimental assessment in animals and humans. Neurosci Biobehav Rev 8:133, 1985.

18. Essig, CF: Nonnarcotic addiction. Newer sedative drugs that can cause states of intoxication and dependence of barbiturate type. JAMA 196:714, 1966.

19. Mohler, H and Okada, T: Demonstration of benzodiazepine receptors in the central nervous system. Science 198:849, 1977.

20. Barnett, A, Iorio, L and Billard, W: Novel receptor specificity of selected benzodiazepines. Clin Neuropharm 8:S8, 1985.

21. Young, WS and Kuhar, JJ: Autoradiographic localisation of benzodiazepine receptors in the brains of humans and animals. Nature 280:393, 1979.

22. Snyder, SH: Basic science of psychopharmacology. In Kaplan, HI and Sadock, BJ (eds): Comprehensive Textbook of Psychiatry/IV, ed 4. Williams & Wilkins, Baltimore, 1985, p 42.

23. Hammer, DW, Skolnick, P and Paul, SM: The benzodiazepine/GABA receptor complex and anxiety. In Meltzer, H (ed): Psychopharmacology: The Third Generation. Raven Press, New York, 1987, p 977.

24. Cook, L and Sepinwass, J: Behavioral analysis of the effects and mechanisms of action of benzodiazepines. In Costa, E and Greengard, P (eds): Mechanism of Action of Benzodiazepine. Raven Press, New York, 1975.

25. Lader, M: Benzodiazepines—the opium of the masses? Neuroscience 3:159, 1978.

26. Busto, U, et al: Withdrawal reaction after long-term therapeutic use of benzodiazepines. N Engl J Med 315:854, 1986.

27. Busto, U, et al: Patterns of benzodiazepine abuse and dependence. Br J Addict 81:87, 1986.

28. Owens, R and Tyrer, P: Benzodiazepine dependence: A review of the evidence. Drugs 25:385, 1983.

29. Khantzian, EJ: Acute toxic withdrawal reactions associated with drug use and abuse. Ann Intern Med 90:361, 1979.

30. Choice of benzodiazepines. The Medical Letter 30:26, 1988.

31. Perry, J and Jacobs, D: Overview: Clinical applications of the amytal interview in psychiatric emergency settings. Am J Psychiatry 139:552, 1982.

32. Anderson, WA and McKeag, DB: The Substance Use and Abuse Habits of College Student-Athletes. Presented to National Collegiate Athletic Association Council. College of Human Medicine, Michigan State University, June, 1985.

33. Elite Women Athletes Survey. Hazelden Health Promotion Services, Minneapolis, January, 1987.

34. Findley, LJ and Calzetti, S: Double-blind controlled study of primidone in essential tremor: Preliminary results. Br Med J 2:608, 1982.

35. Baruzzi, A, et al: Phenobarbital and propanolol in essential tremor: A double-blind controlled clinical trial. Neurology 33:296, 1983.

36. Findley, LJ and Cleeves, L: Phenobarbitone in essential tremor. Neurology 35:1784, 1985.

37. Koller, WL and Royce, VL: Efficacy of primidone in essential tremor. Neurology 36:121, 1986.

38. Koller, W, Biny, N and Cone, S: Disability in essential tremor: Effect of treatment. Neurology 36:1001, 1986.

39. Findley, LJ and Koller, WC: Essential tremor: A review. Neurology 37:1194, 1987.

40. Huber, SJ and Paulson, GW: Efficacy of alprazolam for essential tremor. Neurology 38:241, 1988.

41. Smith, GM and Beecher, HK: Amphetamine sulfate and athletic performance: I. Objective effects. JAMA 197:542, 1959.

42. Ritchie, JM: The aliphatic alcohols. In Gilman, AG, et al (eds): Goodman and Gilman's The Pharmacological Basis of Therapeutics, ed 7. Macmillan, New York, 1985, p 377.

43. Smith, LM and Beecher, HK: Amphetamine, secobarbital and athletic performance: II. Subjective evaluations of performance, mood states, and physical stress. JAMA 172:1502, 1960.

44. Blum, B and Stern, M: A comparative evaluation of the action of depressant and stimulant drugs on human performance. Psychopharm 6:173, 1964.

45. Schroeder, D and Collins, W: Effects of secobarbital and d-amphetamine on tracking performance during angular acceleration. Ergonomics 17:613, 1974.

46. Talland, G and Quarton, G: Methamphetamine and phenobarbital effects on human motor performance. Psychopharm 8:241, 1965.

47. Truijens, C, Trumbo, D and Wagenaar, W: Amphetamine and barbiturate effects on two tasks per-

formed singly and in combination. Acta Psychol 40:233, 1976.

48. Bender, M and O'Brien, F: The influence of barbiturate on various forms of nystagmus. Am J Ophthalmol 29:1541, 1946.

49. Bergman, P, Nathanson, M and Bender, M: Electrical recordings of normal and abnormal eye movements modified by drugs. Arch Neurol Psychiat 67:357, 1952.

50. Norris, H: The time course of barbiturate action in man investigated by measurement of smooth tracking eye movement. Br J Chemother 33:117, 1968.

51. Lader, MH, Curry, S and Baker, WJ: Physiological and psychological effects of clorazepate in man. Br J Clin Pharmacol 9:83, 1980.

52. Ghoneim, MM, Mewaldt, SP and Hinrichs, JV: Memory and performance effects of single and three week administration of diazepam. Psychopharmacology 73:147, 1981.

53. Ghoneim, MM, Mewaldt, SP and Thatcher, JW: The effect of diazepam and fentanyl on mental, psychomotor, and electroencephalographic functions and their rate of recovery. Psychopharm 44:61, 1975.

54. Golombok, S and Lader M: The psychopharmacological effects of premazepam, diazepam, and placebo in healthy human subjects. Br J Clin Pharmacol 18:127, 1984.

55. Korttila, K, et al: Evaluation of instrumental force platform as a test to measure residual effects of anesthetics. Anesthesiology 55:625, 1981.

56. Uhlenhuth, EH, et al: Diazepam: Efficacy and toxicity as revealed by a small sample research strategy. In Sudilovsky, A, Gershon, S and Beer, B (eds): Predictability in Psychopharmacology: Preclinical and Clinical Correlations, Raven Press, New York, 1975, p 105.

57. Aranko, K, Mattila, MJ and Bordignon, D: Psychomotor effects of alprazolam and diazepam during acute and subacute treatment, and during the follow-up phase. Acta Pharmacol Toxicol 56:364, 1985.

58. Borland, RG and Nicolson, AN: Immediate effects on human performance of a 1,5-benzodiazepine (clobazam) compared with the 1,4-benzodiazepines, chlordiazepoxide hydrochloride and diazepam. Br J Clin Pharmacol 2:215, 1974.

59. Clarke, CH and Nicholson, AN: Immediate and residual effects of human performance of the hydrozylated metabolites of diazepam. Br J Clin Pharmacol 4:400, 1977.

60. Clarke, CH and Nicholson, AN: Immediate and residual effects in man of the metabolites of diazepam. Br J Clin Pharmacol 6:325, 1978.

61. Ellinwood, EH, Linnoila, M and Easler, ME: Onset of peak impairment after diazepam and after alcohol. Clin Pharmacol Ther 30:534, 1981.

62. Ellinwood, EH, et al: Profile of acute tolerance to three sedative anxiolytics. Psychopharmacology 79:137, 1983.

63. Haffner, JF, et al: Mental and psychomotor effects of diazepam and ethanol. Acta Pharmacol Toxicol 32:161, 1973.

64. Liljequist, R and Mattila, MJ: Acute effects of temazepam and nitrazepam on psychomotor skills and memory. Acta Pharmacol Toxicol 44:364, 1979.

65. Saario, I: Effect of hypnotics or psychotropic drugs and alcohol on psychomotor skills. Psychiatr Fenn 8:131, 1977.

66. Turner, P: Clinical pharmacological studies on lorazepam. Curr Med Res Med Opinion 1:262, 1973.

67. Berchou, R and Block, RI: Use of computerized psychomotor testing in determining CNS effects of drugs. Percept Mot Skills 57:691, 1983.

68. Hindmarch, I: Some aspect of the effects of clobazam on human psychomotor performance. Br J Clin Pharmacol 7:772, 1979.

69. Linnoila, M and Mattila, MJ: Drug interaction on driving skills as evaluated by laboratory tests and by a driving simulator. Pharmakopsychiatr Neuro-Psychopharmakol 6:127, 1973.

70. Kielholz, P, et al: Driving tests to determine the impairment of driving ability by alcohol, tranquilizers, and hypnotics. Foreign Psychiatry 1:150, 1972.

71. Moser, L, et al: Effects of terfenadine and diphenhydramine alone or in combination with diazepam or alcohol on psychomotor performance and subjective feelings. Eur J Clin Pharmacol 14:417, 1978.

72. Palva, ES, et al: Acute and subacute effects of diazepam on psychomotor skills: Interaction with alcohol. Acta Pharmacol Toxicol 45:257, 1979.

73. Baktir, G, et al: Triazolam concentration-effect relationships in healthy subjects. Clin Pharmacol Ther 34:195, 1983.

74. Malpas, A: Subjective and objective effects of nitrazepam and amylobarbitone sodium in normal human beings. Psychopharmacologia 27:373, 1972.

75. Malpas, A and Joyce, CRB: Effects of nitrazepam, amylobarbitone, and placebo on some perceptual, motor, and cognitive tasks in normal subjects. Psychopharmacologia 14:167, 1969.

76. Moskowitz, H: Attention tasks as skills performance measures of drug effects. Br J Clin Pharmacol 18:51S, 1984.

77. Bond, AJ and Lader, MH: Comparative effects of diazepam and buspirone on subjective feelings, psychological tests and the eeg. Int Pharmacopsychiatry 16:212, 1981.

78. File, SE and Lister, RG: A comparison of the effects of lorazepam with those of propranolol on experimentally-induced anxiety and performance. Br J Clin Pharmacol 19:445, 1985.

79. Kroboth, PD, et al: The effect of four benzodiazepines on psychomotor performance. Drug Intell Clin Pharm 18:502, 1984.

80. Hedges, A, Turner, P and Harry, TVA: Preliminary studies on the central effects of lorazepam, a new benzodiazepine. J Clin Pharmacol 11:423, 1971.

81. Tallone, G, et al: Reaction time to acoustic or visual stimuli after administration of camazepam and diazepam in man. Arzneim Forsch 30:1021, 1980.

82. Subhan, Z, Harrison, C and Hindmarch, I: Alprazolam and lorazepam single and multiple-dose effects on psychomotor skills and sleep. Eur J Clin Pharmacol 29:709, 1986.

83. Liljequist, R, Linnoila, M and Mattila, MJ: Effect of diazepam and chlorpromazine on memory functions in man. Eur J Clin Pharmacol 13:339, 1978.

84. Linnola, M, et al: Effect of treatment with diazepam or lithium and alcohol on psychomotor skills related to driving. Eur J Clin Pharmacol 7:337, 1974.

85. Woods, JH, Katz, JL and Winger, L: Abuse liability of benzodiazepines. Pharmacol Rev 39:251, 1987.

86. Hindmarch, I: Effects of hypnotic and sleep-inducing drugs on objective assessments of human psychomotor performance and subjective appraisals of sleep and early morning behavior. Br J Clin Pharmacol 8:43S, 1979.

87. Peck, AW, Bye, CE and Claridge, R: Differences between light and sound sleepers in the residual effects of nitrazepam. Br J Clin Pharmacol 4:101, 1977.

88. Hauri, P, et al: Sleep laboratory and performance evaluation of midazolam in insomniacs. Br J Clin Pharmacol 16:109S, 1983.

89. McKenzie, R and Elliot, L: Effects of secobarbital with d-amphetamine on performance during a simulated air mission. Aerospace Med 36:774, 1965.

90. Jaffe, JH: Drug addiction and drug abuse. In Gilman, AG, et al (eds): Goodman and Gilman's The Pharmacological Basis of Therapeutics, ed 7. MacMillan, New York, 1985, p 532.

91. Prescribing Benzodiazepines: New Regulations. New York State Department of Health, February, 1988.

CHAPTER 11

Alcohol

HISTORY

And Noah began to be a husband, and he
planted a vineyard:
And he drank of the wine, and was drunken
and he was uncovered within his tent
                                    Genesis 9:20–21[1]

Wine has a "cultural lineage" which parallels that of recorded history.[2] According to Stepto,[3] the Bible cites alcohol's virtues and curses 165 times. Every civilization has had its wine "miracle story." The Hebrews referred to wine as the "foremost medicine"; St. Paul advised Timothy, "Drink no longer water, but use a little wine for thy stomach's sake and thine often infirmities."[4]

It was not until approximately 800 A.D., in Arabia, that the process of distillation was discovered. The word alcohol is derived from the Arabic word *alkuhl* (meaning "essence").[5]

Throughout recorded history, alcohol has been used as a food, as a medicine, as a solvent for therapeutic agents, and as an important element in religious and social life.[2] However, also documented throughout history are the multitude of problems attendant to the excesses of alcohol.

In the United States, approximately 10 million adults (7 percent of the adult population) and 3.3 million youths have alcohol-related problems. As many as 40 million Americans are directly or indirectly affected by alcoholism. Alcohol-related problems account for 12 percent of the nation's total expenditure for health, with direct treatment costs approximating 13.5 billion dollars each year, and total costs, including lost productivity, approximating 117 billion dollars per year. In 1986, there were more than 1.2 million admissions for the treatment of alcoholism, and more than 72 percent were to non-hospital treatment units.[6,6a,6b,7]

Alcohol is a factor in approximately one-half of the 51,000 motor vehicle fatalities per year and plays a role in the 750,000 serious injuries per year from motor vehicle accidents. In total, alcohol abuse accounts for approximately 98,000 deaths annually. In 1 year, the average American consumes over 2 gallons of hard liquor, over 28 gallons of beer, and over 2 gallons of wine.[8] Drinking problems start at a young age: in 1985, nearly 100,000 children 10 and 11 years old reported getting drunk at least once per week. Alcohol is the number one substance of abuse by teenagers.[9]

Despite these alarming statistics, current evidence suggests that drinking patterns are not changing. The University of Michigan drug survey of American high school seniors, college students, and young adults in 1987 found that alcohol use had not changed over a 3-year period. Ninety-two percent of high school seniors have used alcohol, and 66 percent had used it in the 30 days prior to the survey. Five percent of high school seniors are daily drinkers, and 37.5 percent had drunk heavily (more than 5 drinks in a row) in the 2 weeks prior to the survey.[10]

Alcohol has the unique distinction of being the only potent drug in which self-induced intoxication is widely accepted, both legally and socially.

CHEMISTRY AND PHYSIOLOGY

Alcohol (ethanol) is a simple two-carbon structure $-CH_3CH_2OH$ (Fig. 11–1). The central nervous system is the primary target for the clinical manifestations of alcohol ingestion. Like other general anesthetics, ethanol is a general central nervous system depressant.[11] Although no known receptor exists for ethanol, specific regions of the central nervous system appear to show selective sensitivity to ethanol since ethanol is more effective in inhibiting synaptic function rather than impulse propagation.[12-14] The polysynaptic structures in the reticular activating system and certain cortical structures are particularly susceptible and account for the central nervous system excitation that is seen with low doses of ethanol.[15] Although the exact mechanisms of action of ethanol are not un-

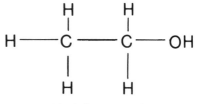

Figure 11–1. Structure of ethanol.

derstood, ethanol has been shown to increase membrane fluidity, and this action correlates well with the known pharmacologic actions of ethanol.[14] In addition, there is evidence that ethanol can cause the following neuronal changes:

1. Reduction of sodium current underlying the action potential[16]
2. Alteration of resting permeability and active transport
3. Stimulation of neurotransmitter release
4. Alteration of postsynaptic excitatory current[17]

Central nervous system effects of alcohol are, in general, proportional to the blood concentration, although not invariably (Table 11–1). Effects correlate better with rapid rises in blood concentration. Acute tolerance may develop, even in naive subjects, secondary to central nervous system adaptation as opposed to altered metabolism.[18]

Chronic alcohol ingestion leads to tolerance and physical dependence, the mechanisms of which are not completely understood. Tolerance appears to be mediated by brain noradrenergic and serotonergic systems. Blockade of either system delays the development of tolerance, and destruction of both completely blocks the development of tolerance.[14] On the other hand, continued exposure to the neuropeptide vasopressin may maintain tolerance despite discontinuation of ethanol exposure.[14]

Dependence may be related to specific receptor changes in the brain. Muscarinic cholinergic receptors increase in the cerebral cortex and hippocampus after prolonged exposure to ethanol and return to normal after the resolution of alcohol withdrawal. The noradrenergic system also appears to play a critical role in the development of dependence.[14]

The metabolite of ethanol, acetaldehyde, may produce toxicity by utilizing nicotin-

Table 11–1. CLINICAL EFFECTS AND BLOOD LEVELS IN ACUTE ALCOHOLISM

Symptoms	Blood Level (mg/dl)
Euphoria, giddiness, verbosity Long reaction time, impaired mental status examination Mild incoordination, nystagmus Hypalgesia to noxious stimuli	25–100
Boisterousness, withdrawal, easily confused Conjunctival hyperemia Ataxia, nystagmus, dysarthria Pronounced hypalgesia	100–200
Nausea, vomiting, drowsiness Diplopia; wide, sluggish pupils Marked ataxia and clumsiness	200–300
Hypothermia, cold sweat, amnesic stupor Severe dysarthria or anarthria Anesthesia Stertor, hypoventilation Coma	>300

From Plum and Posner: The Diagnosis of Stupor and Coma, ed 3. FA Davis, Philadelphia, 1982, p 247, with permission.

Table 11–2. APPROXIMATE BLOOD ALCOHOL CONTENT PER DRINK

Drink	mg per dl
12 oz beer	20 (0.02%)
3 oz wine	20 (0.02%)
1 oz hard liquor (whiskey, vodka)	20 (0.02%)
3.5 oz Martini/Manhattan	40 (0.04%)
4 oz Daiquiri	30 (0.03%)
8 oz Highball	30 (0.03%)

amide adenine dinucleotide (NAD), leading to an increase in the reduced form of nicotinamide adenine dinucleotide (NADH). This, in turn, results in an increased production of lactate and fatty acids and a decrease in the hepatic citric acid cycle metabolism.[19]

Acetaldehyde may link with catecholamine to form tetrahydroisoquinolines, which share an effect in common with opiates on the brain.[20] This action may account for the partial reversal of alcoholic coma by naloxone.[21]

Systemically, alcohol may increase the heart rate without affecting other cardiopulmonary functions. Increased sweating and heat loss occur secondary to enhancement of cutaneous blood flow.

CLINICAL PHARMACOLOGY

Ethanol is rapidly absorbed from the gastrointestinal tract into the circulation. It is widely distributed to all organs and fluid compartments and readily crosses the blood-brain barrier.[19] More than 90 percent is completely oxidized to acetaldehyde, with the remainder being excreted unchanged in the urine. The metabolism of alcohol is little affected by absolute blood levels. Rather, the rate of oxidation is constant with time.[19]

On an empty stomach, peak blood levels may be reached within 45 minutes, although complete absorption may range from 2 to 6 hours in the presence of food or large amounts of alcohol. In nonalcoholics, impairment of sensory perception, cognitive functions, and motor coordination occur with ethanol concentrations of 31 to 65 mg per deciliter (dl).[22] Intoxication occurs with blood concentrations of 50 to 150 mg per dl, and lethargy and coma occur with concentrations greater than 200 mg per dl (see Table 11–1). Legally, intoxication is defined as a blood ethanol concentration greater than 100 mg per dl (0.1%).

On the average, "one drink" (1 ounce of 50 percent hard liquor, 12 ounces of 4 percent beer, or 3 ounces of wine) will result in a maximum blood concentration of 20 mg per dl (Table 11–2). Blood ethanol levels decline at an average rate of 10 to 20 mg per dl per hour.[23] However, blood alcohol levels are considerably influenced by the individual's body weight (Table 11–3).

Clinical Uses

Modern pharmacology has greatly restricted the clinical uses of alcohol. The agent acts as a solvent for the delivery of many drugs. Dehydrated alcohol is useful as a ganglionic blocker for pain relief in disorders

Table 11–3. ESTIMATED PERCENTAGE OF ALCOHOL IN THE BLOOD BY
NUMBER OF DRINKS IN RELATION TO BODY WEIGHT

| Number of Drinks*—Percentage of Blood-Alcohol | | | | | | | | | | | |
| | | | | | | | | | | | |

Body Wt	1	2	3	4	5	6	7	8	9	10	11	12
100 lb	.038	.075	.113	.150	.188	.225	.263	.300	.338	.375	.413	.450
120 lb	.031	.063	.094	.125	.156	.188	.219	.250	.281	.313	.344	.375
140 lb	.027	.054	.080	.107	.134	.161	.188	.214	.241	.268	.295	.321
160 lb	.023	.047	.070	.094	.117	.141	.164	.188	.211	.234	.258	.281
180 lb	.021	.042	.063	.083	.104	.125	.146	.167	.188	.208	.229	.250
200 lb	.019	.038	.056	.075	.094	.113	.131	.150	.169	.188	.206	.225
220 lb	.017	.034	.051	.068	.085	.102	.119	.136	.153	.170	.188	.205
240 lb	.016	.031	.047	.063	.078	.094	.109	.125	.141	.156	.172	.188

*Percent of blood alcohol can be estimated by counting the number of drinks (1 drink = 1 oz 100 proof whiskey, or one 12-oz beer).

Under Number of Drinks and opposite Body Weight, find the percentage of blood-alcohol listed on the chart above. Subtract from this number the average percentage of alcohol "burned up" (.015% per hour) since first drink.

Example: 100 lb person has 4 drinks in 3 hours
.150% minus .045% = .105%
Presumed "Under the influence."

From Epidemic! Kids, Drugs and Alcohol. The Robert Crown Center for Health Education, Hinsdale, Illinois, with permission.

such as trigeminal neuralgia. Alcohol is often used as a "home remedy" for viral syndromes, but its therapeutic value lies in causing drowsiness and encouraging bed rest.[19]

USE IN SPORTS

The athlete has not been immune to the excesses of alcohol and in some ways may be particularly vulnerable. The 1984 Michigan State study[24] of athletes in Division I, II, and III colleges revealed that 88 percent of the 2,039 respondents used alcohol within the prior 12 months, compared with 36 percent who used marijuana or hashish. Twenty-seven percent of those using alcohol had 3 to 5 drinks 2 to 5 times per week, while 23 percent had 6 to 9 drinks at least 2 to 5 times per week. Of those athletes using alcohol, 24 percent indicated they did so in junior high school or before.

In the 1986 Elite Women Athletes Survey, 91 percent of respondents had used alcohol during the prior 12 months, and 76 percent during the 30 days prior to the survey. Twelve percent of respondents reported drinking 5 or more drinks in a row in the prior 2 weeks. Seven percent of respondents used alcohol either before or during competition.[25]

Data are not readily available regarding the incidence of alcohol use and abuse among male professional athletes. Despite the implementation of substance abuse guidelines within many of the professional sports organizations, alcohol has generally not been addressed as a drug of abuse, and professional sports teams rarely test for alcohol abuse. For example, although many feel that the National Basketball Association has the most highly regarded drug abuse program, no provisions are made for alcohol. It was not until 1982 that the National Football League identified alcohol as a drug, but they have since provided treatment options for players with alcohol-related problems.[26] Alcohol is a legal, readily available, and socially acceptable drug, making it difficult to implement strict policy guidelines. A general sense of alcohol abuse denial often exists among players, coaches, and fans, and when a player develops an alcohol-related problem, the incident may be viewed with shock by the fans and coaches.[27]

Attitudes may be changing. In a 14-month period, seven Minnesota Vikings players were charged with driving while intoxicated, which led to a series of mandatory lectures for the players on drinking and driving.[28] Some of the professional football and baseball teams no longer serve alcohol in the clubhouse or on the team airplane. These are small but important steps which reflect attitudinal changes that will hopefully lead to obtaining epidemiologic data and a better understanding of alcohol use among athletes.

Effects on Performance

With regard to acute alcohol ingestion and athletic performance, alcohol is generally not perceived as an ergogenic drug. Studies consistently show significant deterioration in several aspects of psychomotor skills in subjects under the influence of alcohol. Performance decrements correlate with blood alcohol levels. In most subjects, psychomotor impairment begins with blood alcohol levels greater than 35 mg per 100 ml.[29] The following skills are impaired in subjects under the influence of alcohol:

1. Balance and steadiness[30-32]
2. Reaction time[32-36]
3. Fine and complex motor coordination[29,31,33,37,38]
4. Visual tracking[34,38]
5. Information processing[31,37,39,40]

Of note is that static tracking and coordination skills are impaired less than similar tasks performed while the subject is moving.[38]

Amphetamines, taken in combination with alcohol, will lessen the impairment seen in some cognitive tasks, but do not affect the alcohol-induced impairment in balance, reaction time, fine motor coordination, or tracking skills.[41]

Following alcohol administration, a decrease in anaerobic strength tasks may occur,[42-44] although this is not a consistent observation.[33] Endurance, as shown by aerobic capacity, maximum oxygen uptake, and oxygen consumption, is unaffected by alcohol administration.[45-48]

The athlete, especially under the stress of training and performance, may be particularly vulnerable to the after-hours, and perhaps even to the precompetition, calming effects of alcohol.[49] In this regard, a study of the effects of alcohol on airplane pilots is enlightening:[50] pilots were tested under control and hangover conditions in a flight simulator. They performed significantly worse in tasks requiring attention and visual-motor coordination skills 14 hours after ingesting enough alcohol to obtain a blood level between 100 and 125 mg per dl. The study purposefully imitated a typical evening cocktail party in healthy social-drinking pilots, and the findings suggest that the social use of alcohol the evening prior to an athletic event may be detrimental to performance.

Alcohol does not produce a similar deterioration in psychomotor skills among all subjects, and some subjects may perform consistently better following alcohol ingestion.[33] Some authors have even suggested that a finely titrated dose of alcohol may be performance enhancing. In 1892, Kraeplin observed that low doses of alcohol may facilitate short-term memory,[51] an effect which may be secondary to initial cortical excitation due to blockade of norepinephrine reuptake. In a standard textbook of pharmacology, it is stated that the total amount of work accomplished by an individual under the influence of small doses of alcohol may increase secondary to a lessened appreciation of fatigue.[19]

Low-dose alcohol may also have anxiolytic effects which could hypothetically improve athletic performance. Furthermore, Koller and Biary found that alcohol may be better than propranolol in controlling postural essential tremor.[52] In this regard, alcohol use is banned in riflery by the National Collegiate Athletic Association. Breath or blood levels of alcohol may be determined at the request of an individual International Federation for athletes participating in Olympic competition.

The notion that alcohol ingestion consistently can be correlated with impaired performance was similarly challenged by Clark and associates.[53] Studying medical students, they found that 18 percent met the Research Diagnostic Criteria definition of alcohol abusers. On the average, the alcohol-abusing students had better first-year grades and better overall scores than the non–alcohol-abusing students on the National Board of Medical Examiners examination, part I. Their findings were challenged on the basis of improperly defining alcohol abusers.[54] In response, Clark pointed out the fact that he had used a standard textbook definition of alcohol abuse.[55] Challenging physicians to recognize that early alcohol abuse is not necessarily associated with poor performance,

Clark elegantly stated: "It would be foolish to believe that alcohol abuse always translated immediately and directly into intellectual and work impairment. This stereotype about alcoholics, as we emphasize in our article, tends to encourage denial of the prevalence of alcoholism among the professionally competent and gifted, to no one's advantage."[55]

Case Vignette

A 28-year-old male hockey player was brought to the emergency room following a motor vehicle accident. He had been with friends earlier that evening and had drunk several gin and tonics. While driving home, he lost control of the car and hit a tree. He transiently lost consciousness but suffered no other immediate neurological or medical complications.

The patient was observed overnight and was to be discharged in the morning, but he became tremulous and irritable, and an astute house officer placed the patient under one-on-one supervision for impending alcohol withdrawal. He was treated with escalating doses of benzodiazepines as he developed alcoholic hallucinosis. He did not have a seizure, nor did he develop delirium tremens. When he cleared medically, he was transferred to the psychiatric ward at the request of the family and patient.

Further family and social history revealed that the patient's father died of alcoholic cirrhosis and that his sister had a "drinking problem." Two prior marriages ended in divorce. The patient remembers becoming drunk once or twice per week while in high school, and more often in college. Even during the hockey season, he usually drank several beers after practice and still went on drinking binges from time to time. Aside from sometimes feeling hung over, he does not think that alcohol use interfered with his hockey performance.

After a short professional hockey career, he started his own business. Drinking now became more of a daily ritual: two to three drinks during lunch, and several drinks in the evening. He could no longer socialize at home or with friends without first having several drinks, and even when alone he often drank past the point of intoxication. On several occasions, his drinking was asso-

ciated with familial violence, and his two prior wives left him because they were physically abused.

The patient initially insisted he had full control of his drinking habits and adamantly denied being an alcoholic. After several counseling sessions, he agreed that he had an alcohol problem, and he is currently being treated in a rehabilitation center.

ADVERSE EFFECTS

Chronic alcoholic ingestion may cause numerous adverse health effects (Table 11–4),[55a] and the reader is referred to a general textbook of medicine for a more detailed discussion. Many variables, including genetic, nutritional, and general state of health, interact in producing alcohol-related adverse effects, and exact dose relationships do not exist.

Chronic alcohol drinkers are at risk of alcohol withdrawal approximately 8 hours after the last drink. Individuals may progress from simple anxiety and irritability to delirium tremens, a condition with a high morbidity and mortality. Symptoms and signs may evolve as follows:

1. 8 hours: tremors, anxiety, irritability, nausea, vomiting
2. 24 hours: hyperexcitability, insomnia, increased tremors
3. 12 to 48 hours: hallucinations, seizures
4. 2 to 5 days: delirium tremens—confusion, delusions, hallucinations, agitation, autonomic nervous system overactivity, dehydration, fevers, circulatory collapse, death[18,56,57]

Chronic alcohol use causes serious central and peripheral nervous system side effects. Wernicke's encephalopathy and Korsakoff's amnestic syndrome are characterized by a combination of confusion, ophthalmoplegia, ataxia, and a confabulatory amnesia. This is not an uncommon disease and is probably underdiagnosed.[58] Thiamine deficiency plays an important role in this disease, and emergency treatment with thiamine may be life saving.

Alcoholic dementia and cerebellar degeneration may occur separately or together; both are characterized pathologically by brain atrophy. Clinically, individuals may

Table 11–4. ADVERSE EFFECTS OF ALCOHOL

Neurological
  Alcohol withdrawal syndrome
  Wernicke's encephalopathy
  Korsakoff's amnestic syndrome
  Amnestic states (blackouts)
  Dementia
  Cerebellar degeneration
  Peripheral neuropathy
  Myopathy
  Adult-onset epilepsy
  Central pontine myelinolysis
  Nutritional amblyopia

Cardiovascular
  Cardiomyopathy
  Beriberi
  Tachycardia
  Hypertension

Endocrine
  Decreased testosterone
  Increased luteinizing hormone
  Decreased cortisol
  Decreased thyroid hormone
  Vasopressin inhibition
  Testicular atrophy
  Gynecomastia

Metabolic
  Altered lipoprotein metabolism
  Hypertriglyceridemia

Gastrointestinal
  Fatty liver
  Acute alcoholic hepatitis
  Cirrhosis
  Pancreatitis, acute and chronic
  Esophagitis
  Peptic ulcer disease

Hematologic
  Leukopenia
  Pancytopenia
  Folate/vitamin B_{12} deficiency

Psychiatric
  Depression
  Anxiety
  Personality changes

Sexual
  Impotence
  Sexual aggression

Trauma

Dermatologic
  Decreased hair
  Flushing
  Palmar erythema
  Rhinophyma
  Spider angiomata

Fetal Alcohol Syndrome

show subtle cognitive impairment and ataxia, but a progressive dementia and ataxia may occur.[18]

Peripheral neuropathy is quite common among alcoholics and typically manifests as weakness, pain, and paresthesias in the hands and feet.[17] Occasionally, the autonomic nervous system may be involved, leading to vocal cord paralysis, dysphagia, and orthostatic hypotension.[59]

Alcoholic myopathy had been recognized in the 19th century, but its importance among chronic alcohol abusers has long been ignored. Most patients with chronic alcoholism have some abnormalities in electromyography, and almost half have histologic changes of varying severity, including necrosis, acute and chronic inflammation, and interstitial fibrosis. The myopathy leads to progressive muscle wasting and weakness, but in early cases abstinence can reverse the clinical picture.[60] Even acute administration of ethanol can cause skeletal muscle dysfunction by reducing the stimulatory effect of prolonged exercise on glucose uptake.[60]

Alcoholism may be the sole explanation for adult onset epilepsy in 25 percent of newly diagnosed cases. This finding is important since it challenges the ingrained medical perception that seizures related to alcohol occur only in the setting of alcohol withdrawal.[61a]

Rarer neurologic complications of alcoholism include central pontine myelinolysis (a demyelinating disease of the pons) and nutritional amblyopia (visual dysfunction from maculopapillary fiber disease).

Of concern are the adverse effects of ethanol on the developing fetus. The teratogenic effects of ethanol are well documented, and the fetal alcohol syndrome includes characteristic morphologic malformations, growth deficiency, microcephaly, and mental deficiency. Reduction in maternal drinking early in pregnancy can effectively reduce the severity of this syndrome.[19]

The liver is frequently affected in chronic alcohol users. Acutely, alcoholic fatty liver and hepatitis may occur, but chronic use is often associated with cirrhosis, which causes eventual failure of liver function, secondary bleeding varices, clotting abnormalities, and numerous other systemic complications.

Alcohol also alters lipoprotein metabolism. High-density lipoprotein (HDL) is increased (both HDL_2 and HDL_3) in individuals who consume modest amounts (1 to 2 ounces) of alcohol,[62,63] which in turn may reduce the risk of myocardial infarction. However, Hartung and associates[64] found this protective effect only in inactive men and not in runners and joggers.

Alcohol may adversely affect the heart directly or indirectly. Chronic alcohol consumption may be associated with hypertension.[62] In the Western world, alcohol abuse may be the major cause of cardiomyopathy, and cardiac malfunction can be found in most patients with chronic alcoholism.[60] The histopathology and pathogenesis is similar to skeletal muscle myopathy.[60]

Many endocrine changes have been described following alcohol ingestion, as listed in Table 11–4. Of interest is that vasopressin inhibition is largely responsible for the diuretic effect of alcohol intake.

FINAL NOTE

Alcohol is recognized by the National Football League as the most abused drug in football,[26] and the numerous anecdotes in newspapers and journals, plus the well-known national alcohol abuse statistics, suggest that alcohol may be the most abused drug among all athletes. Unlike anabolic steroids and stimulants, however, alcohol serves no readily identifiable ergogenic function. Furthermore, the legal, moral, and social acceptance of alcohol use makes policy guidelines difficult to create and enact.

Nonetheless, the sports community must address the serious philosophical and medical issues of alcohol use and abuse, especially within the context of drug testing for so many other substances. For example, if the sole purpose of drug testing is to detect the use of ergogenic aids, then the NCAA is probably justified in limiting testing for alcohol to competitions such as riflery. If, on the other hand, the principal intent of drug testing is to detect illegal substance abuse, then there would appear to be little reason to test for alcohol. However, since illicit drug abuse and alcohol abuse frequently co-exist, the presence of alcohol in the urine may serve as an indicator of continued illicit drug abuse. Indeed, this concept has been incorporated into the NFL's drug testing program.

The lessons of prohibition remind us that, at least for the foreseeable future, alcohol will remain a legal and socially acceptable drug. Alcohol is ubiquitous in our society, and few would argue against limited social drinking. The difficulty arises when the individual crosses the line from limited social drinking to alcohol abuse and addiction. However, as will be discussed in the chapter "Recognition," the distinction between alcohol use and alcohol abuse is not always clear cut, but is often a subtle continuum.

Recognizing the prevalence of alcohol use and abuse in organized sports underscores the need to better educate the athlete. The primary goal of that education is to prevent the development of alcohol abuse problems. When education fails, mechanisms should be established that will facilitate the early recognition of alcohol abuse and addiction so that proper management can be initiated.

The economic impact of alcohol on both amateur and professional sports cannot be overstated. Beer is perhaps the most important economic contributor to the sports economy. Consider this: Anheuser-Busch spends two thirds of its advertising budget on sports.[65] According to that brewery's executive vice president and director of marketing, Anheuser-Busch will sponsor, in broadcast television, radio, and/or cable:

> 23 of the 24 domestic Major League Baseball teams; 18 of the 28 clubs in the National Football League; 22 of the 23 National Basketball Association franchises; 13 of the 14 domestic National Hockey League teams, and 9 of the 11 Major Indoor Soccer League clubs. That's in addition to various direct, media, or fundraising sponsorships of more than 300 college teams. And Anheuser-Busch will manage or promote about 1,000 secondary and tertiary sporting events—a rate of about three per day—ranging from the Bud Lite Iron Man Triathlon to hydroplane races.[66]

It has been estimated that the average child is exposed to as many as 100,000 beer ads before reaching the legal drinking age.[66] Yet, former U.S. Representative John Sieberling was unable to push through Congress a bill seeking equal television time for messages about the dangers of alcohol abuse because of the intense lobbying against such a measure.[26]

There is no question that a symbiotic relationship exists between the alcohol industry and organized sports. In the center of that relationship is the athlete—the role model. With that in mind, the formal positions of the National Football League and the USOC Sports Medicine Council send an appropriate message for all organized sports.

> NFL players, coaches, and other employees should not endorse or appear in advertisements for alcohol beverages (including beer) or tobacco products.
>
> While fully recognizing that the use of alcohol and tobacco is legal, the NFL nevertheless has long been of the view that participation in ads for such substances by its employees, particularly players, who are prohibited by federal law from appearing in such ads—may have a detrimental effect on the great number of young fans who follow our game. Endorsements or other close identification of NFL players with alcohol or tobacco could convey the erroneous impression that the use of such products is conducive to the development of athletic prowess, has contributed to their success, or at least has not hindered them in their performance.
>
> For the above reasons, players and other club and League employees (including game officials) should not use alcohol or tobacco products while in the playing field area or while being interviewed on television.[67]

The Sports Medicine Council of the U.S. Olympic Committee has discussed the problem of acute and chronic alcohol consumption in the general population and in athletes. While we recognize that moderate alcohol use does not appear to be a health problem, there is no question that both acute alcoholic intoxication and chronic alcohol abuse are significant problems. For many medical and social reasons, the Sports Medicine Council discourages the use of alcohol. In the course of these discussions, we have also considered the concept of advertising for alcoholic beverages by using Olympic athletes, which is a means of enhancing alcohol in the eyes of the person observing the announcement. Since Olympians are much in the public eye and may serve as

role models for young people, we do not believe that the use of the Olympians in advertisements which feature alcoholic beverages is in the best medical interest of the athletes or the public viewing these advertisements.[68]

REFERENCES

1. Greenblatt, RB: A Little Wine. In Search of the Scriptures—A Physician Examines Medicine in the Bible. JB Lippincott, Philadelphia, 1963, p 28.
2. Lucia, SP: Wine: A food throughout the ages. Am J Clin Nutr 25:361, 1972.
3. Stepto, RC: Clinical uses of wine. The New Physician, January, 1968.
4. Lucia, SP: Medicinal values of wine. Med Digest, June 1968, p 40.
5. Goodwin, DW: Alcoholism and alcoholic psychoses. In Kaplan, HI and Sadock, BJ (eds): Comprehensive Textbook of Psychiatry IV, Vol I, Williams & Wilkins, Baltimore, 1985, p 1010.
6. Holden, C: Alcoholism and the medical cost crunch. Science 235:1132, 1987.
6a. Cleary, PD, et al: Prevalence and recognition of alcohol abuse in a primary care population. Am J Med 85:466, 1988.
6b. Gunby, P: Nation's expenditures for alcohol, other drugs, in terms of therapy, prevention, now exceeds $1.6 billion. JAMA 258:2023, 1987.
7. Mello, NK: Alcohol abuse and alcoholism: 1978–1987. In Meltzer, HY (ed): Psychopharmacology: The Third Generation of Progress. Raven Press, New York, 1987, p 1515.
8. ABC's of Drinking and Driving. Nassau County Traffic Safety Board, Mineola, New York, 1971.
9. Smith, DE: Cocaine-alcohol abuse: Epidemiological, diagnostic and treatment considerations. J Psychoactive Drugs 18:117, 1986.
10. Johnston, L and Bachman, J: The Monitoring the Future Study. Institute for Social Research. The University of Michigan, Ann Arbor, 1988.
11. Himwich, H and Callison, D: The effects of alcohol on evoked potentials of various parts of the central nervous system of the cat. In the Biology of Alcoholism, Vol 2, Physiology and Behaviour. Plenum Press, New York, 1972.
12. Ricci, R, Crawford, S and Miner, P: The effect of ethanol on hepatic sodium plus potassium activated ATPase activity in the rat. Gastroenterology 80:1445, 1981.
13. Rabin, R and Molinoff, P: Activation of adenylate cyclase by ethanol in mouse striatal tissue. J Pharmacol Exp Therap 216:129, 1981.
14. Tabakoff, B and Hoffman, PC: Biochemical pharmacology of alcohol. In Meltzer, HY (ed): Psychopharmacology: The Third Generation of Progress. Raven Press, New York, 1987, p 1521.
15. Eisenhofer, G, Lambie, D and Johnson, R: Effects of ethanol on plasma catecholamines and norepinephrine clearance. Clin Pharmacol Ther 34:143, 1983.
16. Wallgren, H and Barry, H: Actions of Alcohol, Vols I & II. American Elsevier Publishing Co, New York, 1970.
17. Zornetzer, S, et al: Neurophysiological changes

produced by alcohol. In Biomedical Processes and Consequences of Alcohol Use. US Department of Health and Human Services, 1982, p 95.

18. Diamond, I and Charness, M: Alcohol neurotoxicity. In Asbury, AK, McKhann, GM and McDonald, WI (eds): Diseases of the Nervous System, Clinical Neurobiology, Vol II. WB Saunders, Philadelphia, 1986, p 1324.
19. Ritchie, JM: The aliphatic alcohols. In Gilman, AG, et al (eds): Goodman and Gilman's The Pharmacological Basis of Therapeutics, ed 7. Macmillan, New York, 1985, p 372.
20. Blum, K: Alcohol and Opiates: A review of common mechanisms. In Mazo, L (ed): Advances in Neurotoxicology. Proceedings of the International Congress of Neurotoxicology. Varese, Italy, September 27–30, 1979. Pergamon Press, Elmsford, NY, 1980.
21. Lyon, L and Anthony, J: Reversal of alcoholic coma by naloxone. Ann Intern Med 96:464, 1982.
22. Goldberg, L: Quantitative studies on alcohol tolerance in man. Acta Physiol Scand 5:1, 1943.
23. Baselt, RC: Disposition of Toxic Drugs and Chemicals in Man, ed 2. Biomedical Publishing, Davis, 1982, p 299.
24. Anderson, WA and McKeag, DB: The Substance Use and Abuse Habits of College Student-Athletes. Presented to National Collegiate Athletic Association Council. College of Human Medicine. Michigan State University, June, 1985.
25. Elite Women Athletes Survey. Hazelden Health Promotion Services, Minneapolis, January 1987.
26. Sullivan, J: Unrestricted drug: Leagues just say no to alcohol-abuse sanctions. Newsday, December 22, 1987.
27. Sexton, J: A local hero's problems cause shock. The New York Times, December 15, 1987.
28. Cowart, VS: Alcohol and athletics don't mix—Can the players now learn to say "nix"? JAMA 258:1571, 1987.
29. Tang, PC and Rosenstein, R: Influence of alcohol and dramamine, alone and in combination, on psychomotor performance. Aerospace Med 38:818, 1967.
30. Begbie, G: The effects of alcohol and of varying amounts of visual information on a balancing test. Ergonomics 9:325, 1966.
31. Pihkanen, TA: Neurological and physiological studies on distilled and brewed beverages. Ann Medicinae Exp et Biol Fenniae 35:7, 1957.
32. Belgrave, BE, et al: The effect of cannabidiol, alone and in combination with ethanol, on human performance. Psychopharm 64:243, 1979.
33. Nelson, DO: Effects of alcohol on the performance of selected gross motor tasks. Res Quart 30:312, 1959.
34. Gustafson, R: Alcohol and vigilance performance: effect of small doses of alcohol on simple visual reaction time. Percept Mot Skills 62:951, 1986.
35. Gustafson, R: Effect of moderate doses of alcohol on simple auditory reaction time in a vigilance setting. Percept Mot Skills 62:683, 1986.
36. Rundell, O and Williams, H: Alcohol and speed accuracy trade-off. Hum Factors 21:433, 1979.
37. Forney, RB, Hughes, FW and Greatbatch, WH: Measurement of attentive motor performance after alcohol. Percept Mot Skills 19:151, 1964.

38. Collins, W, Schroeder, D and Gibson, R: Effects of alcohol ingestion on tracking performance during angular acceleration. J Appl Psychol 55:559, 1971.
39. Moskowitz, H and Burns, M: Effect of alcohol on the psychological refractory period. Quart J Stud Alcohol 32:782, 1971.
40. Huntly, M: Effects of alcohol, uncertainty and novelty upon response selection. Psychopharm 39:259, 1974.
41. Wilson, L, et al: The combined effects of ethanol and amphetamine sulfate on performance of human subjects. Canad Med Assoc J 94:478, 1966.
42. Hebbellinck, M: The effects of a moderate dose of alcohol on a series of functions of physical performance in man. Acta Int Pharmacol 120:402, 1959.
43. Hebbellinck, M: The effects of a small dose of ethyl alcohol on certain basic components of human physical performance. Arch Int Pharmacodyn Ther 143:247, 1963.
44. Williams, M: Effect of selected doses of alcohol on fatigue parameters of the forearm flexor muscles. Res Quart 40:832, 1969.
45. Bobo, W: Effects of alcohol upon maximum oxygen uptake, lung ventilation and heart rate. Res Quart 43:1, 1972.
46. Williams, M: Effect of small and moderate doses of alcohol on exercise, heart rate and oxygen consumption. Res Quart 43:94, 1972.
47. Bond, V, Franks, B and Hawley, E: Effects of small and moderate doses of alcohol on submaximal cardiorespiratory function, perceived exertion and endurance performance in abstainers and moderate drinkers. J Sports Med 23:221, 1983.
48. Blonquist, G, Saltin, B and Mitchell, J: Acute effects of ethanol ingestion on the response to submaximal and maximal exercise in man. Circulation 42:463, 1970.
49. Tennant, FS: Substance abuse in sports. In Biopsychiatric Insights on Substance Abuse (A Symposium), Psychiatric Diagnostic Laboratories of America, Inc., Princeton, 1986, p 35.
50. Yesavage, JA and Leirer, VO: Hangover effects on aircraft pilots 14 hours after alcohol ingestion: A preliminary report. Am J Psychiatry 143:1546, 1986.
51. Ryback, R: Facilitation and inhibition of learning and memory by alcohol. Ann NY Acad Sci 215:187, 1973.
52. Koller, WC and Biary, N: Effect of alcohol on tremors: Comparison with propanolol. Neurology 34:221, 1984.
53. Clark, DC, et al: Alcohol-use patterns through medical school: A longitudinal study of one class. JAMA 257:2921, 1987.
54. Berger, TJ: Alcohol abuse in medical school (letter). JAMA 258:1173, 1987.
55. Clark, DC: Alcohol abuse in medical school (letter). JAMA 258:1173, 1987.
55a. Miller, NS, et al: Alcohol dependence and its medical complications. NY State J Med, September, 1988, p 476.
56. Victor, M and Adams, RD: The effect of alcohol on the nervous system. Res Publ Assoc Nerv Ment Dis 32:526, 1953.
57. Linnoila, M: Alcohol withdrawal and noradrenergic function. Ann Intern Med 107:875, 1987.
58. Harper, C: The incidence of Wernicke's encepha-

lopathy in Australia—A neuropathological study of 131 cases. J Neurol Neurosurg Psychiatry 46:593, 1983.

59. Novak, DJ and Victor, MA: Affection of the vagus and sympathetic nerves in alcoholic polyneuropathy. Arch Neurol 30:273, 1974.

60. Rubin, E: Alcoholic myopathy in heart and skeletal muscle. N Engl J Med 301:28, 1979.

61. Alcoholism linked to adult-onset epilepsy. Am Med News, January 8, 1988, p 46.

61a. Ng, SKC, et al: Alcohol consumption and withdrawal in new-onset seizures. N Engl J Med 319:666, 1988.

62. Klatsky, AL: The relationship of alcohol and the cardiovascular system. In Alcohol and Health Monograph 2: Biomedical Processes and Consequences of Alcohol Use. U.S. Department of Health and Human Services. National Institute on Alcohol Abuse and Alcoholism. Rockville, Maryland, 1982, p 173.

63. Hennekens, CH, et al: Moderate alcohol consumption and risk of myocardial infarction. Circulation 76:IV 501, 1987.

64. Hartung, GH, et al: Effect of alcohol intake on high-density lipoprotein cholesterol levels in runners and inactive men. JAMA 249:747, 1983.

65. Top TV sports advertisers. Sports Inc., February 29, 1988, p 35.

66. Gloede, B: What if beer were banned? Sports Inc., September 5, 1988, p. 14.

67. Drug Policy of the National Football League, 1988.

68. Sportsmediscope. September 1988, p 1.

CHAPTER 12

Tobacco

HISTORY

Like many of the other drugs previously discussed, tobacco—both smoking and smokeless—has experienced the "pendulum swings of fashion."[1] In the 18th century, tobacco smoking in Arabia and Turkey was punishable by torture and death. In the mid-20th century, smoking became equated with maturity and sophistication. By the 1980s, the serious health risks of tobacco had become more publicized, but the glamour and sophistication of tobacco remain strong incentives for its use.

Despite the known health hazards of smoking tobacco, its use is widespread. In 1982, 623 billion cigarettes were sold to 55 million tobacco users in the United States.[2] Currently, 31.5 percent of adult men and 25.7 percent of adult women smoke. Since 1964, smoking has declined 21.4 percent among men and only 5.8 percent in women.[3] It is estimated that 350,000 individuals per year die of tobacco-related deaths. Smoking-related diseases account for $22 billion in annual health care cost and $43 billion in lost productivity.[4]

In the 1980s, anti-smoking movements began to prevail. For example, at the 1988 Olympic Winter Games in Calgary, tobacco smoking was allowed only in designated areas, both indoors and outdoors.[5] A stringent clean air law took effect in New York City in April, 1988. Citywide, smoking became permitted only in designated areas.[6]

Television advertising of cigarettes is banned, but nontelevised cigarette advertising and promotional expenditure reached $2.1 billion in 1984. Much of the advertising is directed at adolescents and teenagers through magazines, and surveys indicate that this age group is considerably influenced by tobacco advertising.[4]

Chewing tobacco was very popular in the United States at the turn of the century, and a communal snuff box remained in Congress until the mid-1930s.[7] The invention of the cigarette-rolling machine, coupled with the discovery that tuberculosis was transmitted through expectoration, led to the replacement of smokeless tobacco with smoking tobacco in the 1920s. However, the mounting health concerns over smoking tobacco and the resurgence of smokeless tobacco use in professional sports in the 1950s led to a nationwide renewed popularity of smokeless tobacco use in the 1970s and 1980s.[8]

Despite the documented health hazards of smokeless tobacco, many users believe it is a safe alternative to smoking tobacco.[8] Of the over 12 million Americans using smokeless tobacco, 3 million are under age 21. Regional surveys indicate that 7 to 36 percent of children and teenagers use smokeless tobacco.[9-11] Prevalence of use among men and women in 1985 was 19 percent and 3 percent, respectively.[12] In one regional survey, 16.9 percent of girls and 9.8 percent of boys reported using smokeless tobacco products.[13]

Tobacco companies have aggressively advertised smokeless tobacco, often using well-known athletes to glamorize their product.[7] In 1980, the United States Tobacco Company, the principal manufacturer of moist snuff, spent over 1 million dollars as an official sponsor of the Winter Olympics. Surveys indicate that television advertisements successfully influence young people to use smokeless tobacco.[8]

CHEMISTRY AND PHYSIOLOGY

Nicotine, a potent alkaloid found in smoking and chewing tobacco, is responsible for the pharmacological effects of tobacco use (Fig. 12–1). Nicotine is a weak base, and at physiologic pH is approximately 69 percent ionized. Diverse effects from nicotine occur as a result of both stimulant and depressant actions on various central and peripheral nervous system pathways.

Dose-dependent, biphasic physiologic changes commonly occur following nicotine intake, leading to a variety of clinical responses. In the peripheral nervous system, low-dose nicotine causes autonomic ganglia stim-

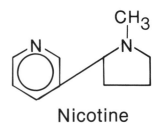

Figure 12–1. Structure of nicotine.

ulation, and high doses lead to ganglionic depression. The adrenal medulla and other organs release catecholamines following nicotine administration, resulting in a sympathetic response. However, larger doses of nicotine may cause inhibition of catecholamine responses from the adrenal medulla.[14] Nicotine may facilitate acetylcholine release at the neuromuscular junction, but large doses may produce neuromuscular blockade because of receptor desensitization.[15] The sympathetic responses of the cardiovascular system from catecholamine release result in heart rate and blood pressure increases. Nicotine may also directly activate chemoreceptors in the aortic and carotid bodies and may cause independent central pressor effects by stimulation of the ventral lateral medulla.[14,16]

In the central nervous system, norepinephrine and dopamine release occurs following nicotine administration,[17] and acetylcholine may increase or decrease, depending on the dose. Nicotine receptors have been identified and are at least in part responsible for the observed neurochemical changes. With regard to acetylcholine, presynaptic nicotinic receptors may enhance its release, but at higher nicotine concentrations, presynaptic muscarinic receptors inhibit acetylcholine release.[2]

Psychic effects of nicotine are varied, but are usually associated with pleasure. Euphorogenic effects similar to those seen following morphine and amphetamine administration may occur.[18] An alerting pattern is seen in the electroencephalogram, and correlates with a sense of increased alertness.[19] Facilitation of memory and attention, sustained vigilance, relaxation, and relief of boredom have all been reported following nicotine intake.[2,20]

Tolerance to many of the sympathetic and

parasympathetic effects of nicotine usually occurs, allowing an increase in dose without the unpleasant side effects that occur in naive subjects. Nicotine is a potent reinforcer in animals and humans.[18,21] Physical dependence occurs among users of smokeless and smoking tobacco,[22,23] and a variable withdrawal syndrome upon tobacco cessation develops. The most consistent symptoms and signs of tobacco withdrawal include tobacco craving, irritability, anxiety, restlessness, difficulty in concentrating, appetite changes, and gastrointestinal complaints.[17]

CLINICAL PHARMACOLOGY

The role of nicotine in tobacco may be likened to the role of ethanol in alcoholic beverages or to delta-9-tetrahydrocannabinol in marijuana.[24] The two major routes of nicotine intake are through smoking and chewing tobacco.

A typical American cigarette contains approximately 10 mg of nicotine. The amount of nicotine delivered to the body is, however, not only determined by the amount of nicotine present in a cigarette but also is a function of the engineering of the cigarette and the manner in which the cigarette is smoked, such as the depth and duration of inhalation (Fig. 12–2). Under standard test conditions using a constant-rate smoking machine, approximately 1 mg of nicotine can be recovered from the absorptive filter.[24]

Smokeless tobacco exists mainly in three popular forms:

1. Loose-leaf tobacco, which is typically sold in foil pouches. A golfball-sized amount is placed between the cheek and lower gum, where it is sucked and chewed; thus its use is termed "chewing."

2. Moist or dry powdered tobacco (snuff), which is typically sold in small round cans. Its use, referred to as "dipping," involves leaving a pinch of the tobacco between the cheek or lip and the lower gum.

3. Compressed tobacco, which is used in pieces, each of which is called a "plug." The

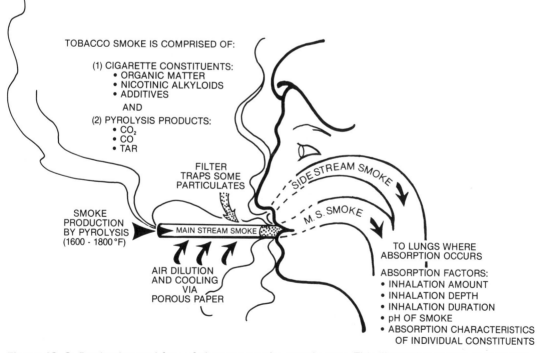

Figure 12–2. Production and fate of cigarette smoke constituents. This illustration shows that nicotine delivery from the cigarette smoking process is complex and that the most fundamental variable to study—dose of the ingested substance—is difficult to measure. (From Henningfield and Nemeth-Coslett,[24] p. 40S, with permission.)

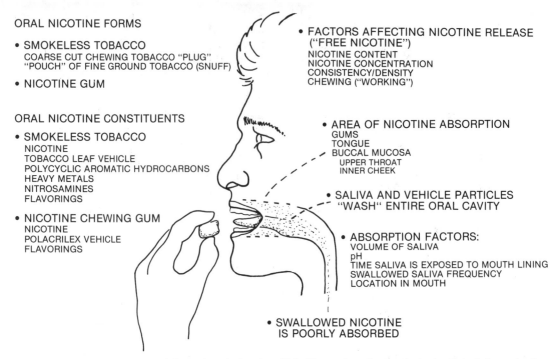

ORAL NICOTINE FORMS

- SMOKELESS TOBACCO
  COARSE CUT CHEWING TOBACCO "PLUG"
  "POUCH" OF FINE GROUND TOBACCO (SNUFF)
- NICOTINE GUM

ORAL NICOTINE CONSTITUENTS

- SMOKELESS TOBACCO
  NICOTINE
  TOBACCO LEAF VEHICLE
  POLYCYCLIC AROMATIC HYDROCARBONS
  HEAVY METALS
  NITROSAMINES
  FLAVORINGS
- NICOTINE CHEWING GUM
  NICOTINE
  POLACRILEX VEHICLE
  FLAVORINGS

- FACTORS AFFECTING NICOTINE RELEASE
  ("FREE NICOTINE")
  NICOTINE CONTENT
  NICOTINE CONCENTRATION
  CONSISTENCY/DENSITY
  CHEWING ("WORKING")

- AREA OF NICOTINE ABSORPTION
  GUMS
  TONGUE
  BUCCAL MUCOSA
  UPPER THROAT
  INNER CHEEK

- SALIVA AND VEHICLE PARTICLES
  "WASH" ENTIRE ORAL CAVITY

- ABSORPTION FACTORS:
  VOLUME OF SALIVA
  pH
  TIME SALIVA IS EXPOSED TO MOUTH LINING
  SWALLOWED SALIVA FREQUENCY
  LOCATION IN MOUTH

- SWALLOWED NICOTINE
  IS POORLY ABSORBED

Figure 12–3. Absorption and fate of oral nicotine. This illustration shows that nicotine delivery in the form of a chewing gum presents a similar set of problematic issues as those encountered with cigarette smoking. Factors such as chewing intensity, pH level, and amount of saliva produced and/or swallowed are all determinants in how much nicotine is actually absorbed. (From Henningfield and Nemeth-Coslett,[24] pp. 40S–41S, with permission.)

user bites or whittles off a small piece and places it in the mouth in a manner similar to dipping.[7]

Nicotine gum is another form of oral nicotine intake, but is used primarily by those trying to quit tobacco smoking.[25] Oral nicotine absorption is considerably influenced by the vehicle of delivery, the manner in which the tobacco is chewed, and by local factors in the mouth (Fig. 12–3).

Plasma nicotine levels in chronic smokeless tobacco users (dippers, snuffers, or chewers) and smoking tobacco users are similar, and range from 5 to 30 ng per ml. Nicotine is extensively metabolized in the liver, and to a lesser extent, kidney and lung.[2] The half-life averages 2 hours, and the major metabolites, cotinine and nicotine-N-oxide, are without known biologic activity.[2]

Clinical Uses

Smoking and smokeless tobacco use have no role in clinical medicine. Nicotine chewing gum in appropriate doses may be helpful to persons who are attempting to stop smoking.[25]

USE IN SPORTS

Although no firm data exist regarding the incidence of tobacco use among professional athletes, its widespread presence and influence in the sports world are indisputable. It is difficult to watch a professional baseball game without seeing the traditional puffed-out cheek and spitting ritual characteristic of chewing tobacco. During the fifth game of the 1986 World Series, Jones noted a total of 23 minutes and 55 seconds of perceptible chewing tobacco use on television.[26]

A recent survey of 7 major league baseball teams indicates that 34 percent of respondents currently use smokeless tobacco, and 17 percent reported past use. The product most frequently used contained the highest level of nicotine bioavailability in comparison to other available products. Among current users, 38 percent have noticed gum or mouth sores. Fifty-two percent use the product to help them relax, and 28 percent admit to being unable to stop smokeless tobacco use.[8]

In the 1984 Michigan State Study of National Collegiate Athletic Association athletes, 20 percent of respondents had used smokeless tobacco in the prior 12 months, and 5 percent had smoked cigarettes in the same time period. Forty percent of baseball players and 30 percent of football players polled had used smokeless tobacco regularly.[27] It has been reported that in Texas, approximately one third of varsity football and baseball players use smokeless tobacco.[28] In the 1986 Elite Women Athletes Survey, 16 percent of Olympic-caliber respondents had smoked cigarettes during the prior 30 days; 20 percent had used smokeless tobacco in their lifetime.[29]

Effects on Performance

Although some may argue that smokeless tobacco use among athletes is simply a cultural phenomenon, its use may also be secondary to perceived ergogenic effects. General alerting mechanisms and improvement in information-processing tasks[2,30,31] may be beneficial to the athlete. Performance decrements during sustained vigilance tasks are less after nicotine, and visual information-processing tasks are increased.[2]

Nicotine may potentially improve psychomotor performance through its calming effects, as demonstrated in animal models.[32,33] The performance of complex swimming acts by rats is improved following nicotine administration,[34] but endurance per se, as measured by swimming to exhaustion, is decreased.[35]

Nicotine ergogenicity, vis-à-vis the athlete, has not been clearly established. Some may use the drug for its calming effects, and others for its stimulatory effects.[15] Nicotine may reduce appetite, and in this regard may be used as an aid for weight control. Some athletes may have begun using nicotine for social reasons, but became dependent on the drug to prevent symptoms of withdrawal. Edwards and associates[36] studied the effects of smokeless tobacco on three perceptual motor tasks (reaction time, movement time, total response time). No discernible acute beneficial effects were noted in individuals (both athletes and nonathletes) who used

oral nicotine compared to those who did not. Heart rate, however, was consistently elevated above baseline for those who were given oral tobacco. Dose of tobacco and potential bioavailability of nicotine are not mentioned in the study.

Impaired oxygen transport secondary to increases in carboxyhemoglobin,[37,38] and increases in minute ventilation during submaximal exercise[39] may cause some performance impairment in smokers. No similar clear-cut detrimental effects have been shown following smokeless tobacco use, although the associated tachycardia may decrease physical work capacity.[40]

Case Vignette

A 26-year-old male baseball player was evaluated for severe periodontal disease.

The patient began smoking cigarettes at age 14 and by age 15 he smoked 10 to 20 cigarettes per day. He quit cigarette smoking at age 16 because he felt that his endurance was suboptimal. Soon after quitting smoking tobacco, however, he noticed increased anxiety, jitteriness, and irritability. A friend recommended chewing tobacco as a supplement, and he remembers having felt relaxed and somewhat euphoric after his first use of chewing tobacco.

He was quite talented as a baseball player, and he enjoyed playing under the influence of nicotine. Typically, he titrated the amount of chewing tobacco used and changed the way in which it was chewed according to both how he felt and to the tempo of the play. Before batting, he always used a large amount of fresh tobacco in order to achieve a "surge" of alertness. While sitting in the dugout, he usually chewed the tobacco slowly and used smaller amounts. If he felt bored or inattentive in the outfield, he again used a large amount of fresh tobacco and usually felt more alert and less fatigued after doing so.

Chewing tobacco became a routine for the patient, both on and off the field. He estimated that he chewed tobacco 6 to 10 hours daily. He drank alcohol rarely, maintained his abstinence from smoking tobacco, and used no illicit drugs.

He presented to the dental clinic with complaints of a persistent white patch on the lower gums. Exam revealed edematous gums with some sloughing and several patches of whitish discoloration. Biopsy showed no evidence of malignancy, but a diagnosis of leukoplakia was made. The patient was advised to discontinue chewing tobacco and was warned of the malignant potential of leukoplakia. Despite several attempts, the patient was unable to tolerate the tobacco craving and jitteriness that he experienced after discontinuing the drug, and he resumed his habit against medical advice.

ADVERSE EFFECTS

Smoking is the chief single avoidable cause of death in our society.[41] Adverse health effects of smoking and smokeless tobacco are shown in Tables 12–1 and 12–2, respectively. It is noteworthy that cigarette smoking alone causes more premature deaths than all of the following together: acquired immunodeficiency syndrome (AIDS), cocaine, heroin, alcohol, fire, automobile accidents, homicide, and suicide.[41] The life expectancy gain from a tobacco-free society would be equivalent to the life expectancy gain that would be achieved by the complete elimination of all cancers not caused by tobacco.[41]

Although lung cancer is the best known of smoking tobacco–related cancers, a variety of other neoplasms have been implicated.[42] Smoking is a major risk factor in the development of atherosclerosis, with resultant coronary artery and cerebrovascular disease. Tobacco smoke has direct toxic effects on the bronchi and lung parenchyma, leading to various respiratory disorders including chronic obstructive pulmonary disease.

Of concern are the adverse effects of maternal smoking on pregnancy outcome. In addition to the placental transfer of nicotine to the fetus, maternal smoking has been shown to have deleterious effects on maternal oxygenation and uteroplacental perfusion, all of which can result in fetal hypoxemia. Cigarette smoking is a major cause of intrauterine growth retardation.[42a]

Smokeless tobacco is an increasing major health concern because of its rapidly developing popularity among the young. Severe periodontal disease may develop, including oral cancer. The American Academy of Oral Medicine recognizes the severity of the problem, and has adopted the following position:

> The American Academy of Oral Medicine agrees that the use of smokeless tobacco poses potentially significant oral and systemic health hazards. Such prod-

---

Table 12–1. ADVERSE EFFECTS OF CHRONIC SMOKING TOBACCO USE

Neoplasms	*Respiratory Disease*
Lung	Pneumonia
Trachea	Bronchitis
Bronchi	Chronic obstructive pulmonary disease
Lip	
Oral cavity	*Gastrointestinal Disease*
Pharynx	Peptic ulcer
Esophagus	
Larynx	*Neuropsychiatric*
Stomach	Addiction/withdrawal
Pancreas	
Cervix	*Maternal-Induced Neonatal Disease*
Bladder	Short gestation
Kidney	Low birthweight
	Respiratory distress syndrome
Cardiovascular Disease	? Sudden infant death syndrome
Hypertension	
Coronary artery disease	
Cardiac arrest	
Cerebrovascular disease	
Aortic aneurysm	

Table 12–2. ADVERSE EFFECTS
OF CHRONIC SMOKELESS
TOBACCO USE

Periodontal destruction
Teeth abrasion
Oral mucosa hyperkeratosis
Gingival inflammation
Leukoplakia
Decreased taste perception
Squamous cell carcinoma of oral cavity
Addiction/withdrawal
Halitosis
Dysgeusia
Dysosmia

ucts have a high variability in constituents
and may include nicotine, salt, sugar,
heavy metals, radioisotopes and potentially carcinogenic chemicals. Chronic use
of these products may induce carcinoma,
periodontal pathosis, and dental caries.
The high nicotine content can be addictive
and a high sodium content has shown adverse effects on the cardiovascular system.
These products may induce or enhance
halitosis, dysgeusia, and dysosmia.
Smokeless tobacco is not an innocuous
substitute for cigarette smoking. Its use
should be recognized as potentially hazardous and therefore discouraged by all
health professionals.[43]

On May 20, 1984, United States Surgeon
General C. Everett Koop, M.D., issued a call
for a smoke-free society by the year 2000.
The goal has been upgraded to a tobacco-free
society,[41] especially given the addicting potential of tobacco. In the 20th report of the
Surgeon General of the Public Health Service on the health consequences of tobacco,
Dr. Koop notes the following:

1. Cigarettes and other forms of tobacco
are addicting.
2. Nicotine is the drug in tobacco that
causes addiction.
3. The pharmacologic and behavioral processes that determine tobacco addiction are
similar to those that determine addiction to
drugs such as heroin and cocaine.[44]

FINAL NOTE

Tobacco and sports are so interlinked that
it is difficult to imagine certain sporting
events without visualizing tobacco products.
Benson and Hedges sponsors golf tournaments, Virginia Slims sponsors the women's
tennis circuit, and cigarette billboards appear
in the background of televised sporting
events. Baseball and smokeless tobacco have
become an accepted marriage.

Tobacco, however, is a potent drug which
is responsible for 1000 deaths per day in the
United States. Since athletes serve as highly
visible role models, the encouragement of tobacco to the young carries with it serious
consequences. Tobacco use raises another interesting question: some evidence suggests
that the effects of nicotine may be ergogenic.
Although the data are less convincing than
for amphetamines, they seem at least as convincing as for phenylpropanolamine and
ephedrine. If all pharmacologic ergogenic
aids are to be banned from athletic competition, then shouldn't one seriously consider
banning tobacco. The sports community may
not be ready for such a bold move, but the
health and ergogenic aspects of tobacco use
among athletes deserve serious discussion.

REFERENCES

1. Marks, J: Opium, the religion of the people. Lancet 1:1439, 1985.
2. Jones, RT: Tobacco dependence. In Meltzer, HY (ed): Psychopharmacology: The Third Generation of Progress. Raven Press, New York, 1987, p 1589.
3. Fielding, JE: Smoking and women: Tragedy of the majority. N Engl J Med 317:1343, 1987.
4. Davis, RM: Current trends in cigarette advertising and marketing. N Engl J Med 316:725, 1987.
5. McGinn, PR: Anti-smoking movement advances; Canada bans smoking at Olympics, plans laws. Am Med News, Mar 11, 1988, p 3.
6. Coburn, MR: Anti-smoking movement advances; New York City enacts stringent clean air law. Am Med News, Mar 11, 1988, p 3.
7. Glover, E, et al: Implications of smokeless tobacco use among athletes. Phys Sportsmed 14(12):95, 1986.
8. Connolly, GN, Orleans, CT and Kogan, M: Use of smokeless tobacco in Major League Baseball. N Engl J Med 318:1281, 1988.
9. Smokeless tobacco use has increased markedly in U.S. Oncology Times, October 1987, p 19.
10. Smokeless tobacco use rising among school-age children. Oncology Times, February 1987, p 4.
11. Torres, M and Brecher, DB: Smokeless tobacco: A new health hazard. Medical Times 115:73, 1987.
12. Leads from the MMWR. Smokeless tobacco use in the United States—Behavioral risk factor surveil-lance system, 1986. JAMA 258:24, 1987.
13. Leads from the MMWR. Smokeless tobacco use in rural Alaska. JAMA 257:1861, 1987.
14. Taylor, P: Ganglionic stimulating and blocking

agents. In Gilman, AG, et al (eds): Goodman and Gilman's The Pharmacological Basis of Therapeutics, ed 7. Macmillan, New York, 1985, p 215.

15. Lombardo, J: Stimulants and athletic performance: Cocaine and nicotine. Phys Sportsmed 14(12):85, 1986.

16. Tseng, LJ and Robertson, D: The pressor effect of nicotine in the ventral lateral medulla of the rat. Circulation 76(5):IV-303, 1987.

17. Jaffe, JH: Drug addiction and drug abuse. In Gilman, AG, Goodman, LS, Rall, TW, et al (eds): Goodman and Gilman's The Pharmacological Basis of Therapeutics, ed 7. Macmillan, New York, 1985, p 215.

18. Henningfield, J, Miyasto, K and Jasinski D: Cigarette smokers self administer intravenous nicotine. Pharm Biochem Behav 19:887, 1983.

19. Domino, E: Neuropsychopharmacology of nicotine and tobacco smoking. In Dunn, W (ed): Smoking Behavior: Motives and Incentives. VH Winston and Sons, Inc., Washington, D.C., 1973, p 5.

20. Jaffe, J and Jarvik, M: Tobacco use and tobacco. In Lipton, M, DiMascio, A and Killam, K (eds): Psychopharmacology: A Generation of Progress. Raven Press, New York, 1978, p 1665.

21. Goldberg, S, Spealman, R and Goldberg, D: Persistent behavior at high rates maintained by intravenous self-administration of nicotine. Science 214:573, 1981.

22. Glover, E: Conducting smokeless tobacco clinics. Am J Public Health 76:207, 1986.

23. U.S. Department of Health and Human Services, Public Health Service: The Health Consequences of Using Smokeless Tobacco: A Report of the Advisory Committee to the Surgeon General. National Institute of Health, Bethesda, MD, April 1986, Publication No. 86-2874.

24. Henningfield, JE and Nemeth-Coslett, R: Nicotine dependence: Interface between tobacco and tobacco-related disease. Chest 93:375, 1988.

25. Tonnesen, P: Effect of nicotine chewing gum in combination with group counseling on the cessation of smoking. N Engl J Med 318:15, 1988.

26. Jones, RB: Use of smokeless tobacco in the 1986 World Series. N Engl J Med 316:952, 1987.

27. Anderson, WA and McKeag, DB: The Substance Use and Abuse Habits of College Student-Athletes. Presented to National Collegiate Athletic Association Council by College of Human Medicine, Michigan State University, June, 1985.

28. Lombardo, JA: Stimulants. In Strauss, RH (ed):

Drugs and Performance in Sports. WB Saunders, Philadelphia, 1987, p 69.

29. Elite Women Athletes Survey. Hazelden Health Promotion Services, Minneapolis, January, 1987.

30. Battig, K: Behavioral Effects of Nicotine. S Karger, Basel, 1978.

31. Warburton, DM and Wesnes, K: Drugs as research tools in psychology: Cholinergic drugs and information processing. Neuropsychobiology 11:121, 1984.

32. Bovet, D, Bovet-Nitti, F and Oliverio, A: Action of nicotine on spontaneous and acquired behavior in rats and mice. Ann NY Acad Sci 142:261, 1967.

33. Morrison, C: Effect of nicotine on operant behavior of rats. Int J Neuropharmacol 7:229, 1967.

34. Battig, K Von: Differential effect of nicotine and tobacco smoking alkaloids on swimming endurance in the rat. Psychopharm 18:330, 1970.

35. Bhagat, B and Wheeler, W: Effect of nicotine on the swimming endurance of rats. Neuropharmacol 12:1161, 1973.

36. Edwards, SW, Glover, ED and Schroeder, KL: The effects of smokeless tobacco on heart rate and neuromuscular reactivity in athletes and nonathletes. Phys Sportsmed 15(7):141, 1987.

37. Rode, A and Shephard, R: The influence of cigarette smoking upon the oxygen cost of breathing in near maximal exercise. Eur J Appl Physiol 51:371, 1983.

38. Klausen, K, Anderson, S and Nandrup, S: Acute effects of cigarette smoking and inhalation of carbon monoxide during maximal exercise. Eur J Appl Physiol 51:371, 1983.

39. Maksud, MC and Baron, A: Physiological responses to exercise in chronic cigarette and marijuana users. Eur J Appl Physiol 43:127, 1980.

40. Sepponen, A: Physical work capacity in relation to carbon monoxide inhalation and tobacco smoking. Ann Clin Res 9:269, 1977.

41. Wainer, KE: Health and economic implications of a tobacco-free society. JAMA 258:2080, 1987.

42. Leads from the MMWR: Smoking-attributable mortality and years of potential life lost—United States, 1984. JAMA 258:2648, 1987.

42a. Charlton, VE: The small-for-gestational-age infant. In Rudolph, AM: Pediatrics, ed 18. Appleton & Lange, East Norwalk, CT, 1987, p 144.

43. Eskow, RN: Hazards of smokeless tobacco. N Engl J Med 317:1229, 1987.

44. Surgeon General emphasizes nicotine addiction in annual report on tobacco use, consequences. JAMA 259:2811, 1988.

CHAPTER 13

Marijuana

HISTORY

Thousands of years ago, the cultivation of hemp, *Cannabis sativa*, gradually moved westward from China. Originally used for weaving, the plant's prominent medicinal and mind-altering properties were noted in early Chinese history. In 2657 B.C., the Emperor Shen-Nung recommended hemp as a cure for "gout, rheumatism, malaria, beriberi, constipation, and absentmindedness." By 100 B.C., the Chinese used hemp juice to derive psychic pleasure.[1]

Ancient India's major interest in marijuana was in the resin derived from the female flower for its mind-altering effects. Referred to as "bhang," stories related to this form of marijuana were woven into Indian legend, religion, and history.

As cannabis moved westward, methods to enhance its psychic effects evolved. The inhalation of the fumes of hemp seeds thrown on hot bricks dates back to fifth century B.C. Greek history. The hashish pipe of the Middle East had its roots in African customs of the thirteenth century A.D. These devices were used to cool the hot fumes of the burning cannabis resin, hashish.

Because central European weavers used flax rather than hemp, marijuana was not known to Europe until the nineteenth century, when seafarers brought it from Africa. In early American history, the hemp plant principally served as an important source of fiber. It has been suggested that the hemp grown at that time in relatively cool climates such as the United States probably had small amounts of psychoactive material. As hemp was replaced by cotton, the hemp plant in the United States became primarily a weed.

South of the border, however, in the warm

climate of Mexico, the psychoactively rich hemp plant played a major role in Aztec history. During World War I, Mexican workers brought their cannabis with them, as did sailors from other warm-climate countries such as Jamaica. The Harrison Act of 1914, which outlawed heroin and cocaine, did not prohibit marijuana;[2] by the 1920s, a substantial market existed in the United States for the drug. Its connection with crime resulted in the Marijuana Tax Act, which outlawed marijuana everywhere in the United States by 1937.[2]

Following World War II, an increasing demand developed for marijuana, which accelerated during the Vietnam War years. Intensive research into the effects and health hazards of marijuana followed.[3]

Marijuana smoking is the most frequent form of illicit drug use in America today,[4] and the consequences of marijuana use may be serious: a California study revealed that one-third of fatal automobile accidents involve drivers under the influence of marijuana.[5] The use of this drug among youth and young adults escalated rapidly during the 1970s. In 1979, the annual prevalence for marijuana use peaked among high school seniors at 50.8 percent, and has since declined steadily to the 1987 figure of 36.3 percent. The 30-day prevalence use peaked in 1978 at 37.1 percent and similarly has declined to the 1987 rate of 21.0 percent. Daily marijuana use among high school seniors was 10 percent in the late 1970s and 3.3 percent in 1987. As the perception among students that marijuana use may be harmful has grown, usage has decreased.[6,7]

CHEMISTRY AND PHYSIOLOGY

Marijuana is derived from the herbaceous plant *Cannabis sativa*. There are over 400 chemical entities in the plant, approximately 60 of which are biologically active.[1,8] Cannabinoids are 21-carbon compounds, most of which are biologically inactive. The principal active constituent of marijuana is delta-9-tetrahydrocannabinol (delta-9-THC). The effects of delta-8-THC are similar to those of delta-9-THC; however, it occurs only in minute amounts in marijuana.[10] Delta-9-THC primarily affects the central nervous system,

influencing diverse neurochemical pathways. To date, no specific receptor site has been discovered for cannabis or delta-9-THC.[9,10] Although the data are somewhat conflicting,[9,11–13] the following brain neurochemical changes seem to occur after THC blood-brain barrier penetration:

1. An increase in catecholamine synthesis[12,13]
2. An alteration of norepinephrine and serotonin uptake at the synaptic level in the hypothalamus, as well as dopamine and GABA synaptic uptake changes in the striatum and cerebral cortex, respectively[14]
3. A dose-related decrease in acetylcholine synthesis and release, most pronounced in the hippocampus[15]

The acute behavioral changes following marijuana intake include decreased attention span and concentration ability, decreased memory, euphoria, excitement, a feeling of calm, dissociation of ideas, relaxation, anxiety, distortion of time, distortion of visual perception, and a decrement in psychomotor performance.[10,16] Acute changes vary among individuals and range from feeling pleasantly relaxed with stream-of-consciousness thought, to feeling anxious, paranoid, and delusional.

Specific behavioral-biochemical associations are difficult to ascertain due to the multitude of effects on various neurochemical pathways in response to delta-9-THC. However, two biochemical effects stand out as important mediators of behavior:

1. Serotonin potentiation and subsequent euphoria and distortion of time and space[17,18]
2. Hippocampal cholinergic changes which may be linked to memory and perceptual dysfunction[19]

Marijuana differs from many other drugs in that it produces both central nervous system excitation and depression, expressed both behaviorally and neurophysiologically.[20–22] The multitude of effects on brain neurochemicals may be, in part, responsible for observed biphasic responses. Additionally, direct neuronal depressive effects may occur independently of the neurochemical changes.[23]

Chronic marijuana use is associated with the development of tolerance,[24] and the user

Table 13-1. SYMPTOMS AND
SIGNS OF MARIJUANA
WITHDRAWAL

Anorexia	Restlessness
Anxiety	Irritability
Agitation	Tremor/tremulousness
Depression	Insomnia
Sweating	Cannabinoid craving

may have the tendency to increase both the dose and frequency of drug use.[4] Tolerance may lead to psychological dependence and in some cases physical dependence.[25] Marijuana is not self-administered with the same intensity as amphetamines, cocaine, or opiates in the animal, but self-administration has been documented in monkeys and rats.[26] In humans, physical dependence in frequent users is associated with symptoms and signs of withdrawal upon discontinuation[25] (Table 13-1). Withdrawal symptoms and signs begin 10 hours after discontinuation, and peak at about 48 hours. Physical dependence and withdrawal, however, are not as consistently observed in animals and man, and the overall evidence for such physiologic changes is less compelling than for other drugs, such as ethanol and opiates.[10]

CLINICAL PHARMACOLOGY

Cannabis sativa is a tall, green, strong-smelling, dioecious plant. It is the female plant which is of interest to the marijuana grower. Typically, the shredded brown mixture referred to as marijuana consists of dried hemp flowers, seeds, leaves, and small stems. The stems and seeds are discarded prior to smoking. In part, the concentration of delta-9-THC depends on the ratio of leaves to flowers. Hashish is derived from the resin of the female flowers. Even more potent than solid hashish is an extract known as hashish oil, which is made by "percolating" cannabis flowers through a fatty solvent. Although marijuana is most commonly smoked, it may be taken orally. When marijuana is smoked, the efficiency of the delivery of delta-9-THC is approximately 20 percent, whereas the systemic bioavailability

following oral administration is about 6 percent.[27,28] Blood levels occur within minutes after the inhalation of a marijuana cigarette; following oral administration, blood levels may not peak for several hours. Peak physiologic and subjective effects occur within 20 to 30 minutes of smoking marijuana, and the subjective effects often last 2 to 4 hours. Following oral ingestion, the onset of subjective effects can be delayed from 30 minutes to as long as 2 hours, and may persist for 3 to 5 hours.[3] Delta-9-THC and the other cannabinoids are highly lipid soluble, rapidly entering the brain and other tissues, particularly adipose tissue. Consequently, blood levels fall very rapidly, reaching levels of 5 to 10 percent of their initial levels in a 1-hour period. Because of its redistribution in the body, the terminal half-life of delta-9-THC in blood is about 20 hours.[16] In the initial distribution phase, blood levels of delta-9-THC and other cannabinoids do not reflect brain levels, but following redistribution, brain levels parallel those in blood.

Delta-9-THC is rapidly metabolized to 11-hydroxytetrahydrocannabinol (THC-OH), which in turn is quickly converted to tetrahydrocannabinol-11-carboxylic acid (THC-COOH) or 8,11-dihydroxytetrahydro-cannabinol (THC-DI-OH). A minority of delta-9-THC is converted to cannabinol. The three significant metabolites found in urine are THC-OH, THC-COOH, and THC-DI-OH.[29] Delta-9-THC and its metabolites are slowly released from the fat depots into the circulation. The half-life of these metabolites is 50 hours or more, with up to 20 percent of the metabolites remaining in the body for 1 week. Complete elimination may take up to 1 month.[16]

Marijuana today is 5 to 10 times more potent than that which was commonly smoked 10 years ago. Hashish may contain 20 to 30 times the amount of delta-9-THC as marijuana per se,[16] and hashish oil may contain substantially higher concentrations of delta-9-THC than hashish.[3,30]

An analysis of the pharmacology of illicit marijuana is complicated by the variations in dosage as well as by the presence of numerous additives and adulterants, for example, phencyclidine (PCP).[3] Similarly, the effects of marijuana on various organ systems are complicated by the presence of contaminants such as paraquat (causing pulmonary fibrosis), insects, aspergilla, and salmonella.[3,31]

Clinical Uses

The therapeutic potential of marijuana has been widely investigated. Marijuana is an effective bronchodilator, decreases intraocular pressure, reduces muscle spasm, and reduces nausea and vomiting in patients receiving chemotherapy. However, other medications are at least as efficacious as marijuana. Synthetic THC has been approved as a Class II drug with antiemetic indications.[32]

USE IN SPORTS

Although marijuana is not perceived as an ergogenic aid, it is the most widely used of all the illicit drugs. In 1975, it was reported that the incidence of marijuana use in athletes was the same as in the general population.[33] In the 1984 Michigan State survey of college athletes, 36 percent of respondents had used marijuana or hashish during the previous year; 54 percent had used the drug at least sometimes with teammates.[34] In the 1986 Elite Women Athletes Survey, 17 percent of responders had used marijuana during the preceding 12 months; 3 percent of Olympic-caliber athletes used marijuana before competition.[35]

Effects on Performance

Many of the acute effects of marijuana are deleterious to athletic performance. Marijuana impairs skills requiring eye-hand coordination and fast reaction time[36-49] and reduces motor coordination, tracking ability, and perceptual accuracy.[2] Additionally, the altered perception of time common with marijuana usage, primarily that time appears to move more slowly,[9] may adversely affect performance. Difficulty in concentrating and dreamlike states are common features of acute marijuana usage,[3] which similarly may impair peak performance. Amphetamines taken in combination with marijuana do not override the adverse psychomotor effects.[50,51]

Although the acute effects of marijuana have been reported to last only 4 hours,[52] Yesavage and associates[53] demonstrated impairment in airplane flying skills for as long as 24 hours after marijuana intoxication, despite the fact that the subjects did not perceive any impairment. This study cast doubt on the commonly held belief that the social use of marijuana the evening prior to an athletic event will not affect performance.

Tachycardia, primarily mediated through changes in vagal tone,[54] is a predictable occurrence following marijuana usage and, acutely, may be deleterious to athletic endurance.[55,56] Although marijuana-induced tachycardia has been implicated as a mechanism to explain the decrease in observed maximal work capacity, other factors must be invoked to explain this decrease. For example, it has been demonstrated that at work loads in excess of 80 percent of maximum effort, no significant difference exists in the heart rates between marijuana users and control subjects.[57] Marijuana induces an increase in metabolic rate which is paralleled by changes in minute ventilation.[31,57]

Marijuana is known to induce bronchodilatation which can last for at least 60 minutes, but this provides no athletic advantage since there is no further bronchodilatation above and beyond that which is normally induced by exercise.[57] However, extensive marijuana smoking has been associated with mild airway obstruction.[31]

Although muscle strength is said to be decreased following marijuana usage,[3,9] specific data relative to athletic performance are lacking.

The "amotivational syndrome" remains one of the most controversial issues surrounding chronic marijuana usage.[3,58] Its potential implications relative to athletic performance are clear. Apathy, impaired judgment, loss of ambition, and an inability to carry out long-term plans characterize the amotivational syndrome. The evidence for a cause-and-effect relationship has been refuted by a number of investigators who contend that such a symptom complex develops only in susceptible individuals.[59-61]

Marijuana is not on the list of substances banned by the International or United States Olympic Committee. The United States Olympic Committee will screen for marijuana when requested by a National Governing Body. Marijuana is banned by the National Collegiate Athletic Association. Collegiate athletes who test positive for marijuana in urine drug screens are subject to penalties for first-time offenses.[62]

Case Vignette

A 19-year-old male college wrestler presented to the emergency room for treatment of a right shoulder dislocation. During a match, the individual uncharacteristically found himself in a quite vulnerable position, and his attempt to remedy the situation led to the acute problem. A friend who observed the match commented that the final move lacked good judgment, which was also uncharacteristic for this particular wrestler. Upon hearing this comment, the wrestler began to cry, and the following story unfolded.

Although always hardworking and intense, he responded negatively to external pressures from coaches, teachers, and his father. His own self-discipline and independence allowed him to achieve relatively good success academically and athletically.

He started smoking marijuana at age 16, and he remembers feeling particularly calm during his first "high." Although he initially smoked only with friends, and only during the weekends, at age 17 he started smoking when alone. Initially, he smoked alone only after working out and completing his studies. Frequently he wrote poetry or read novels while high, and he felt removed from any perceived external pressures.

During the last few months of his senior year in high school, he began smoking marijuana during the day, and he noticed no decrement in his academic or athletic performance. Frequently he smoked half a marijuana cigarette in the morning and at lunch, and another cigarette after dinner. Although he particularly enjoyed the feeling of calm and inner creativity associated with marijuana use, he avoided becoming so high as to lose self-control. Friends, however, began to comment that he was becoming more withdrawn and self-centered.

He continued to smoke during his freshman year in college, including before wrestling practice and matches. The high associated with marijuana smoking seemed to give him a protective bubble in which the external world could not harm him, and he felt

pleasantly "in touch" with his inner feelings. Soon he realized that he spent his entire waking hours under the influence of marijuana, but he rationalized that he felt better able to function, and he felt that he could easily discontinue smoking at any time.

On the day of his injury, he smoked a particularly potent marijuana cigarette, and he felt distinctly uncertain of his visual perceptions and sense of timing. He panicked during the match, and his more experienced opponent easily took advantage of the situation. An ill-fated attempt to escape being pinned led to the shoulder separation.

After spending considerable time with a psychiatrist, the individual agreed to continue outpatient psychotherapy. He not only wanted to discontinue his marijuana habit but also agreed that he needed to understand and deal more effectively with the insecurity of facing the world while not intoxicated.

ADVERSE EFFECTS

The issues relative to the adverse health effects of marijuana have too often been clouded by the commingling of emotion and science. Hollister's "Health aspects of cannabis"[3] is an excellent review of this subject. Table 13–2 summarizes the adverse effects of marijuana usage.

Acute behavioral manifestations following marijuana use have included paranoia, panic attacks, delirium, and psychoses.[3] Neuroleptics and hospitalization may be required, but the behavioral changes are felt to be reversible. The amotivational syndrome, described previously, probably occurs only in susceptible individuals. A report describing cerebral atrophy in chronic marijuana users[63] has been refuted by Co and associates.[64]

Rhinitis, pharyngitis, bronchitis, and bronchospasm have been documented in marines who smoked hashish. Symptoms may be present in up to 75 percent of frequent users, but may be related to the high combustion temperature with hashish usage.[65] Chronic inhalation of marijuana may cause both bronchitis and squamous metaplasia,[66] but to date there is no documented case of associated lung cancer. Marijuana impurities such

Table 13–2. ADVERSE EFFECTS OF MARIJUANA

Neuropsychiatric	*Immunological*
Panic attack	Impaired cell-mediated immunity
Delirium	Impaired monocyte maturation
Psychosis	
?Amotivational syndrome	*Endocrine*
	Decreased sperm production
Respiratory	Inhibition of ovulation
Rhinitis	Gynecomastia
Pharyngitis	
Bronchitis	*Cardiovascular*
Bronchospasm	Tachycardia
Bronchial squamous metaplasia	Orthostatic hypotension
Pulmonary fibrosis	Increased carboxyhemoglobin
Pneumomediastinum	

as paraquat may result in pulmonary fibrosis.[3] Holding marijuana smoke in the lungs at total lung capacity has caused pneumomediastinum.[66] Compared with cigarette smoking, smoking marijuana is associated with a threefold increase in the amount of tar (insoluble particulate) inhaled, and a one-third increase in respiratory tract retention of that tar.[67]

Cell-mediated immunity may be impaired from marijuana usage, but the clinical significance of the immune impairment is not clear.[3] Marijuana may stimulate the development of immature monocytes but appears to block the development of fully mature cells.[68]

Decreased sperm production and inhibition of ovulation may occur following marijuana use, but infertility has not been substantiated.[3] Gynecomastia has been documented in male marijuana users and is reversible upon discontinuation of the drug.[69]

Tachycardia and orthostatic hypotension may develop acutely after marijuana ingestion, but tolerance to these effects may develop with chronic use.[3] Carboxyhemoglobin saturation increases nearly threefold after smoking a marijuana cigarette, which is a five-fold greater increment than from smoking a single filter-tipped tobacco cigarette.[67]

Though the debate regarding the medical risks of marijuana usage and its sociologic implications continues, the athlete should bear in mind that the potential contaminants and adulterants in marijuana may exceed even the most deleterious effects of the cannabinoids themselves.[3]

FINAL NOTE

Presumably marijuana is banned by the National Collegiate Athletic Association, certain National Governing Bodies, and by some professional sports organizations on the basis that it is an illegal substance, and one can argue that all illegal activities should be banned from sports. Marijuana has no ergogenic potential and therefore ergogenicity can not be advanced as a basis for banning its use. Banning the use of marijuana in order to protect the health and well-being of the athlete is a less compelling argument, unless similar rules are made for alcohol and tobacco. Credibility dictates that the basis for banning marijuana be clearly articulated.

REFERENCES

1. Stwertka, E and Stwertka, A: Marijuana, ed 2. A First Book, New York, 1986.
2. Polich, JM, et al: Strategies for Controlling Drug Abuse. The Rand Corporation, Santa Monica, CA, 1984.
3. Hollister, L: Health aspects of cannabis. Pharmacol Rev 38:1, 1986.
4. Mendelson, JH: Marijuana. In Meltzer, HY (ed): Psychopharmacology: The Third Generation of Progress. Raven Press, New York, 1987, p 1565.
5. Gallagher, W: Marijuana. American Health, March 1988, p 92.
6. Johnston, L and Bachman, J: The Monitoring The

Future Study. Institute for Social Research. The University of Michigan, 1988.

7. Semlitz, L and Gold, MS: Adolescent Drug Abuse: Diagnosis, Treatment, and Prevention. Psychiatr Clin North Am 9:455, 1986.

8. Tuner, V: Marihuana and cannabis: Research: Why the conflict? In Harvey, DJ (ed): Marihuana '84. IRL Press, Oxford, 1985, p 31.

9. Jaffe, JH: Drug addiction and drug abuse. In Gilman, AG, et al (eds): Goodman and Gilman's The Pharmacological Basis of Therapeutics, ed 7. Macmillan, New York, 1985, p 532.

10. Dewey, W: Cannabinoid pharmacology. Pharmacol Rev 38:151, 1986.

11. Maitre, L, Staehelin, M and Bein, H: Effect of an extract of cannabis and some cannabinols on catecholamine metabolism in rat brain and heart. Agents Action 1:136, 1970.

12. Bloom, A, Johnson, K and Dewey, W: The effects of cannabinoids on body temperature and brain catecholamine synthesis. Res Commun Chem Path Pharmacol, 20:51, 1978.

13. Bloom, A and Kiernan, C: Interaction of ambient temperature with the effects of delta-9-tetrahydrocannabinol on brain catecholamine synthesis and plasma corticosterone levels. Psychopharm 67:215, 1980.

14. Banerjee, S, Snyder, S and Mechoulam, R: Cannabinoids: Influence on neurotransmitter uptake in rat brain synaptosomes. Pharm Exp Ther 194:74, 1975.

15. Tripathi, H, Vocci, F and Dewey, W: Effect of cannabinoids on cholinergic systems in various regions of the mouse brain. Fed Proc 38:590, 1979.

16. Jones, R: Marijuana: Health and treatment issues. Psychiatr Clin North Am 7:703, 1984.

17. Johnson, K, Dewey, W and Harris, L: Some structural requirements for inhibition of high-affinity synaptosomal serotonin uptake by cannabinoids. Mol Pharmacol 12:345, 1976.

18. Carpenter, M and Sutin, J: Human Neuroanatomy. Williams & Wilkins, Baltimore, 1983, p 406.

19. Domino, E, Donelson, A and Tuttle, T: Effects of delta-9-tetrahydrocannabinol on regional brain acetylcholine. In Jenden, DJ (ed): Cholinergic Mechanism and Psychopharmacology. Plenum Publishing Co., New York, 1978, p 673.

20. Karler, R and Turkanis, S: The cannabinoids as potential antiepileptics. J Clin Pharmacol 21:4375, 1981.

21. Paton, W: Pharmacology of marijuana. Ann Rev Pharmacol 15:191, 1975.

22. Turkanis, S and Karler, R: Electrophysiologic properties of cannabinoids. J Clin Pharmacol 21:4495, 1981.

23. Turkanis, S and Karler, R: Electrophysiologic mechanisms and loci of delta-9-tetrahydrocannabinol caused CNS depression. In Harvey, D (ed): Marihuana '84. IRL Press, Oxford, 1985, p 233.

24. McMillan, DE, et al: Tolerance to active constituents of marijuana. Arch Int Pharmacolyn Ther 198:132, 1972.

25. Tennant, FS: The clinical syndrome of marijuana dependence. Psychiatric Annals 16:226, 1986.

26. Kaymakcalan, S: The addictive potential of cannabis. Bull Narc 33:21, 1981.

27. Lindgren, J, et al: Clinical effects of plasma levels of delta-9-tetrahydrocannabinol in heavy and light users of cannabis. Psychopharmacol 74:208, 1980.

28. Ohlsson, A, et al: Plasma delta-9-tetrahydrocannabinol concentration and clinical effects after oral and intravenous administration and smoking. Clin Pharmacol Ther 28:409, 1980.

29. Moyer, TP: Laboratory medicine. Marijuana testing—How good is it? Mayo Clin Proc 62:413, 1987.

30. Kulberg, A: Substance abuse: Clinical identification and management. Pediatr Clin North Am 33:325, 1986.

31. Biron, S and Well, J: Marijuana and its effect on the athlete. Athlete Training, Winter, 1983, p 295.

32. From the FDA: Dronabinol, a synthetic THC, approved as a class II drug with antiemetic indication. JAMA 256:817, 1986.

33. Corder, B, Dezelsky, T and Tochey, J: Trends in drug abuse behavior at ten central Arizona high schools. Ariz Health Phys Ed Recreat 19:10, 1975.

34. Anderson, WA and McKeag, DB: The Substance Use and Abuse Habits of College Student Athletes. Research Paper no. 2. General Findings. Presented to NCAA Drug Education Committee by the College of Human Medicine, Michigan State University, June, 1985.

35. Elite Women Athletes Survey. Hazelden Health Promotion Services, Minneapolis, January, 1987.

36. Borg, J: The effects of smoked marijuana on human cognitive and motor functions. Psychopharm 29:159, 1973.

37. Clark, L: Behavioral effects of marijuana: Experimental studies. Arch Gen Psychiatry 28:193, 1970.

38. Dornbush, R: Marijuana, memory, and perception. Am J Psychiatry 128:194, 1971.

39. Moskowitz, H: Effect of marijuana on the psychological refractory period. Percept Mot Skills 38:959, 1974.

40. Peeke, S: Effects of practice on marijuana-induced changes in reaction time. Psychopharm 48:159, 1976.

41. Milstein, S: Marijuana-produced impairments in coordination. Nervous Ment Dis 161:26, 1975.

42. Kiplinger, G: Dose-response analysis of the effects of tetrahydrocannabinol in man. Clin Pharmacol Ther 12:650, 1971.

43. Abel, E: Effects of marijuana on the solution of anagrams, memory, and appetite. Nature 231:260, 1971.

44. Abel, E: Marijuana and memory. Nature 227:1151, 1970.

45. Belmore, S and Miller, L: Levels of processing and acute effects of marijuana on memory. Pharm Biochem Behav 13:199, 1980.

46. Dittrich, A: Effects of (−) delta-9-tetrahydrocannabinol on memory, attention and subjective state. Psychopharm 33:369, 1973.

47. Casswell, S and Marks, D: Cannabis induced impairment of performance of a divided attention task. Nature 241:60, 1973.

48. Jones, R and Stone, G: Psychological studies of marijuana and alcohol in man. Psychopharm 18:108, 1970.

49. Sharma, S and Moskowitz, H: Effects of two levels of attention demand on vigilance performance under marijuana. Percept Mot Skills 38:967, 1974.

50. Forney, R, et al: The combined effect of marihuana

and dextroamphetamine. Ann NY Acad Sci 281:162, 1976.

51. Evans, M, et al: Effects of marijuana-dextroamphetamine combination. Clin Pharmacol Ther 20:350, 1976.

52. Janowski, D, et al: Marijuana effects on simulated flying ability. Am J Psychiatry 133:384, 1976.

53. Yesavage, J, et al: "Hangover" effects of marijuana intoxication on aircraft pilot performance. Am J Psychiatry 142:1325, 1985.

54. Clark, S, et al: Cardiovascular effects of marijuana in man. Am J Psychiat 142:1325, 1985.

55. Aronow, W and Cassidy, J: Effect of marijuana and placebo marijuana on angina pectoris. N Engl J Med 291:65, 1974.

56. Shapiro, B: Cardiopulmonary effects of marijuana smoking during exercise. Chest 70:441, 1976.

57. Renaud, A and Cornmier, Y: Acute effects of marihuana smoking on maximal exercise performance. Med Sci Sports Exer 18:685, 1986.

58. Smith, D: The acute and chronic toxicity of marijuana. Psychedelic Drugs 2:347, 1968.

59. Carter, W and Doughty, P: Social and cultural aspects of cannabis use in Costa Rica. Ann NY Acad Sci 282:2, 1976.

60. Coitas, L: Cannabis and work in Jamaica: A refutation of the amotivational syndrome. Ann NY Acad Sci 282:24, 1976.

61. Mellinger, G, et al: The amotivational syndrome and the college student. Ann NY Acad Sci 282:37, 1976.

62. NCAA and USOC Rule differences. Sports Mediscope 7:4, 1988.

63. Campbell, A: Cerebral atrophy in young cannabis smokers. Lancet 2:1219, 1971.

64. Co, B, et al: Absence of cerebral atrophy in chronic cannabis users: Evaluation by computerized transaxial tomography. JAMA 237:1229, 1977.

65. Fisher, M and Glassroth, J: The respiratory effects of marijuana and hashish. Int Med 9:140, 1988.

66. Henderson, R, Tennant, F and Guerney, R: Respiratory manifestations of hashish smoking. Arch Otolaryngol 95:248, 1972.

67. Wu, TC, et al: Pulmonary hazards of smoking marijuana as compared with tobacco. New Engl J Med 318:347, 1988.

68. Stockwell, S: Marijuana's ability to impair immune system is clarified. Oncology Times 10(1):1, 1988.

69. Bracker MD, et al: College wrestler with unilateral gynecomastia. Phy Sportsmed 15(12):115, 1987.

CHAPTER 14

Narcotics

HISTORY

Opium, derived from the poppy plant, *Papaver somniferum*, is one of the oldest substances known to mankind. Ideographs of the ancient Sumerians suggest that its psychologic effects may have been known around 4000 B.C. The Egyptians described the medicinal value of the opium poppy in 1552 B.C. However, the first reference to the actual juice of the poppy appeared in the 3rd century B.C. writings of Theophrastus. The term opium is derived from the Greek word for juice and refers to the juice of the poppy capsule.[1,2,2a]

In the 8th and 9th centuries A.D., Arabian traders introduced opium to the Orient, where it was frequently used to control dysentery. However, its medical use could never be completely separated from its "recreational" use. Opium made its appearance in Western Europe in the 11th and 12th centuries. It was in 1520 that Paracelsus was credited with compounding laudanum—a mixture of opium, wine, and spices. Laudanum, in one form or another, is still used today to treat a variety of ailments.[2a]

For as many as 800 years after its introduction into China, opium, taken orally, was used almost exclusively as a pain killer and as a treatment for dysentery. However, by the end of the 18th century, the smoking of opium for its psychic effect became commonplace. Soon China's demand for opium grew. The demand was met by English traders who initially traded opium for Chinese tea, and later traded it for silver. Large quantities of opium flooded China, large quantities of silver left, and opium smoking escalated. These events soon led to the famous Opium Wars, in which Western nations tried to maintain their lucrative "right" to supply opium to China.[2a]

While opium was smoked in China, opium eating and opium drinking (laudanum) became the way of the middle class in England. Supplies of opium were virtually unlimited, and the medical community was divided about any potential harm that might result from opium use. Like cocaine, opium was found in patent medicines and even in food-stuffs. As with cocaine, there were authors and poets who proclaimed that opium enhanced the creative process. Samuel Taylor Coleridge's "The Rime of the Ancient Mariner" and "Kubla Khan" were written while he was under the influence of laudanum, as was Wilkie Collins's classic detective novel, *The Moonstone*.[2a]

Opium smoking in the United States was initially believed to be a problem limited to Oriental immigrants. However, opium eating and opium drinking, and even opium cultivation, became commonplace in 19th century America. Again, like cocaine, opium was readily available in drug stores. The 1897 edition of the Sears and Roebuck catalogue even advertised laudanum for 6 cents an ounce.[1,2,2a]

In 1803, Freidrich Sertuner isolated morphine, the primary active ingredient of opium. Morphine is named after Morpheus, the Greek god of dreams. Like opium, morphine was incorporated into a variety of patent medicines. However, it was the invention of the hypodermic syringe in 1856 that paved the way for the development of morphine addiction, one legacy of the Civil War. As syringes became increasingly available, both the use of morphine and the problem of morphine addiction increased.[1,2,2a]

By 1898, the problem of narcotic addiction was compounded by the discovery of heroin (diacetylmorphine), a semisynthetic opiate more potent than morphine. At the time of its introduction into clinical medicine, heroin, like other narcotics that followed, was heralded for its potency and its lack of addictive qualities.[3] However, heroin proved to be significantly more addicting than morphine itself.[2a]

Recognizing the problem of opiate addiction, the United States enacted the Harrison Narcotics Act of 1914. This congressional act prohibited opium, heroin, and morphine, as well as other drugs such as cocaine, from nonprescription preparations. Additionally,

it made the possession of opium or its derivatives without a prescription a criminal offense.[2a]

Heroin use in the United States surged in the late 1960s, and by the 1970s had spread to suburbia.[4] By 1982, the trend had reversed and heroin was being used by young adults less frequently (1.2 percent tried it at least once as contrasted with 3.5 percent in 1979). Among high school seniors in 1987, the annual prevalency rate of heroin use was 0.5 percent, and for other opiates 5.0 percent.[5] However, such statistics do not necessarily reflect the reality of inner-city opiate use. In New York State alone there are 285,000 regular heroin abusers. It is estimated that there are over one-half million untreated heroin addicts nationwide.[6] Intravenous heroin use carries with it a major societal threat: in New York City, 50 to 60 percent of intravenous drug abusers are thought to be seropositive for human immunodeficiency virus.[7]

In 1983, the three most commonly prescribed drugs requiring use of the triplicate prescription procedure of New York State were narcotics: oxycodone (Percodan), meperidine (Demerol), and hydromorphone (Dilaudid).[6] In New York State, codeine, one of the most frequently prescribed narcotics, does not require a triplicate prescription.

CHEMISTRY AND PHYSIOLOGY

Morphine is representative of the narcotic analgesics and is one of approximately 20 alkaloids derived from opium. The complex structure of morphine prevented its elucidation until 1925, and its synthesis until 1952.[4]

Morphine exerts its primary effects on the central nervous system and the gastrointestinal tract,[4] both mediated through specific opioid receptors. The concept of opioid receptors, and subclasses of opioid receptors, led to the discovery of multiple endogenous opioids located in various regions of the central nervous system[8] (Table 14–1). Morphine-like drugs thus appear to take advantage of an innate central nervous system complex which modulates pain, emotions, and other functions.

The subclasses of opioid receptors correlate with some of the known endogenous opioids (Table 14–2). For example, the mu 1 receptor is a high-affinity, nonselective opioid receptor which binds morphine-like drugs as well as the endogenous opioids. Mu

Table 14–1. SOME ENDOGENOUS
OPIATE PEPTIDES

Leu-enkephalin
Met-enkephalin
Beta-endorphin
Dynorphin A
Dynorphin B
Alpha-neo-endorphin
Beta-neo-endorphin

In the central nervous system, opioid receptors are localized almost exclusively in the gray matter. The greatest concentration of receptors occurs in the periaqueductal gray, limbic cortex, hypothalamus, and the basal ganglia.[8]

Morphine and the opioids do not alter the threshold of responsivity of afferent peripheral nerve endings to noxious stimuli, nor do they impair the conduction of nerve impulses. Rather, alterations probably occur at the various levels of sensory integration, beginning in the spinal cord. Through receptor binding, the central release of neurotransmitters can be altered, with subsequent attenuation in pain perception.[11]

Morphine and other narcotics primarily cause analgesia, euphoria or dysphoria, drowsiness, mental clouding, and decreased bowel motility. In higher doses, muscular ri-

2 preferentially binds morphine rather than enkephalins. The selectivity of the delta receptor is for endogenous enkephalins and enkephalin-like drugs.[8,9] Both spinal and supraspinal receptor sites exist in the CNS, the delta site being an example of a primary spinal receptor.[10]

Table 14–2. TENTATIVE CLASSIFICATION OF OPIATE RECEPTOR SUBTYPES
AND ACTIONS*

Subtype	Prototypic Drugs	Proposed Actions
mu		
mu_1	Opiates and most opioid peptides	Supraspinal analgesia: including periaqueductal gray, nucleus raphe magnus, and locus coeruleus Prolactin release Free feeding and deprivation-induced feeding Acetylcholine turnover in the brain Catalepsy
mu_2	Morphine sulfate	Respiratory depression Growth hormone release (?) Dopamine turnover in the brain Gastrointestinal tract transit Guinea pig ileum bioassay Feeding Most cardiovascular effects
delta	Enkephalins	Spinal analgesia Dopamine turnover in the brain Mouse vas deferens bioassay Growth hormone release (?) Feeding
kappa	Ketocyclazocine and dynorphin	Spinal analgesia Inhibition of antidiuretic hormone release Sedation Feeding
epsilon	β-Endorphin	Rat vas deferens bioassay Hormone (?)
sigma	N-allylnormetazocine (SKF 10,047)	Psychotomimetic effects Linked to N-methyl-D-aspartate

*From Pasternak, GW: Multiple morphine and enkephalin receptors and the relief of pain. JAMA 259:1364, 1988, with permission.

Table 14–3. OPIATE
WITHDRAWAL SYNDROME

Purposeful drug-seeking behavior
Lacrimation
Rhinorrhea
Yawning
Sweating
Restlessness
Mydriasis
Tremor
Nausea
Vomiting
Diarrhea
Tachycardia
Hypertension
Piloerection
Muscle cramps/spasms
Generalized CNS hyperexcitability
Potential cardiovascular collapse

Table 14–4. EXAMPLES OF
NARCOTIC AGONIST AND MIXED
AGONIST-ANTAGONIST DRUGS

Narcotic Agonists
Morphine
Heroin
Hydromorphone (Dilaudid)
Codeine
Oxycodone (Percocet, Percodan)
Levorphanol (Levo-Dromoran)
Meperidine (Demerol)
Methadone
Propoxyphene (Darvon)

Mixed Narcotic Agonist-Antagonists
Pentazocine (Talwin)
Nalbuphine (Nubain)
Butorphanol (Stadol)

gidity, respiratory depression, and hypotension can occur.[12] The primary clinical effects correlate well with the concentration of receptors in the periaqueductal gray, limbic cortex, and gastrointestinal tract.

The specificity of certain receptors allows for the possibility of developing selectively acting analgesic drugs, thereby minimizing or eliminating unwanted side effects. It also allows for the possibility of using multiple drugs in the treatment of chronic pain on a rotating basis, thereby avoiding the development of tolerance.[13]

Reinforcing effects of opiates may be receptor dependent. For example, mu agonist compounds are likely to be self-administered in animals, but kappa agonists fail to maintain such reinforced behavior.[14] Tolerance may develop quickly with frequent opiate use, necessitating an increase in dosage in order to obtain the desired clinical effect. Repeat administration of opiate compounds is associated with physiologic dependence.[4] Once dependence occurs, discontinuation of opiates leads to withdrawal symptoms and signs (Table 14–3). Opiate withdrawal may be fatal if significant dehydration and autonomic hyperexcitability occur.

CLINICAL PHARMACOLOGY

Narcotics may be pure agonists or both agonist-antagonists (Table 14–4). The available prescription narcotics in the United States do not currently take advantage of opioid receptor site selectivity, so analgesia is accompanied by side effects such as mental clouding and potential respiratory depression.

The more commonly used oral narcotics for mild to moderate pain are shown in Table 14–5, along with the equianalgesic doses of commonly used oral non-narcotics.[15]

The time of peak analgesia following oral narcotic use ranges from 1 to 2 hours, and the duration of action is generally from 3 to 6 hours.[12,16] With the narcotics enumerated in Table 14–5, tissue buildup normally does not occur, but in others, such as methadone (half-life 15 to 30 hours) and levorphanol (Levo-Dromoran) (half-life 12 to 16 hours), accumulation may occur, leading to untoward effects of sedation and respiratory depression with repetitive dosing.[12,16]

Metabolism of the opioids primarily occurs in the liver through conjugation with glucuronic acid, with excretion largely in the urine in the conjugated form.[15] N-demethylation is also a significant biotransformation step for many opiate drugs, most notably meperidine and propoxyphene.[12]

Clinical Uses

Narcotics have their principal clinical use in the management of moderate to severe pain. The opiates remain among the most effective agents available for suppressing

Table 14–5. EQUIANALGESIC **ORAL** DOSE OF SOME COMMONLY USED NARCOTIC AND NON-NARCOTIC DRUGS

Drug	Equianalgesic Oral Dose
Narcotic	
Morphine	6 mg
Codeine	32–65 mg
Propoxyphene	65–130 mg
Oxycodone	5 mg
Meperidine	50 mg
Pentazocine	50 mg
Non-Narcotic	
Aspirin	650 mg
Acetaminophen	650 mg
Ibuprofen	200–400 mg

cough and diarrhea. They serve as useful adjuncts in the management of the dyspnea associated with acute left ventricular failure (pulmonary edema). Their effectiveness in this setting, although not entirely clear, probably relates to allaying anxiety, relieving pain, and causing venous pooling.[12,17] Methadone is used in the management of heroin addiction.

USE IN SPORTS

Narcotics are not perceived as ergogenic drugs. However, their use, misuse, and abuse potential in sports may be high because of pressures on the athlete to perform competitively despite varied musculoskeletal injuries. In the 1984 Michigan State study of NCAA athletes, 28 percent of respondents had used "major pain medications" within the prior 12 months. Most often these medications were obtained from a team physician (31 percent) or another physician (46 percent). Twelve percent received these drugs from a coach or a trainer, and 10 percent from a teammate or a friend. The vast majority (67 percent) stated that they used these drugs for sports-related injuries, and 27 percent used it for injuries unrelated to sports. Only 1 percent used these drugs in an effort to enhance performance, and 6 percent claimed they use "major pain medications" for "social or personal reasons."[18] In the 1986 Elite Women Athletes Survey, 11 percent of responders reported using narcotics

either during the sports season or off-season.[19]

Effects on Performance

Although, a priori, it would seem that chronic narcotic usage would lead to an impairment of athletic skills, the available evidence does not necessarily support this assumption. In chronic abusers of narcotics, several studies have failed to demonstrate a significant difference between age-matched controls and addicts with regard to motor strength, rapid alternating movements, eye-hand coordination, visual perception, and cognitive skills.[20–22] The effects of narcotics on endurance have not been specifically assessed. Other studies have shown that when standard clinical doses of narcotics are used chronically, no significant changes are seen in cognition, memory, visual-perceptual-spatial skills, or in motor function tasks.[23,24]

In a comparative study between narcotic addicts and long-term benzodiazepine users, significant cognitive impairment was noted in the benzodiazepine users when compared to both the narcotic addicts and controls.[25]

Used acutely in naive subjects, the narcotic analgesics share with morphine the ability to produce a number of adverse psychomotor effects. Generally dose related, these include, but are not limited to, sedation, drowsiness, clouding of the sensorium, changes in mood, difficulty in mentation, apathy, euphoria, dysphoria, reduced visual acuity, nausea, and vomiting.[12,16,17,26] Though it would appear that these acute adverse effects would adversely affect athletic performance, no studies have reported on this issue.

In individuals taking narcotics chronically, tolerance is well known to occur within days of the initial treatment[27] and can lead to escalating doses and eventual addiction. On the other hand, narcotic dependence, both physical and psychological, is very unlikely following the short-term use of even high doses of narcotics when they are used for the management of severe pain.[17,27] The issues of tolerance and dependency may be obviated by the use of equianalgesic doses of nonsteroidal anti-inflammatory drugs for the treatment of pain associated with musculoskeletal strains and sprains and related problems.[28–30] If a decision, whatever the reason, is made to treat acute pain with a narcotic, the dose can be minimized when the narcotic is used in conjunction with non-narcotic or adjuvant analgesic drugs.[27,31,32]

As is true with the use of narcotics in general and perhaps even more so with athletes intent on performing in the face of injury, narcotics may serve to mask serious mechanical and medical problems resulting in more serious long-term sequelae.[33]

Codeine is banned by the United States Olympic Committee but not by the National Collegiate Athletic Association.[33] Heroin and other narcotics are banned by some professional sports organizations (see Appendices).

Table 14–6. ADVERSE EFFECTS OF NARCOTICS

Nausea
Vomiting
Dizziness
Mental clouding
Dysphoria
Pruritus
Constipation
Delirium
Addiction/withdrawal
Seizures
Parkinsonism (MPTP)

Case Vignette

A 38-year-old male weight lifter presented to the physician's office with complaints of right arm pain and a lump in the region of the biceps muscle.

The patient had been a bodybuilder for several years, and he had used anabolic steroids for approximately 6 years, although he denied any anabolic steroid use during the prior 3 years. He dedicated 2 to 3 hours daily to various exercises, and he lifted weights 3 times per week.

For 1 year the patient noticed right shoulder pain which was made worse with shoulder movement or right arm weight bearing. He responded well initially to nonsteroidal anti-inflammatory drugs, but the pain became more intense during the 2 months prior to evaluation. He began taking acetaminophen with codeine and alternated this with nonsteroidal anti-inflammatory drugs. Although the pain persisted, he was able to continue his weight-training routine.

During the month prior to evaluation, the patient ingested 1,200 to 1,600 mg per day of ibuprofen, 2,600 mg per day of acetaminophen, and 240 to 480 mg per day of codeine. Despite the drug regimen, the pain persisted. The patient was determined to continue lifting weights, so he usually took Tylenol #4 (acetaminophen 325 mg plus codeine 60 mg), 3 to 4 tablets just prior to and after his weight-lifting workout. This drug regimen allowed him to complete a full workout with minimal pain. On the day of evaluation, he developed acute pain in the right biceps region along with a sensation of a "pop." Clinical evaluation revealed a rup-

ture of the long head of the right biceps tendon.

ADVERSE EFFECTS

Adverse effects of narcotics are listed in Table 14–6. Acute effects in naive subjects may include nausea, vomiting, dizziness, mental clouding, dysphoria, pruritus, constipation, and delirium.[12,34,35] Chronic narcotic use leads to addiction, and discontinuation may cause withdrawal symptoms and signs. Accumulation of N-demethylated metabolites may result in central nervous excitation and seizures.[12] Recently, a new synthetic meperidine analogue, 1-methyl-4-phenyl-1,2,3,6-tetrahydropyridine (MPTP) has appeared in the illicit drug market. Its frighteningly adverse effect is to produce destructive lesions of the substantia nigra and locus ceruleus, leading to severe parkinsonism.[36–39]

FINAL NOTE

The issues of performance enhancement and pleasure seeking have been less dramatized with respect to narcotic use among competitive athletes. The potential abuse, nonetheless, of narcotic analgesics among athletes is a serious concern. Musculoskeletal injuries are commonplace, and the need to perform despite pain is a pressure felt by almost all athletes. It is in this setting that narcotic analgesics may potentially ruin an athlete's career. Decreased awareness and concern for pain are the desired clinical effects of narcotics but can cause a feeling of invincibility, which in turn can lead to serious misuse of the body. Athletes, coaches, trainers, and team physicians need to be aware of the seriousness of masking pain perception in order to continue athletic performance.

The rationale for drug testing for both illicit and licit narcotic drugs must be clearly defined. As with other illicit drugs, their use, per se, can understandably be a justification for drug testing. On the other hand, if the prevention of enhanced performance through the reduction of pain is to be the basis for drug testing, then this needs to be considered within the context of other pain relief methods, for example, the use of anti-inflammatory drugs and the use of injectable anesthetics. The United States Olympic Committee has addressed the latter issue, and prohibits the use of intravenous, intramuscular, or intra-articular anesthetic injections.

REFERENCES

 1. Polich, JM, et al: Strategies for Controlling Drug Abuse. The Rand Corporation, Santa Monica, CA, 1984.
 2. Jaffe, JH: Opioid dependence. In Kaplan, HI and Saddock, BJ (eds): Comprehensive Textbook of Psychiatry IV, ed 4. Williams & Wilkins, Baltimore, 1985, p 1008.
2a. Levinthal, CF: Messengers of Paradise—Opiates and the Brain. Anchor Press, Doubleday, New York, 1988.
 3. Gomez, L: Cocaine—America's 100 Years of Euphoria and Despair. Life Magazine, May 1984.
 4. Jaffe, JH: Drug addiction and drug abuse. In Gilman, AG, et al (eds): Goodman and Gilman's The Pharmacological Basis of Therapeutics, ed 7. Macmillan, New York, 1985, p 532.
 5. Johnston, L and Bachman, J: The Monitoring the Future Study. Institute for Social Research. The University of Michigan, Ann Arbor, 1988.
 6. Kreek, MJ: Multiple drug abuse patterns and medical consequences. In Meltzer, HY (ed): Psychopharmacology: The Third Generation of Progress. Raven Press, New York, 1987, p 1597.
 7. Jordan, KG: Coping with AIDS. The special problems of New York City. New Engl J Med 317:1469, 1987.
 8. Pasternak, G and Childers, S: The actions of opioids and opioid peptides. In Recent Advances in Clinical Pharmacology, vol 3. Churchill Livingstone, New York, 1983, p 253.
 9. Pasternak, G: High and low affinity opioid binding sites: Relationship to mu and delta sites. Life Sciences 31:1303, 1982.
10. Ling, G and Pasternak, G: Spinal and supraspinal

opioid analgesia in the mouse: The role of subpopulations of opioid bindings sites. Brain Res 271:152, 1983.
11. Payne, R: Anatomy and physiology of cancer pain. In Management of Cancer Pain, Syllabus of Postgraduate Course. Memorial Sloan Kettering Cancer Center, New York, 1985, p 1.
12. Jaffe, JH and Martin, WR: Opioid analgesics and antagonists. In Gilman, AG, et al (eds): Goodman and Gilman's The Pharmacological Basis of Therapeutics, ed 7. Macmillan, New York, 1985, p 491.
13. Pasternak, G: Neuropharmacology of pain. In Management of Cancer Pain, Syllabus of Postgraduate Course. Memorial Sloan Kettering Cancer Center, New York, 1985, p 111.
14. Woods, JH and Winger, G: Opioids, receptors, and abuse liability. In Meltzer, HY (ed): Psychopharmacology: The Third Generation of Progress. Raven Press, New York, 1987, p 1555.
15. Inturrisi, C: Non-Narcotic and narcotic analgesics: Principles. In Management of Cancer Pain, Syllabus of Postgraduate Course. Memorial Sloan Kettering Cancer Center, New York, 1985, p 111.
16. Inturrisi, CE: Role of opioid analgesics. Am J Med (Suppl) 77:27, 1984.
17. American Medical Association Department of Drugs, Division of Drugs and Technology: General Analgesias. In AMA Drug Evaluations, ed 6. WB Saunders, Philadelphia, 1986, p 53.
18. Anderson, WA and McKeag, DB: The Substance Use and Abuse Habits of College Student Athletes. Research Paper No. 2. General Findings. Presented to NCAA Drug Education Committee, College of Human Medicine, Michigan State University, June, 1985.
19. Elite Women Athletes Survey. Hazelden Health Promotion Services, Minneapolis, January, 1987.
20. Rounsaville, B, et al: Neurophysiological functioning in opiate addicts. J Nervous Mental Dis 170:209, 1982.
21. Brown, R and Partington, J: A psychometric comparison of narcotic addicts with hospital attendants. J Gen Psychol 27:71, 1942.
22. Bruhn, P and Maage, N: Intellectual and neuropsychological functions in young men with heavy and long-term patterns of drug abuse. Am J Psychiatry 132:397, 1975.
23. Ghoneim, M, Mewaldt, S and Thatcher, J: The effect of diazepam and fentanyl on mental, psychomotor and electroencephalographic functions and their rate of recovery. Psychopharm 44:61, 1975.
24. Lombardo, W, Lombardo, B and Goldstein, A: Cognitive functioning under moderate low dose methadone maintenance. Int J Addict 2:389, 1976.
25. Hendler, N, et al: A comparison of cognitive impairment due to benzodiazepines and to narcotics. Am J Psychiatry 137:828, 1980.
26. Inturrisi, CE: Narcotic drugs. Med Clin North Am 66:1061, 1982.
27. Foley, K: The practical use of narcotic analgesics. Med Clin North Am 1976:389, 1982.
28. Indelicato, P: Comparison of diflunisal and acetaminophen with codeine in the treatment of mild to moderate pain due to strains and sprains. Clin Ther 8:269, 1986.
29. Aghababian, RV: Comparison of diflunisal and ac-

etaminophen with codeine in the management of grade 2 ankle sprain. Clin Ther 8:520, 1986.

30. Indelicato, PA: Efficacy of diflunisal versus acetaminophen with codeine in controlling mild to moderate pain after arthroscopy. Clin Ther 8:164, 1986.
31. Beaver, WT: Combination analgesics. Am J Med (Suppl) 77:38, 1984.
32. Kantor, TG: Control of pain by nonsteroidal anti-inflammatory drugs. Med Clin North Am 66:1053, 1982.
33. NCAA and USOC rule differences. Sports Mediscope 7:4, 1988.
34. Khantzian, EJ and McKenna, GJ: Acute toxic and withdrawal reactions associated with drug use and abuse. Ann Intern Med 90:361, 1979.
35. Gold, MS and Estroff, TW: The comprehensive evaluation of cocaine and opiate abusers. In Hall, RCW

and Beresford, R (eds): Handbook of Psychiatric Diagnostic Procedures, vol. 2. Spectrum Publications, Inc., Englewood Cliffs, 1984, p 213.

36. Ziporyn, T: A growing industry and menace: Makeshift laboratory's designer drugs. JAMA 265:3061, 1986.
37. Burns, RS, et al: The clinical syndrome of striatal dopamine deficiency. Parkinsonism induced by 1-methyl-4-phenyl-1,2,3,6-tetrahydropyridine (MPTP). N Engl J Med 312:1418, 1985.
38. Ballard, PA, Tetrud, JW and Langston, JW: Permanent human parkinsonism due to 1-methyl-4-phenyl-1,2,3,6-tetrahydropyridine (MPTP): Seven cases. Neurology 35:949, 1985.
39. Forno, LS, et al: Locus ceruleus lesions and eosinophilic inclusions in MPTP-treated monkeys. Ann Neurol 20:449, 1986.

CHAPTER 15

Miscellaneous

BETA BLOCKERS

Adrenergic receptors are classified into two types: alpha receptors and beta receptors. The beta receptors, in turn, are divided into beta-1 and beta-2 receptors. In general, the beta-1 receptor mediates the cardiac effects (tachycardia), and the beta-2 receptor is responsible for bronchodilatation and peripheral vasodilatation. "Beta-adrenergic blockers" (beta blockers) refers to a group of drugs that produce blockade of the beta-adrenergic receptors. Beta blockers are divided into two groups. The nonselective beta-blocking drugs produce blockade of both beta-1 and beta-2 receptors, whereas the selective beta-blocking drugs only block beta-1 receptors (Table 15–1). A knowledge of the function of major beta-adrenergic receptors (see Table 6–1) allows one to deduce the clinical effects of beta blockers. For example, in low doses, selective beta-1 blockers inhibit beta-1 activity in the heart and cause bradycardia, without associated bronchospasm; at higher doses, however, the drugs are less beta-1 selective, and bronchospasm may occur in susceptible individuals.[1] Nonselective beta blockers cause bradycardia and inhibit bronchodilatation and peripheral vasoconstriction.

Beta blockers are commonly used in the treatment of hypertension, angina, and certain cardiac arrhythmias.[2] They also serve as a primary treatment agent for migraine prophylaxis[3,4] and for control of essential tremor.[5] Beta blockers may alleviate symptoms of anxiety disorders and stage fright,[6,7] and may be useful as adjuncts to control sympathetic overactivity in pheochromocytoma,[8] thyrotoxicosis,[9] and alcohol withdrawal.[10]

Table 15–1. PHARMACOLOGY OF SOME REPRESENTATIVE BETA BLOCKERS

Generic Name	Brand Name	Half-life (Hours)	Average Oral Adult Daily Maintenance Dose for Hypertension
Nonselective			
Propranolol	Inderal	4	40 mg tid/60 mg bid
	(Inderal LA)	10	120 mg qd
Timolol	Blocadren	4–5	10 mg bid
Nadolol	Corgard	20–24	40 mg qd
Labetalol*	Normodyne; Trandate	6–8	200 mg bid
Pindolol†	Visken	3–4	5 mg bid
Beta₁-selective			
Acebutolol†	Sectral	3–4	400 mg qd
Atenolol	Tenormin	6–7	50 mg qd
Metoprolol	Lopressor	3–7	100 mg qd

*Plus alpha$_1$-selective blockade.
†Plus intrinsic sympathomimetic activity.

Effects on Performance

In normal individuals, beta blockade has been shown to adversely affect the following variables of relevance to the athlete:[11]

1. Anaerobic endurance, as measured both by the average power during a maximal 30-second cycle exercise, and by static endurance time at 65 percent of maximal voluntary contraction force
2. Aerobic power, measured as:
   a. $\dot{V}O_2$max
   b. endurance, measured as time to fatigue
   c. time for a 2000-meter run

$\dot{V}O_2$max is similarly affected by both nonselective and selective beta-1 blockade, whereas aerobic endurance is adversely affected to a greater extent by nonselective blockade. Muscle strength appears to be unaffected by both nonselective and beta-1 selective blockade.[11]

The anxiolytic, bradycardic, and antitremor effects of beta blockers are the basis for their use by athletes participating in events such as riflery and archery. Because of their potential ergogenic effect in sporting events in which hand/arm steadiness is crucial, beta blockers are banned by both the International Olympic Committee and the National Collegiate Athletic Association.[12,13]

Adverse Effects

Adverse effects of beta blockers are primarily related to the blockade per se.[2] Cardiac depression and secondary congestive heart failure usually develop only in individuals with pre-existing cardiac dysfunction. Beta blockers, particularly the nonselective ones, are contraindicated in asthmatics because of the likelihood of precipitating bronchospasm. Because propranolol (Inderal) is highly lipophilic and therefore easily crosses the blood-brain barrier, it may cause central nervous system depressive symptoms such as insomnia, nightmares, and depression. Sexual dysfunction (impotence, poor erection) may develop in males who use beta blockers.

DIURETICS

Diuretics are drugs that increase the rate of urine formation. In general, the diuretics act directly on the kidney tubules to produce the desired clinical effects. Clinically, diuretics are used to control hypertension, to reduce edema, and as an adjunct in treating congestive heart failure.[14] Representative diuretics are listed in Table 15–2.

Effects on Performance

Athletes use diuretics primarily for two reasons: (1) to achieve rapid weight loss—

Table 15–2. PHARMACOLOGY OF SOME REPRESENTATIVE DIURETICS

Type	Generic Name	Brand Name	Mechanism of Action	Average Adult Daily Dose
Osmotic	Mannitol	Osmitrol	Osmotic diuresis	50–200 gm IV
Carbonic Anhydrase Inhibitor	Acetazolamide	Diamox	Inhibit carbonic anhydrase, increase urine concentration of HCO_3^- and NA^+	250–500 mg PO/IV
Benzothiazides	Hydrochlorothiazide	Hydrodiuril	Increase urine concentration of Na^+	25–100 mg PO
	Chlorthiazide	Diuril		500–2000 mg PO
High Ceiling (Loop) Diuretic	Furosemide	Lasix	Inhibit electrolyte resorption in loop of Henle	20–80 mg PO/IV
	Ethacrynic Acid	Edecrin		50–200 mg PO/IV
Aldosterone Antagonists	Spironolactone	Aldactone	Competitive antagonism of aldosterone	25–200 mg PO

"make weight"—in sports where weight categories are involved; and (2) to reduce the concentration of drugs in the urine through rapid diuresis, thereby decreasing the likelihood of detection of banned drugs in urine testing.

It is not uncommon for jockeys and other athletes involved in weight category sports, such as wrestling, boxing, and judo to deliberately lose as much as 3 to 5 percent of body weight 1 to 2 days prior to competition. This is achieved through some combination of heat exposure (e.g., sauna), exercise, food and water restriction, self-induced vomiting, laxatives, and diuretics, despite evidence that hypohydration limits physical performance.[15–19] Diuretics are also sometimes used by female athletes involved in individual effort sports such as gymnastics and dancing.[19a] In this setting, the diuretics are used in conjunction with strict dieting which can lead to anorectic behavior manifested as a compulsive effort to remain thin.[20] Diuretics are often used to manage premenstrual fluid retention.[19a]

No study has documented athletic performance enhancement following diuretic intake. Caldwell and associates compared three commonly used methods of hypohydration—diuretics, sauna, and exercise—and measured various parameters of relevance to the athlete.[21] Diuretic therapy caused a mean weight loss of 4.1 percent over 24 hours. Significant decreases were noted in $\dot{V}O_2max$, work load in maximal exercise, and blood lactate levels. Similarly, sauna treatment caused significant performance deterioration. Exercise-induced weight loss, on the other hand, was associated with less performance decremental effects than the other two methods of forced hypohydration.

In the Position Stand of the American College of Sports Medicine (ACSM) on "Weight Loss in Wrestlers," it is noted that the practice of making weight is generally associated with:

1) a reduction in muscular strength, 2) a decrease in work performance times, 3) lower plasma and blood volumes, 4) a reduction in cardiac functioning during submaximal work conditions, which is associated with a higher heart rate, smaller stroke volume and reduced cardiac output, 5) a lower aerobic capacity, especially with food restriction, 6) impairment of body temperature regulation, 7) a decrease in blood flow to the kidney and in the volume of fluid being filtered by the kidney, 8) a depletion of liver glycogen stores and 9) an increase in electrolyte loss.[22]

With regard to the practice of using diuretics to dilute urine drug concentrations, the International Olympic Committee Medical Commission and the National Collegiate Athletic Association include diuretics on the list of banned classes of drugs.[23]

Table 15–3. ADVERSE EFFECTS
OF DIURETICS

Type	Some Adverse Effects
Hyperosmolar	Headache, nausea, vomiting, hypovolemia, muscle cramps
Carbonic Anhydrase Inhibitors	Drowsiness, paresthesias, calculus formation, hypovolemia, muscle cramps
Benzothiazides	Hypokalemia, hypercalcemia, hypophosphatemia, hyperglycemia, hypovolemia, muscle cramps, sun sensitivity, rash, hyperuricemia
Loop Diuretics	Hypokalemia, hyperuricemia, allergic interstitial nephritis, deafness, hypovolemia, muscle cramps, sun sensitivity, rash, hyperuricemia
Aldosterone Inhibitors	Hyperkalemia, gynecomastia, hypovolemia, muscle cramps

Adverse Effects

Aside from the detrimental effects listed above in the Position Stand of the ACSM, diuretics may be associated with other adverse health effects (Table 15–3). Dehydration, hypovolemia, muscle cramps, and orthostatic hypotension are potential side effects with all diuretics, especially when used in the heat. Biochemical changes, especially hypokalemia and, on occasion, hyperkalemia, may be life-threatening when the changes are severe. Athletes, trainers, and physicians must realize that diuretics, except under circumstances of strict medical control and for medical indications, have no role in athletic competition.

NONSTEROIDAL ANTI-INFLAMMATORY DRUGS

Nonsteroidal anti-inflammatory drugs (NSAIDs) have analgesic, anti-inflammatory, and antipyretic properties. They are the mainstay of pharmacologic therapy for rheumatic conditions and for the treatment of soft-tissue athletic injuries. Nonsteroidal anti-inflammatory drugs cause various effects on several biologic systems, including kinins, complement, coagulation, and fibrinolysis.[24] The inhibition of prostaglandin synthesis following NSAID use plays an important role in their anti-inflammatory effect.

The pharmacology of NSAIDs is summarized in Table 15–4. All NSAIDs are capable of relieving pain and stiffness, reducing swelling, and improving the function of inflamed joints. Low doses of these drugs produce analgesic effects while higher doses reduce inflammation.[25] Individual variation in response to the drug is the major factor in determining the observed clinical effects of the various agents.[24] NSAIDs are available in long-acting and short-acting forms and present no risk of dependence or tolerance.

Effects on Performance

The athlete frequently uses NSAIDs for the following conditions:[25]

1. Acute injuries, such as ligament sprains, muscle strains, contusions, fractures, and cartilage damage
2. Chronic injuries, such as tendinitis, tenosynovitis, bursitis, fasciitis, compartment syndromes, and stress fractures
3. Other conditions, such as osteoarthritis of weight-bearing joints

When added to such traditional care of acute injuries as rest, ice, compression, and elevation, NSAIDs may hasten return to competition because of enhanced pain relief and swelling reduction.[26,27] Some studies suggest that the NSAIDs other than aspirin may be superior to aspirin in relieving pain and hastening recovery for soft tissue injuries,[28,29] although high-dose aspirin (3,000 mg per day) has a similar analgesic and anti-inflammatory effect to the other NSAIDs.[24] In chronic overuse injuries, Noble found that training reduction plus an NSAID hastens recovery when compared to training reduction alone.[30]

In addition to their use as anti-inflammatory agents, NSAIDs are widely used for the treatment of menstrual cramps.

Nonsteroidal anti-inflammatory drug use is not banned by the International Olympic Committee, the National Collegiate Athletic Association, or by other amateur and professional sports organizations. This raises an in-

Table 15–4. PHARMACOLOGY OF NONSTEROIDAL ANTI-INFLAMMATORY DRUGS

Generic Name	Brand Name	Half-life (Hours)	Average Oral Adult Daily Dosage for Anti-Inflammatory Effect	
Salicylates				
Acetylsalicylic acid (aspirin)	Ascriptin, Bayer, Bufferin, Ecotrin, Excedrin	0.25*	300–600 mg.	q4 h
Salsalate	Disalcid	Variable	500–1000 mg	bid–tid
Choline magnesium trisalicylate	Trilisate	Variable	500–1500 mg	bid
Diflunisal	Dolobid	8–15	250–500 mg	bid
Indoles				
Indomethacin	Indocin	2–3	25–50 mg	tid
Sulindac	Clinoril	16–20	150–200 mg	bid
Tolmetin	Tolectin	1–2	200–400 mg	tid–qid
Pyrazoles				
Phenylbutazone	Butazolidin	50–80	100 mg	bid–qid
Oxyphenbutazone	Tandearil	50	100 mg	bid–qid
Mefenamic Acid				
Mefenamic Acid	Ponstel	4–6	250 mg	qid
Meclofenamate	Meclomen	2–3	100 mg	tid–qid
Proprionic Acid Derivatives				
Ibuprofen	Motrin, Advil, Nuprin, Medipren, Haltran	2–3	400–600 mg	qid
Naproxen	Naprosyn	12–15	375–500 mg	bid
Fenoprofen	Nalfon	2–3	200–600 mg	tid–qid
Pyroxicans				
Piroxicam	Feldene	45	20 mg	qd
Phenylacetic Acid				
Diclofenac	Voltaren	2	50–75 mg	bid–tid

*Rapidly hydrolyzed to salicylic acid, which has a biologically active half-life of 2–3 hours with low-dose aspirin and 12 hours with anti-inflammatory doses.

teresting philosophical issue about the use of therapeutic drugs by athletes. In the athlete with a mild soft tissue or bony injury, NSAID use is ergogenic in that performance is less pain-limited. Although one cannot directly compare the performance-enhancing effects of NSAIDs in an injured patient to those of therapeutic doses of phenylpropanolamine or ephedrine in a patient with upper respiratory symptoms, one may well ask if the drug policy guidelines for these two classes of therapeutic drugs, vis-à-vis potential ergogenicity, are consistent.

Adverse Effects

Serious side effects are unusual with NSAIDs, but less serious adverse effects, especially gastric irritability and potential gastrointestinal bleeding, are common to virtually all of these agents.[24] They include rash, tinnitus, edema, bronchospasm, and, in susceptible individuals, hypertension and congestive heart failure.[31] Blood dyscrasias may occur rarely, and diarrhea is a potentially serious side effect of meclofenamate (Meclomen).[25] Nonspecific complaints such as headaches and dizziness have also been reported.[24] When an injury is serious enough to cause bleeding into soft tissue, a minimum of 24 hours should elapse between the injury and the start of NSAID therapy. Taking NSAIDs sooner may considerably increase bleeding into the soft tissue.[25]

Although concerns have been raised that the analgesic effects of NSAIDs for arthritic conditions may lead to progressive "analgesic arthropathy" due to joint overuse, it is doubtful that the judicious use of these agents causes enough analgesia to accelerate the progression of traumatic osteoarthritis.[25]

VITAMINS AND MINERALS

Vitamins are organic compounds that are required for the maintenance of normal metabolic functions within the cell, but which are not synthesized in the body and therefore are essential in the diet. Some substances that have activities which are related to vitamins, but which have no known nutritional value in humans, have been dubbed "pseudovitamins." Examples of pseudovitamins include para-aminobenzoic acid (PABA), choline, and inositol.[32] Nonvitamins are substances that may naturally occur in foods and similarly have no demonstrated nutritional value in humans.[32] Examples of these substances include bioflavonoids ("vitamin P") and pangamic acid ("vitamin B$_{15}$").

Pangamic acid is actually not a well-defined pharmacologic entity, since it is a nonregulated mixture of various substances ranging from lactose and methionine[33] to potentially carcinogenic substances such as dimethylglycine and diisopropylamine.[34] Minerals are nonorganic substances (e.g., calcium, zinc, copper, iron) required for metabolic functions in the body.

Effects on Performance

Vitamin and mineral supplements are perceived as ergogenic aids by many athletes,[32] and consequently their use has become widespread. However, there is no firm scientific evidence to show that athletic performance is enhanced when vitamins and minerals are taken in quantities greater than the recommended daily allowance[32,35,35a] (Table 15–5). Similarly, substances such as brewer's yeast—a good source of B vitamins and some minerals—have not been shown to have ergogenic properties.[36]

A daily multivitamin is recommended to avoid the development of a deficiency state when individuals are not eating regular, well-balanced meals. No vitamin or mineral supplementation is necessary in athletes ingesting a well-balanced diet.[36a] Supplementation in excess of the daily recommended allowance has not been shown to improve strength, to increase endurance, to increase

Table 15–5. RECOMMENDED DAILY DIETARY ALLOWANCE

Vitamins	Men	Women	Boys	Girls
Fat-soluble				
Vitamin A	1000 μg	800 μg	700–1000 μg	700–800 μg
Vitamin D	5.0–7.5 μg	5.0–7.5 μg	10 μg	10 μg
Vitamin E	10 mg	8 mg	7–10 mg	7–8 mg
Vitamin K	10–140 μg	70–140 μg	30–100 μg	30–100 μg
Water-Soluble				
Vitamin C	60 mg	60 mg	45–60 mg	45–60 mg
Thiamine	1.4–1.5 mg	1.0–1.1 mg	1.2–1.4 mg	1.2–1.4 mg
Riboflavin	1.6–1.7 mg	1.2–1.3 mg	1.4–1.7 mg	1.3–1.4 mg
Niacin	18–19 mg	13–14 mg	16–18 mg	14–16 mg
Vitamin B$_6$	2.2 mg	2.0 mg	1.6–2.0 mg	1.6–2.0 mg
Folacin	400 μg	400 μg	300–400 μg	300–400 μg
Vitamin B$_{12}$	3.0 μg	3.0 μg	3.0 μg	3.0 μg
Biotin	100–200 μg	100–200 μg	100–200 μg	100–200 μg
Pantothenic Acid	4–7 mg	4–7 mg	4–7 mg	4–7 mg

Table 15–6. ADVERSE EFFECTS OF VITAMINS

Vitamin	Toxic Dose	Adverse Effects
Vitamin A	>200,000 μg adult, >60,000 μg child (single dose)	acute hydrocephalus
	6000–20,000 μg daily	pseudotumor cerebri cirrhosis bone resorption hypercalcemia hypertriglyceridemia teratogenic effects
Vitamin D	>1250 μg daily	hypercalcemia apathy/headache anorexia hypertension/cardiac arrhythmias bone pain/ectopic calcification
Vitamin E	>150 mg daily	weakness/fatigue headache/nauea/diarrhea phlebitis hypercholesterolemia
Pyridoxine (Vitamin B_6)	>200 mg daily	sensory neuropathy
Niacin	100 mg (single dose) variable dose	urticaria/flushing/bronchospasm hyperuricemia/hyperglycemia hepatitis hypertension
Vitamin C	>2000 mg daily	diarrhea/nausea vitamin B_{12} destroyed

peak running speed, or to enhance other psychomotor skills of relevance to the athlete. Additionally, no improvement has been demonstrated in $\dot{V}O_2$max, blood lactate turnpoint, or peak postexercise blood lactate level.[35a]

Adverse Effects

Physicians, trainers, and athletes should all be aware that excessive vitamin intake is well documented in the medical literature to cause various neurologic and systemic disorders[37–43] (Table 15–6). The potential side effects and lack of ergogenicity of vitamins and minerals should be emphasized, as many athletes have a ritualistic dependency on these substances, and tremendous marketing efforts have been directed at athletes stressing both the benign nature of these substances as well as their performance-enhancing qualities.

AMINO ACIDS AND PROTEIN

Amino acids are compounds utilized by the body in various ways, including protein synthesis, neurotransmitter function, and energy production. Protein consumed in the diet is enzymatically hydrolyzed in the alimentary tract to amino acids, which then pass into the blood.[44] Individual amino acids may also be ingested in commercially produced pills or tablets. Essential amino acids (Table 15–7) are not synthesized in the body and must be ingested, whereas nonessential amino acids can be made within the body from carbon and nitrogen precursors. A diet containing the recommended daily protein requirements supplies the necessary essen-

Table 15–7. DAILY
REQUIREMENTS OF ESSENTIAL
AMINO ACIDS (mg/kg)

Amino Acid	Adolescent	Men	Women
Histidine	—	—	—
Isoleucine	28	10–11	10
Leucine	49	11–14	13
Lysine	59	9–12	10
Methionine/			
Cysteine	27	11–14	13
Phenylalanine/			
Tyrosine	27	14	13
Threonine	34	6	7
Tryptophan	4	3	3
Valine	33	14	11

tial amino acids (Table 15–8). However, veg-
etarians who eat no milk or egg products
must either mix grains and vegetables, since
the former are low in lysine and the latter are
low in methionine, or eat adequate amounts
of soy, which is a complete protein.[45]

Effects on Performance

Athletes may ingest large quantities of
protein or amino acid supplements in the belief they are ergogenic aids, despite lack of
evidence to support such a practice. Some
believe that amino acids increase muscle
bulk, others believe they increase efficient
energy utilization, and still others use amino
acids in an attempt to stimulate endogenous
growth hormone release.

Controversy exists regarding daily protein
requirements for the athlete. Some investigators argue that exercise may have little effect on total protein requirements,[46] whereas
others recommend that endurance and
power athletes increase protein intake two to

Table 15–8. RECOMMENDED
SAFE DAILY PROTEIN INTAKE
(gm/kg)

	Males	Females
Adolescent	0.9–1.0	0.8–1.0
Adult	0.75	0.75

threefold.[47,48] Still others state that protein intake should be increased, but only as part of
a well-balanced diet in which total calories
are increased in an individual with greater
daily caloric demands.[49,50,50a] Athletes, however, often consume diets that are disproportionately high in proteins,[46,51] despite the lack
of evidence to support the claim that additional protein or amino supplementation increases growth or energy utilization.[46,50]

Protein supplements are a popular method
of increasing total protein intake, and gelatin
is often the major advertised protein source
in these products. Gelatin, however, is a very
poor-quality protein that is deficient in several amino acids.[49] Although gelatin contains
glycine—a nonessential amino acid which is
a precursor of phosphocreatine—no evidence supports the claim that it is ergogenic.[52] Spirulina, another advertised protein
supplement, has no ergogenic properties despite claims to the contrary, and may be contaminated with toxic bacteria and insect
filth.[53]

Arginine and ornithine are two nonessential amino acids that may stimulate endogenous growth hormone release (see chapter
5), and for this reason athletes may ingest
these substances in order to achieve supraphysiologic growth hormone levels. However, the stimulatory effects are transient,[54]
and the effects of chronic exposure to arginine and ornithine are unknown.

Adverse Effects

Amino acid supplements have never been
demonstrated to benefit endurance athletes
or bodybuilders who are otherwise in good
health and eating a well-balanced diet.[46] Furthermore, excessive amino acid intake may
cause dehydration, gout, liver damage, kidney damage, excessive loss of urinary calcium, and impaired essential amino acid
absorption.[46,49] Because of a lack of data
regarding specific amino acid supplementation (e.g., arginine), no guidelines for a margin of safety are available to the athlete.

CARNITINE

L-carnitine is a compound found in human
heart and skeletal muscle. It is a nonprotein
amino acid, and is not a vitamin.[55] *L*-carni-

tine is the substrate for a number of enzymes known as carnitine acyltransferases, and its primary function is to transport long-chained fatty acids into the mitochondria, thereby facilitating fatty acid metabolism. The average daily American diet contains about 100 to 300 mg of *l*-carnitine, most of which is concentrated in red meat and dairy products.[56] Carnitine deficiency can be acquired as a result of diets low in carnitine and low in one of the essential nutrients required for carnitine biosynthesis—lysine, methionine, ascorbic acid, iron, vitamin B_6, or niacin.[56] Carnitine deficiency can also be an inheritable disorder secondary to a deficiency in carnitine palmitoyl transferase.[60]

Effects on Performance

Manifestations of *l*-carnitine deficiency include progressive myopathic weakness, cardiomyopathy, and intermittent hypoglycemia, all of which may respond to carnitine supplementation.[57,58] Extrapolating from these observations, endurance athletes have taken carnitine supplements in efforts to enhance performance by improving fatty acid metabolism. However, no study has substantiated any benefit from carnitine supplementation.[56,57]

Adverse Effects

When commercially available *dl*-carnitine ("Vitamin B_T") is taken as a supplement, the *d*-isomer may inhibit the activities of the *l*-isomer, thereby producing a functional carnitine deficiency state characterized by myopathic weakness.[59] One patient with a partial carnitine deficiency secondary to muscle carnitine palmitoyl transferase deficiency developed severe rhabdomyolysis following ibuprofen therapy, presumably because the ibuprofen somehow disrupted the patient's muscle uptake or retention of carnitine.[60]

BICARBONATE DOPING

Bicarbonate doping refers to the practice of ingesting sodium bicarbonate (baking soda) prior to athletic competition. The rationale for bicarbonate doping is to raise muscle pH in order to rid the muscle more rapidly of hy-drogen ions (lactic acid), thereby delaying hydrogen ion–induced muscle fatigue.

Lactic acid production depends on several variables, including the amount of anaerobic expenditure and the amount of stored muscle glycogen. Typically, endurance (aerobically trained) athletes have primarily type I muscle fibers—slow twitch, tonic fibers with a high oxidative capacity. Sprint-trained athletes and power lifters (anaerobically trained) have primarily type II fibers—phasic fast twitch with a greater phosphorylase content, which metabolizes glycogen to lactate for immediate ATP needs. An elite sprinter's muscle glycogen content is about 400 gm, from which 4,444 mmol of lactic acid can be produced,[61] whereas a nonathlete's muscle glycogen is about 150 gm, which can produce 1,667 mmol of lactic acid.[62]

Effects on Performance

Hermansen and Medbo[63] demonstrated that blood pH acutely falls to 7.06 ± 0.01, with a concomitant blood lactate increase to 17.0 ± 1.2 mmol following 1 minute of maximal exercise in sprint-trained athletes, compared to a pH of 7.17 ± 0.01 and blood lactate of 12.6 ± 0.04 mmol in endurance trained athletes. Such exercise-induced physiologic changes led to experimentation with sodium bicarbonate in an effort to buffer acidosis, thereby potentially delaying the onset to fatigue.

Robinson and Verity noted that sodium bicarbonate does not significantly affect the normal rise in lactic acid in individual rowers performing 1-mile workouts, and they concluded that bicarbonate must not be ergogenic.[64] Klein and associates[65] noted no performance-enhancing effect among athletes who trained on an arm-crank cycle ergometer during a 2-minute power test. Hooker and co-workers[66] studied 6 male runners during a 10-kilometer treadmill maximal effort run to exhaustion, and found that bicarbonate ingestion did not change $\dot{V}O_2$max, nor did it prolong the time to exhaustion. Taken as a group, the above studies indicate that bicarbonate doping has no significant effect on aerobic activities or on upper body anaerobic activities.

Gledhill,[67] however, states that bicarbonate doping is only useful in anaerobic situations, and especially for events which rely on leg performance, since the lower body—given the greater muscle mass—is more susceptible than the upper body to the buildup of hydrogen ions. Wilkes, Gledhill, and Smyth[68] compared the effects of sodium bicarbonate, calcium carbonate, and placebo taken just prior to racing 800 meters. Six trained runners ingested 300 mg per kg sodium bicarbonate 30 minutes prior to the race, and pre-race blood pH was significantly higher (7.49 ± 0.004) when compared with the 2 other treatment groups. The average racing time improved 2.9 seconds in this group, and post-race blood pH and lactate were both significantly higher. According to Costill,[68a] bicarbonate doping has no effect on short duration sprints, but does lead to improved times for interval training with rest periods in between sprints. The above data raise the possibility that bicarbonate doping may be ergogenic under specific circumstances. The mechanism of ergogenicity may be an increase in extracellular buffering, which facilitates hydrogen ion efflux from the cells of the working muscle, thereby delaying the decrease in intracellular pH and postponing fatigue.[68]

Bicarbonate doping is not specifically banned by any amateur or professional sports organization, and aside from an increase in urinary pH, no urine test can detect the use of sodium bicarbonate. Urinary pH may not be valid, since some antacids may similarly affect the urine.[68]

Adverse Effects

No serious adverse effects have been reported with bicarbonate doping. Large quantities of sodium bicarbonate can cause diarrhea and/or gastric distress, and chronic use can cause disturbances in body sodium and water balance.[68a] In cases of massive bicarbonate ingestion, profound metabolic alkalosis may result, leading to apathy, confusion, stupor, and tetany.

ANALGESIC INJECTIONS

Clinically, lidocaine and similar local anesthetics are often injected in conjunction with corticosteroids into the joint space, the peritendon region, or paraspinal region of an injured individual.

Effects on Performance

Under specific conditions, and in well-trained hands, such injections may serve a useful purpose by alleviating pain and promoting a regional anti-inflammatory effect. When used in this manner, analgesic injections may be ergogenic because athletic performance is not impaired by pain. Analgesic injections may be used to treat arthritis, bursitis, tendinitis, sciatica, and other tendon-ligament-joint injuries. When used, intra-articular injections should be part of a broad management plan which may include nonsteroidal anti-inflammatory drugs, local cold treatment, rest, and graduated physical therapy. The individual should be advised against vigorous physical activity for 2 to 3 weeks following intra-articular, peritendon, or other similar injections.[69]

The USOC bans the use of intramuscular or intravenous corticosteroid and injectable anesthetics. Intra-articular or superficial skin injections may be used if the following conditions are met: (1) the injections are not used in conjunction with epinephrine or cocaine; (2) they must be medically justified, without risk of injury to the athlete; and (3) medical officials must be notified of the diagnosis; the name, site, and route of administration of drug used; and the date of injection.[70]

Adverse Effects

Intra-articular injections may cause serious adverse effects. The immediate pain relief may provide sufficient analgesia to allow an athlete to compete despite a severe injury, thereby leading to more serious damage, such as acute tendon rupture. Repeated injections may cause a local arthropathy,[71] and corticosteroid-induced collagen inhibition may delay normal wound healing.[69]

PHOSPHATE LOADING

The ingestion of phosphate within 1 week of an athletic event has been employed in an attempt to improve oxygen delivery. The physiologic change accounting for improved oxygen delivery is an increase in red blood cell 2,3-diphosphoglyceride (2,3-DPG), which in turn shifts the hemoglobin-oxygen dissociation curve to the right, thereby permitting greater oxygen unloading to tissues.

Effects on Performance

At high altitudes, plasma phosphate and 2,3-DPG levels normally increase in individuals, permitting an appropriate adaptation with better oxygen unloading.[72,73] Several authors have demonstrated an increase in 2,3-DPG following phosphate loading,[74,75,76,77] and this may occur in addition to the normal physiologic adaptive response that occurs at high altitudes.[77] The addition of other agents, such as sodium bicarbonate, vitamin C, and pyruvate, does not increase the 2,3-DPG levels any further.[76]

Jain and colleagues[77] studied 36 healthy men in a double-blind fashion to determine the physiologic effects of phosphate loading at a high altitude. After airlifting subjects to an altitude of 3500 meters, half were given 500 mg of sodium hydrogen phosphate (3.2 mmol), and the other half placebo. The dose of drug was repeated daily for the next 3 days. Subjects were examined on the 3rd, 7th, 14th, and 21st days of their altitude stay. Significant and comparable increases in both groups occurred in the following measures: hemoglobin, red blood cell count, hematocrit, and reticulocyte count. On day 3, plasma phosphate and 2,3-DPG levels in the phosphate-treated group increased significantly compared with the placebo group. In addition, learning efficiency was significantly better in the phosphate-treated group. Significant differences were no longer present between the two groups by day 7. Plasma phosphate and 2,3-DPG levels returned to baseline after discontinuing phosphate supplementation.

The above study and those of other authors indicate that 2,3-DPG levels can be increased from phosphate supplementation. The improved mental task efficiency seen in Jain's study for phosphate-treated subjects suggests that the rightward shift in the oxygen dissociation curve due to increased 2,3-DPG levels results in better oxygen delivery

to tissues, including the brain. The overall effect on athletic performance is unknown and should be addressed in well-designed double-blind crossover studies for endurance athletic events.

Adverse Effects

Adverse effects of short-term phosphate loading are unclear, but hyperphosphatemia has been well reported to cause metastatic calcifications in soft tissues. Amateur and professional organizations do not test for phosphate supplementation in athletes.

REFERENCES

1. Choice of a beta-blocker. The Medical Letter 28:20, 1986.
2. Weiner, N: Drugs that inhibit adrenergic nerves and block adrenergic receptors. In Gilman, AG, et al (eds): Goodman and Gilman's The Pharmacological Basis of Therapeutics, ed 7. Macmillan, New York, 1985, p 181.
3. Weber, RB and Reinmuth, OM: The treatment of migraine with propranolol. Neurology 22:366, 1972.
4. Ziegler, DK, et al: Migraine prophylaxis: A comparison of propranolol and amitriptyline. Arch Neurol 44:486, 1987.
5. Findley, LJ and Koller, WC: Essential tremor: A review. Neurology 37:1194, 1987.
6. Brantigan, CO, Brantigan, TA and Joseph, N: Effect of beta blockade and beta stimulation on stage fright. Am J Med 72:88, 1982.
7. Drug may help the overanxious on SAT's. New York Times, October 22, 1987.
8. Northfield, TC: Cardiac complications of phaeochromocytoma. Br Heart J 29:588, 1967.
9. Das, G and Krieger, M: Treatment of thyrotoxic storm with intravenous propranolol. Ann Intern Med 70:985, 1969.
10. Kraus, ML, et al: Randomized clinical trial of atenolol in patients with alcohol withdrawal. N Engl J Med 313:905, 1985.
11. Kaiser, P: Physical performance and muscle metabolism during β-adrenergic blockade in man. Acta Physiol Scand 536 (Suppl):1, 1984.
12. US Olympic Committee, Division of Sports Medicine and Science: Drug Education & Control Policy. Colorado Springs, 1988.
13. The NCAA Drug Testing Program 1988–89. Mission, Kansas, NCAA Publishing, Sept., 1988.
14. Weiner, IM and Mudge, GH: Diuretics and other agents employed in the mobilization of edema fluid. In Gilman, AG, et al (eds): Goodman and Gilman's The Pharmacological Basis of Therapeutics, ed 7. Macmillan, New York, 1985, p 887.
15. Bock, W, Fox, EL and Bowers, R: The effects of acute dehydration upon cardio-respiratory endurance. J Sports Med Phys Fitness 7:67, 1967.

16. Horstman, DH and Horvath, SM: Cardiovascular adjustments to progressive dehydration. J Appl Physiol 35:501, 1973.

17. Nielsen, B, et al: Physical work capacity after dehydration and hyperthermia: A comparison of the effect of exercise versus passive heating and sauna and diuretic dehydration. Scand J Sports Sci 3:2, 1981.

18. Ribisl, PM and Hervert, WG: Effects of rapid weight reduction and subsequent rehydration upon the physical working capacity of wrestlers. Res Quart 41:536, 1970.

19. Saltin, B: Aerobic work capacity and circulation at exercise in man with special reference to the effect of prolonged exercise and/or heat exposure. Acta Physiol Scand 230(Suppl):1, 1964.

19a. Rosen, LW and Hough, DO: Pathogenic weight-control behaviors of female college gymnasts. Phys Sportsmed 16(9):140, 1988.

20. Katz, JL: Eating disorders. In Shangold, M and Mirkin, G (eds): Women and Exercise: Physiology and Sports Medicine, FA Davis Company, Philadelphia, 1988, p 252.

21. Caldwell, JE, Ahonen, E and Nousiainen, U: Differential effects of sauna-, diuretic-, and exercise-induced hypohydration. J Appl Physiol 57:1018, 1984.

22. Position Stand: Weight Loss in Wrestlers. American College of Sports Medicine, Indianapolis, 1976.

23. IOC: Statement of Diuretics. Sports Mediscope 6:5, 1987.

24. Given, WP: Nonsteroidal anti-inflammatory drugs, a review. North Shore Univ Hosp Clin J 7:15, 1984.

25. Calabrese, LH and Rooney, TW: The use of non-steroidal anti-inflammatory drugs in sports. Phys Sportsmed 14(2):89, 1986.

26. Santelli, H, Tuccimei, V and Cannestra, FM: Comparative study with piroxicam and ibuprofen versus placebo in the supportive treatment of minor sports injuries. J Int Med Res 8:265, 1980.

27. Krishan, G: A placebo-controlled double-blind trial of benoxylate tablets in the treatment of bursitis and synovitis due to sports injuries. Rheumatol Rehab 16:186, 1977.

28. Muckle, DS: Comparative study of ibuprofen and aspirin in soft tissue injuries. Rheumatol Rehab 13:141, 1974.

29. Muckle, DS: A double blind trial of flubiprofen and aspirin in soft tissue trauma. Rheumatol Rehab 16:58, 1977.

30. Noble, C: Fenbufen in the treatment of overuse injuries in long distance runners. S A Med J 5:387, 1981.

31. Radack, KL, Deck, CC and Bloomfield, FF: Ibuprofen interferes with the efficacy of antihypertensive drugs. Ann Intern Med 107:628, 1987.

32. Grandjean, A: Vitamins, diet, and the athlete. Clin Sports Med 2:105, 1983.

33. Gonzalez, ER: Medical news: Vitamin B15—Whatever it is, it won't help. JAMA 243:2473, 1980.

34. Herbert, V: Pangamic acid ("vitamin B15"). Am J Clin Nutr 32:1534, 1979.

35. Recommended Dietary Allowances, ed 9. National Academy of Sciences, Washington, D.C., 1980.

35a. Weight, LM, Myburgh, KH, and Noakes, TD: Vitamin and mineral supplementation. Effect on the running performance of trained athletes. Am J Clin Nutr 47:192, 1988.

36. Ergogenic aid of the month: Brewer's yeast. Sports Med Digest 9:7, 1987.

36a. Weight, LM, et al: Vitamin and mineral status of trained athletes including the effects of supplementation. Am J Clin Nutr 47:186, 1988.

37. Toxic effects of vitamin overdose. The Medical Letter 26:73, 1984.

38. Gerhardt, AL: Vitamin megadoses: Use, abuse, and toxicity. Consultant 28:151, 1988.

39. Albin, RL, et al: Acute sensory neuropathy—Neuronopathy from pyridoxine overdose. Neurology 37:1729, 1987.

40. Schaumburg, H, et al: Sensory neuropathy from pyridoxine abuse: A new megavitamin syndrome. N Engl J Med 309:445, 1983.

41. Parry, GJ and Bredesen, DE: Sensory neuropathy with low-dose pyridoxine. Neurology 35:1466, 1985.

42. Ahlskoy, JE and O'Neill, BP: Pseudotumor cerebri. Ann Intern Med 97:249, 1982.

43. Rush, JA: Pseudotumor cerebri: Clinical profile and visual outcome in 63 patients. Mayo Clin Proc 55:541, 1980.

44. Munro, HN and Crim, MC: The proteins and amino acids. In Shils, ME and Young, VR (eds): Modern Nutrition in Health and Disease, ed 7. Lea and Febiger, Philadelphia, 1988, p 1.

45. Energy and protein requirement. Report of Joint FAO/WHO/UNU Expert Consultation. Technical report series 724, WHO, Geneva, 1985, p 121.

46. Slavin, JL, Lanners, G and Engstrom, MA: Amino acid supplements: Beneficial or risky? Phys Sportsmed 16(3):221, 1988.

47. Lemon, PW, Yarasheski, KE and Dolny, DG: The importance of protein for athletes. Sports Med 1:474, 1984.

48. Brotherhood, JR: Nutrition and sports performance. Sports Med 1:350, 1984.

49. Ergogenic aid of the month: Protein supplements. Sports Med Digest 9:6, 1987.

50. Hecker, AL: Nutrition and physical performance. In Strauss, RH (ed): Drugs & Performance in Sports, WB Saunders, Philadelphia, 1987, p 23.

50a. Layman, DK: How much protein does an athlete need? Phys Sportsmed 15(12):181,1987.

51. Short, SH and Short, WR: Four-year study of university athletes' dietary intake. J Am Diet Assoc 82:632, 1983.

52. Fad of the month: Gelatin and glycine. Sports Med Digest 10:6, 1988.

53. Ergogenic aid of the month: Spirulina. Sports Med Digest 9:7, 1987.

54. Macintyre, JG: Growth hormone and athletes. Sports Med 4:129, 1987.

55. Dipalma, JR: L-Carnitine: Its therapeutic potential. American Family Physician 34:127, 1986.

56. Borum PR: Carnitine in human nutrition. Nutrition and the M.D. 9:1, 1982.

57. Carnitine. The Medical Letter 28:88, 1986.

58. Rebouche, CJ and Engel, AG: Carnitine metabolism and deficiency syndromes. Mayo Clin Proc 58:533, 1983.

59. Keith, R: Symptoms of carnitine like deficiency in a trained runner taking DL-carnitine. JAMA 255:1137, 1986.

60. Ross, NS and Hoppel, CL: Partial muscle carnitine palmitoyltransferase-A deficiency: Rhabdomyolysis associated with transiently decreased muscle carnitine content after ibuprofen therapy. JAMA 257:62, 1987.

61. Hultman, E: Muscle glycogen synthesis in relation to diet studied in normal subjects. Acta Med Scand 182:109, 1967.

62. Halperin, M and Fields, LA: Review: Lactic acidosis: Emphasis on the carbon precursors and buffering of the acid load. Am J Med Sci 289:154, 1985.

63. Hermansen, L and Medbo, JI: The relative significance of aerobic and anaerobic processes during maximal exercise of short duration. Med Sport Sci 17:56, 1984.

64. Robinson, K and Verity, LS: Effect of induced alkalosis on rowing ergometer performance (rep) during repeated 1-mile work-outs. Med Sci Sports Exerc 19(suppl):S68, 1987.

65. Klein, L, Berger, R and Kearney, JT: The effect of bicarbonate ingestion on upper body power in trained athletes. Med Sci Sports Exerc 19(suppl):S67, 1987.

66. Hooker, S, Morgan, C and Wells, C: Effect of sodium bicarbonate ingestion on time to exhaustion and blood lactate of 10k runners. Med Sci Sports Exerc 19(suppl):S67, 1987.

67. Groves, D: Studies: Bicarbonate doping has no benefits. Phys Sportsmed 15(12):51, 1987.

68. Wilkes, K, Gledhill, N and Smyth, R: Effect of acute induced metabolic alkalosis on 800-m racing time. Med Sci Sports Exerc 15:277, 1983.

68a. Costill, DL: Exercise physiology: Is sodium bicarbonate an aid to sprint performance? Sports Medicine Digest 10:4, 1988.

69. Stanitski, CL: Pharmacological adjuncts to the management of musculoskeletal injuries in sports. In Strauss, RH (ed): Drugs & Performance in Sports, WB Saunders, Philadelphia, 1987, p 173.

70. US Olympic Committee, Division of Sports Medicine and Science: Drug Education & Control Policy. United States Olympic Committee, Colorado Springs, 1988.

71. Haynes, RC and Murad, F: Adrenocorticotropic hormone; Adrenocortical steroids and their synthetic analogs; Inhibitors of adrenocortical steroid biosynthesis. In Gilman, AG, et al (eds): Goodman and Gilman's The Pharmacological Basis of Therapeutics, ed 7. Macmillan, New York, 1985, p 1459.

72. Eaton, JW, Brewer, GJ, and Grover, EF: Role of red cell 2,3-diphosphoglycerate in the adaptation of man to altitude. J Lab Clin Med 73:603, 1969.

73. Dempsey, JA, et al: Muscular exercise, 2,3-DPG and oxy-hemoglobin affinity. Int J Physiol 30:34, 1971.

74. Brain, MC and Card, RT: Effect of inorganic phosphate on red cell metabolism—in vitro and in vivo studies. In Brewer, GJ (ed): Haemoglobin and Red Cell Structure and Function. Plenum Press, New York, 1972, p 145.

75. Moore, LG, et al: Pharmacologic stimulation of erythrocyte 2,3-diphosphoglycerate production in vivo. J Pharmacol Exp Ther 203:722, 1977.

76. Moore, LG, and Brewer, GJ: Beneficial effect of rightward hemoglobin-oxygen dissociation curve shift for short term high altitude adaptation. J Lab Clin Med 98:145, 1981.

77. Jain, SC, et al: Effect of phosphate supplementation on oxygen delivery at high altitude. Int J Biometeor 31:249, 1987.

CHAPTER 16

Blood Doping and Erythropoietin

HISTORY

Blood Doping

Blood doping refers to the practice of intravenously infusing blood into an individual in order to induce erythrocythemia. The procedure may be autologous (one's own blood) or homologous (donated blood). Reports of blood doping in a controlled scientific setting first appeared in 1947.[1] In 1966, Ekblom[2] began a series of studies addressing the question of improved aerobic capacity following blood doping. In the 1976 Olympic Games, reports began to circulate which suggested that the procedure was used by athletes as an ergogenic aid.[3] Several U.S. cyclists admitted to blood doping for the 1984 Summer Olympics,[4] and common knowledge suggests that blood doping by athletes is often done for endurance events.[5]

Erythropoietin

Erythropoietin is a naturally occuring glycoprotein hormone that originates in the kidneys. Erythropoietin production leads to stimulation of certain bone marrow stem cells which will differentiate into red blood cells. Erythropoietin is now potentially available in mass quantities through the process of genetic engineering.[6] In 1987, Eschbach and associates[7] reported the clinical usefulness of recombinant human erythropoietin in the correction of the anemia of end-stage renal disease. Analysts speculate that the potential use—and abuse—of erythropoietin may be enormous.[8,9]

PHYSIOLOGY

Blood Doping

Blood doping is used by athletes engaged in aerobic athletic activities, for example, long-distance running, cross-country skiing, and cycling. The expressed purpose is to increase their total aerobic power by increasing the transport of oxygen to the contracting muscle.

Adenosine triphosphate (ATP) is the energy source for all biologic work, including muscle contraction. In the absence of oxygen—anaerobic metabolism—ATP generation is relatively inefficient. For example, for every 180 grams of glycogen metabolized by anaerobic metabolism, only 3 moles of ATP are formed. On the other hand, in the presence of oxygen—aerobic metabolism—every 180 grams of glycogen yields 39 moles of ATP. Aerobic metabolism can utilize glycogen, fatty acids, and protein as sources of fuel and can produce unlimited ATP without fatiguing by-products such as lactic acid. Consequently, the aerobic system is particularly suited for manufacturing ATP during prolonged, endurance activities. During a marathon race, for example, 150 moles of ATP are produced and utilized through aerobic metabolic pathways.[10]

The amount of oxygen required to fully oxidize 180 grams of glycogen is 192 grams, or 134.4 liters. Once inspired, the oxygen must be transported to the working muscle to generate ATP. Oxygen is primarily transported to the muscle in chemical combination with hemoglobin. Specifically, each gram of hemoglobin can maximally combine with 1.34 ml oxygen. Assuming a sea-level hemoglobin concentration of 15 gm per 100 ml blood, then 100 ml blood can transport 20.1 ml oxygen ($1.34 \times 15 = 20.1$).

Blood doping represents a method of increasing the hemoglobin concentration of the blood in order to increase the amount of oxygen that can be transported to the working muscle. For example, raising the hemoglobin concentration to 16 gm per 100 ml produces 21.44 ml oxygen per 100 ml blood ($1.34 \times 16 = 21.44$). Improved oxygen delivery yields more energy-rich ATP and theoretically can enhance aerobically dependent endurance activities.

Stated differently, it has been estimated that 500 ml of whole blood, or 275 ml of packed red blood cells, can add about 100 ml of oxygen to the total oxygen-carrying capacity of the blood. Because an athlete's total blood volume circulates 5 to 6 times each minute in maximal exercise, the potential extra oxygen available to the tissues from red cell reinfusion is about 0.5 liters per minute.[11]

Endurance performance enhancement derived from blood doping presumes no adverse effects on blood viscosity from the increased red cell concentration in the circulating blood. Theoretically, a sufficiently large blood transfusion increases blood viscosity, which can then decrease cardiac output, decrease blood flow velocity, and reduce peripheral blood oxygen concentration—all of which can reduce aerobic capacity. However, viscosity effects are probably small at hematocrit levels of 50 percent or less.[12]

Normally, blood doping is followed by certain compensatory physiologic adjustments that preserve the sought-after beneficial aerobic effect. Most notably, immediately following blood doping, there is a shift of plasma from the intravascular space to the extravascular space, thereby restoring the blood volume to normal,[13] ensuring no significant alteration in cardiac output, and increasing total oxygen delivery secondary to increased hemoglobin concentration.[12,14] The affinity of the red blood cell for oxygen, as measured by 2,3-diphosphoglycerate and P_{50}, is unaffected by blood doping, indicating there is no change in the affinity of the red cell for oxygen.[15-17]

Debate has often centered on whether the limiting factor in endurance exercise capacity is oxygen delivery or the inherent oxidative capacity of the muscle.[12,18] Ekblom and associates[19] have demonstrated that both the oxygen uptake and the oxidative capacity of the muscle are not adversely affected with induced erythrocythemia. Following induced erythrocythemia, there is not only an increase in the amount of oxygen delivered to the working muscles, but oxygen used by the working muscle also increases.[20] Robertson and co-workers[21] have demonstrated that both the volume of oxygen delivered by the left ventricle and the volume of oxygen actually used during maximal exercise are significantly increased following induced erythrocythemia (Fig. 16–1).

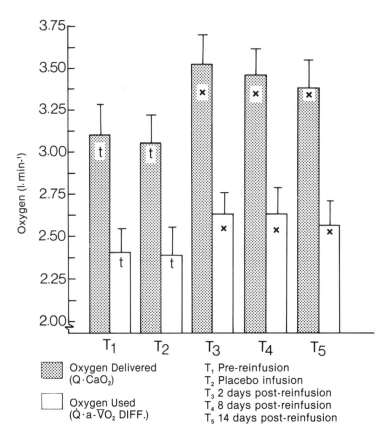

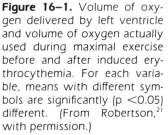

Figure 16–1. Volume of oxygen delivered by left ventricle and volume of oxygen actually used during maximal exercise before and after induced erythrocythemia. For each variable, means with different symbols are significantly ($p < 0.05$) different. (From Robertson,[21] with permission.)

Oxygen Delivered ($\dot{Q} \cdot CaO_2$)

Oxygen Used ($\dot{Q} \cdot a \cdot \bar{V}O_2$ DIFF.)

T_1 Pre-reinfusion
T_2 Placebo infusion
T_3 2 days post-reinfusion
T_4 8 days post-reinfusion
T_5 14 days post-reinfusion

Procedure for Blood Doping

The procedure that has been utilized for blood doping is as follows:[2,15,22,23]

1. Four to 8 weeks prior to the anticipated athletic event for which blood doping is desired, 2 units of blood are removed from the individual.

2. The red blood cells are separated from the plasma, then preserved via glycerol freezing, allowing preservation for an indefinite period of time.

a. Alternatively, the red blood cells may be refrigerated, but the maximal storage time is decreased to only 3 weeks. Since prephlebotomy hemoglobin levels are usually not achieved in just 3 weeks, the full benefit of reinfused red blood cells is not realized. Therefore, this method has fallen out of favor.

b. If homologous transfusions are to be given, storage of the individual's blood for the purpose of auto-transfusion is not necessary.

3. The individual retrains to full aerobic capacity during the 4 to 8 weeks postphlebotomy.

4. At the time of reinfusion, the frozen red blood cells are thawed and reconstituted with a physiologic saline solution, then infused intravenously over 1 to 2 hours. Reinfusion is usually done 1 to 7 days prior to the desired athletic event.

Erythropoietin

Under normal conditions, humans maintain a constant red blood cell mass. Red blood cells are formed and destroyed at approximately the same rate—2 to 3 million per second.[24] The rate of formation of red blood cells is determined largely by erythropoietin,[24] which serves as one limb in an oxygen-mediated feedback loop.[8]

Eschbach and colleagues[7] demonstrated that exogenous administration of recombinant human erythropoietin may increase the hematocrit 35 percent or more in chronic renal failure patients. At doses of 50 units per kilogram or higher, consistent dose-dependent increases in the rate of rise in hematocrit were seen, and a sustained reticulocytosis occurs for at least 7 months.[7]

The long-term clinical utility of erythropoietin in the treatment of the anemia of chronic renal failure and the future use of erythropoietin for the treatment of other anemias are at present unknown.

USE IN SPORTS

No data exist regarding the incidence of blood doping among endurance athletes, although anecdotal stories abound. It is not unusual for a runner or cyclist who performs unexpectedly well to be accused of blood doping.[20,25] In 1984, Ireland's John Treacy stated that he saw an entire national team injecting themselves with a blood-colored liquid prior to the world cross-country championship. The 1984 United States cycling team admitted to blood doping following their impressive showing at the Olympics.[20] Dr. Robert Voy,[5] director of science for the United States Olympic Committee, says that blood doping among athletes has gotten "completely out of control." Dr. Voy further suggests that when a country comes out of nowhere to world prominence in an endurance event, the international athletic community nods knowingly and thinks blood doping.[5]

Effects on Performance

In a 1973 article, Williams[26] noted that the bulk of evidence did not support the contention that blood doping improved endurance performance. Since then, however, the technique of blood doping has been perfected, and conclusions that blood doping is not ergogenic can be attributed to flaws in blood doping technique.

Gledhill[27] notes that critical technical factors are total volume of red cells withdrawn and reinfused, the time interval between withdrawing and reinfusing blood, and the method used to store the blood. Specifically, about 900 ml of whole blood should be withdrawn and then frozen for storage. Reinfusion should be done about 6 to 10 weeks later, in order to allow baseline hemoglobin levels to be achieved before reinfusion.

Following the principles outlined by Gledhill, recent studies have clearly supported the contention that blood doping improves endurance performances.[14–17,28] The improvements have a clear-cut practical meaning: statistically significant differences are noted in race times, using the athlete as his or her own control. Endurance capacity may improve up to 25 percent following blood doping. Some modifying factors exist. For example, Sawka and associates[28] state that the magnitude of increase in maximal oxygen uptake is related to the individual's initial aerobic fitness. Individuals in moderately good physical condition experience twice the increase in maximal oxygen uptake as individuals of greater or lesser fitness. The total amount of blood needed to be removed and reinfused to achieve a maximal effect has not been clearly established, although Spriet and co-workers[14] note that the aerobic power of working muscles was not surpassed following 3 units of autologous blood transfusions in 4 highly trained endurance runners.

Blood doping is banned by the National Collegiate Athletic Association (NCAA) and the International Olympic Committee (IOC). The American College of Sports Medicine views blood doping for ergogenic purposes as unethical and unjustifiable.[29] Evidence confirming blood doping leads to punitive actions according to NCAA and IOC guidelines, but no urine or blood test accurately detects blood doping. Berglund and associates[30] addressed this latter issue in 6 cross-country skiers. A combination of an increase in serum hemoglobin, bilirubin, and iron coupled with a decrease in the serum erythropoietin level is supportive evidence, and a second comparison serum sample may give further supportive evidence. However, this procedure is invasive, has not been validated, and at present can detect only 50 to 67 percent of blood-doped individuals.

Erythropoietin "doping" by athletes has not been reported, but there have been speculations about its potential abuse.[9] The physiologic principles of induced erythrocythemia by exogenous erythropoietin administration may be similar to those of blood doping. Erythropoietin is an investigational drug for patients with chronic renal failure, and its use in the future will probably be limited to patients with other chronic disease-induced anemia or chemotherapy-induced anemia. The effects of erythropoietin in normal individuals have not been tested, but the drug is discussed with blood doping since the athletic community must be prepared to deal with the possibility of a black market for this drug.

ADVERSE EFFECTS

Homologous blood transfusions are now rarely given for blood doping, and the risk is clearly substantial. Three percent of such transfusions are complicated by immune side effects such as fever, urticaria, and, more rarely, severe hemolytic reactions and anaphylactic shock. Viral infections are well known to occur and include hepatitis and the acquired immunodeficiency syndrome (AIDS).

Autologous blood transfusions appear safe when performed by trained personnel, using approved techniques, and with storage and labeling in a registered blood bank.[12] Any flaw in technique may lead to complications ranging from bacterial infections to fatal reactions due to blood mislabeling.

Eschbach[7] observed no organ dysfunction or other toxic effects of recombinant erythropoietin among the chronic renal failure patients studied.

It should be noted that any form of induced erythrocythemia carries with it the potential medical complications which have been well described with polycythemia, including hypertension, congestive heart failure, and stroke.

FINAL NOTE

It can be argued that blood doping does not represent drug use or abuse per se since blood is not a drug in the traditional sense. But the fact is that blood is a drug. As Klein states: "Collection, storage, and compatibility testing of blood for transfusion are carefully prescribed by the Food and Drug Administration. Facilities for blood collection and transfusion are registered, licensed, and inspected for compliance. Like other drugs, blood should be given only for medical indications."[12]

Blood doping represents a particularly challenging problem for the sports community. Of all the drugs discussed in this book, blood doping is the most unequivocally ergogenic under specified conditions, yet deception transcends the technologic ability to detect its use. Recombinant erythropoietin may one day present a similar dilemma. Blood doping is unique in that the inability to detect its use, coupled with its clear-cut ergogenic potential, demands from the individual athlete a more profound ethical and moral decision. As with other drugs and methods of deception which are always available, the athlete is left with a choice— to embrace the meaning of the essence of sport, or to participate in the practice of winning at any cost. With blood doping, the ethical stakes are particularly high.

REFERENCES

1. Pace, N, et al: The increase in hypoxia tolerance of normal men accompanying the polycythemia induced by transfusion of erythrocytes. Am J Physiol 148:152, 1947.
2. Ekblom, B: Blood doping, oxygen breathing, and altitude training. In Strauss, RH (ed): Drugs & Performance in Sports. WB Saunders, Philadelphia, 1987, p 53.
3. Gledhill, N, et al: Blood doping and related issues: A brief review. Med Sci Sports Exerc 14:193, 1982.
4. Jeansonne, J: The controversy surrounding blood doping. Newsday, April 15, 1988.
5. Blood doping: The coming issue. New Haven Journal Courier, Jan 4, 1988.
6. Strick, D: The hormone that's making Amgen grow. Business Week, March 16, 1987, p 96.
7. Eschbach, JW, et al: Correction of the anemia of end-stage renal disease with recombinant human erythropoietin. Results of a combined phase I and II clinical trial. N Engl J Med 316:73, 1987.
8. Erslev, A: Erythropoietin coming of age. N Engl J Med 316:101, 1987.
9. Walker, R and Brown, A: Test drug surpassed doping. Calgary Herald, Feb 17, 1988.
10. Fox, EL: Sports Physiology, ed 2. Saunders College Publishing, New York, 1984, p 9.
11. McCardle, WD, Katch, FI and Katch, VL: Exercise Physiology—Energy, Nutrition, and Human Performance. Lea and Febiger, Philadelphia, 1981, p 305.
12. Klein, HG: Blood transfusions and athletics. Games people play. N Engl J Med 312:854, 1985.
13. Williams, MH, et al: Effect of blood reinjection upon endurance capacity and heart rate. Med Sci Sports 5:181, 1973.
14. Spriet, LL, et al: Effect of graded erythrocythemia on cardiovascular and metabolic responses to exercise. J Appl Physiol 61:1942, 1986.
15. Brien, AJ and Simon, TL: The effects of red blood

cell infusion on 10-km race time. JAMA 257:2761, 1987.

16. Buick, FJ, et al: Effect of induced erythrocythemia on aerobic work capacity. J Appl Physiol 48:636, 1980.

17. Williams, MH, et al: The effect of induced erythrocythemia upon 5-mile treadmill run time. Med Sci Sports Exerc 13:169, 1981.

18. Gollnick, PD, et al: Enzyme activity and fiber composition in skeletal muscle of untrained and trained men. J Appl Physiol 33:312, 1972.

19. Ekblom, G, Golbard, A and Gullbring, B: Response to exercise after blood loss and reinfusion. J Appl Physiol 33:175, 1972.

20. Higden, H: Blood doping among endurance athletes: rationalizations, results, and ramifications. Am Med News, Sept 27, 1985, p 37.

21. Robertson, RJ, et al: Hemoglobin concentration and aerobic work capacity in women following induced erythrocythemia. J Appl Physiol 57:568, 1984.

22. Eichner, ER: Blood doping: Implications of recent research. Sports Med Digest 9(3):4, 1987.

23. Wilmore, JH: Blood doping. Sports Med Digest 9(11):6, 1987.

24. McBride, G: Just a laboratory curiosity. Medicine on the Midway. Winter, 1988, p 7.

25. O'Brien, R, Schlesinger, D and Hirsch, GA: Special report: Foreign intrigue. Runners World, June, 1988, p 62.

26. Williams, MH, et al: Effect of blood reinjection upon endurance capacity and heart rate. Med Sci Sports 5:181, 1973.

27. Gledhill, N: Blood doping and related issues: A brief review. Med Sci Sports Exerc 14(3):183, 1982.

28. Sawka, MN, et al: Erythrocyte reinfusion and maximal aerobic power: An examination of modifying factors. JAMA 257:1496, 1987.

29. American College of Sports Medicine Position Stand: Blood Doping as an Ergogenic Aid, Indianapolis, 1987.

30. Berglund, B, Hemmingsson, P and Birgegard, G: Detection of autologous blood transfusions in cross-country skiers. Int J Sports Med 8:66, 1987.

PART III

Recognition and Management of Drug Abuse in the Athlete

CHAPTER 17

Recognition

INTRODUCTION

Recognizing drug abuse in a blatantly intoxicated individual is as easy for the layperson as it is for the professional. However, in a society where the use of certain substances to modify mood or behavior is often regarded as "normal and appropriate,"[1] the recognition of drug abuse can be much more difficult. Drug abuse can be extremely subtle and often defies recognition even by the health care professional. This is not at all surprising given the variety and dosages of substances that are abused, the settings in which they are abused, the episodic nature of drug abuse, and the personality characteristics of the abuser, as well as the individual abuser's sensitivity and tolerance to abused substances.

Any discussion of the diagnosis of drug abuse must begin with a review of terms used in the literature. It should be emphasized that most of the terminology in the drug abuse field pertains to psychoactive substances and not to performance-enhancing drugs, although there are clearly areas of overlap, for example, cocaine and amphetamines.

DEFINITIONS

Drug Abuse

Drug abuse as defined by the World Health Organization (WHO) in 1969 is persistent or sporadic excessive drug use inconsistent with or unrelated to acceptable medical practice.[2] Included in the WHO definition of drug abuse is the concept that the abuse of drugs may not only be deleterious to the individual but it may have deleterious consequences to society.[3] The term "misuse," as contrasted with the term "abuse," suggests more of a quantitative rather than an actual qualitative difference. At any given time, drug misuse can be as destructive as drug abuse, whether as a result of physical illness, psychotic reaction, destructive behavior, or suicide.

Drug Dependence

Drug dependence has been defined as "a state, psychic and sometimes also physical, resulting from the interaction between a living organism and a drug, characterized by behavioral and other responses that always include a compulsion to take the drug on a continuous or periodic basis in order to experience its psychic effects and sometimes to avoid the discomfort of its abstinence."[2] Such drug use can continue despite the development of adverse consequences.

Drug dependence has been divided into two broad categories: physical dependence and psychological dependence.

Physical Dependence

Much of the early work on the subject of physical dependence pertained to opiate analgesics. This class of drugs had been demonstrated, in both animal models and humans, to produce a withdrawal syndrome following the cessation of repeated drug administration. Specific withdrawal symptoms and signs vary from drug to drug. Narcotic withdrawal symptoms and signs are related to the degree of dependence and the length of time of abstinence. Initially, the individual may develop lacrimation, yawning, excessive perspiration, and dilated pupils. As the length of abstinence increases, tremor, piloerection, muscle twitching, intense abdominal, leg and back cramps, progressive restlessness, vomiting, and diarrhea may all appear. Withdrawal symptoms and signs peak between 36 and 48 hours, and can remain at maximal intensity for 72 hours before gradually subsiding during the next 5 to 10 days.[2]

In addition to narcotics, marked physiologic signs of withdrawal are common with alcohol, sedatives, and anxiolytics. Physiologic signs of withdrawal are less apparent with amphetamines, cocaine, nicotine, and marijuana; however, there may be intense subjective symptoms associated with withdrawal from the use of these substances. The use of some drugs such as hallucinogens is not associated with any withdrawal symptoms.[1]

Intimately related to the concept of physical dependence is the concept of tolerance. Tolerance refers to the "declining effect of the same dose of a drug when it is administered repeatedly over a period of time."[2] Alternatively stated, tolerance occurs when increasing doses of a drug are required in order to achieve the same or lessening effects. The degree to which tolerance develops varies with the class of substance that is abused. Cross-tolerance results when the use of one drug leads an individual to require greater than the usual doses of another drug to obtain a desired effect. One consequence of cross-tolerance is death resulting from multiple drug ingestions while attempting to achieve a desired psychic effect.

Psychological Dependence

Physical dependence is not necessary for an individual to develop psychological dependence. Inherent in the concept of psychological dependence is an individual's reliance on a drug to produce an altered state of consciousness or affect. The psychologically dependent drug abuser, even when recognizing that the use of a substance is excessive, is unable to reduce or control its use and may spend a great deal of time in activities directed at obtaining the substance. Continued use occurs despite the impairment of social, recreational, and occupational activities, and despite the development of psychological and physical symptoms.[1]

The American Psychiatric Association has developed diagnostic criteria for Psychoactive Substance (Drug) Dependence (Table 17–1). These criteria refer to the "maladaptive behavior associated with more or less regular use of (psychoactive) substances."[1] Complementing this diagnostic category is another diagnostic category, Psychoactive Substance Abuse (Table 17–2). This category pertains to maladaptive patterns of psychoactive substance use which fail to meet the rigorous diagnostic criteria for actual dependency. Both of these categories are separate and distinct from the Psychoactive Substance-Induced Organic Mental Disorders, which define the direct and specific acute

Table 17–1. DIAGNOSTIC CRITERIA FOR PSYCHOACTIVE SUBSTANCE
DEPENDENCE

A. At least three of the following:
    1. substance often taken in larger amounts or over a longer period than the person intended
    2. persistent desire or one or more unsuccessful efforts to cut down or control substance use
    3. a great deal of time spent in activities necessary to get the substance (e.g., theft), taking the substance (e.g., chain smoking), or recovering from its effects
    4. frequent intoxication or withdrawal symptoms when expected to fulfill major role obligations at work, school, or home (e.g., does not go to work because hung over, goes to school or work "high," intoxicated while taking care of his or her children), or when substance use is physically hazardous (e.g., drives when intoxicated)
    5. important social, occupational, or recreational activities given up or reduced because of substance use
    6. continued substance use despite knowledge of having a persistent or recurrent social, psychological, or physical problem that is caused or exacerbated by the use of the substance (e.g., keeps using heroin despite family arguments about it, cocaine-induced depression, or having an ulcer made worse by drinking)
    7. marked tolerance: need for markedly increased amounts of the substance (i.e., at least a 50% increase) in order to achieve intoxication or desired effect, or markedly diminished effect with continued use of the same amount
    Note: The following items may not apply to cannabis, hallucinogens, or phencyclidine (PCP):
    8. characteristic withdrawal symptoms (see specific withdrawal syndromes under Psychoactive Substance-induced Organic Mental Disorders)
    9. substance often taken to relieve or avoid withdrawal symptoms
B. Some symptoms of the disturbance have persisted for at least one month, or have occurred repeatedly over a longer period of time.

Criteria for Severity of Psychoactive Substance Dependence
    Mild: Few, if any, symptoms in excess of those required to make the diagnosis, and the symptoms result in no more than mild impairment in occupational functioning or in usual social activities or relationships with others.
    Moderate: Symptoms or functional impairment between "mild" and "severe."
    Severe: Many symptoms in excess of those required to make the diagnosis, and the symptoms markedly interfere with occupational functioning or with usual social activities or relationships with others.*
    In Partial Remission: During the past six months, some use of the substance and some symptoms of dependence.
    In Full Remission: During the past six months, either no use of the substance, or use of the substance and no symptoms of dependence.

*Because of the availability of cigarettes and other nicotine-containing substances and the absence of a clinically significant nicotine intoxication syndrome, impairment in occupational or social functioning is not necessary for a rating of severe nicotine dependence.
From Diagnostic and Statistical Manual of Mental Disorders, ed. 3, revised. American Psychiatric Association, Washington, DC, 1987, with permission.

Table 17–2. DIAGNOSTIC CRITERIA FOR PSYCHOACTIVE SUBSTANCE **ABUSE**

A. A maladaptive pattern of psychoactive substance use indicated by at least one of the following:
    1. continued use despite knowledge of having a persistent or recurrent social, occupational, psychological, or physical problem that is caused or exacerbated by use of the psychoactive substance
    2. recurrent use in situations in which use is physically hazardous (e.g., driving while intoxicated)
B. Some symptoms of the disturbance have persisted for at least one month, or have occurred repeatedly over a longer period of time
C. Never met the criteria for Psychoactive Substance Dependence for this substance

From Diagnostic and Statistical Manual of Mental Disorders, ed. 3, revised. American Psychiatric Association, Washington, DC, 1987, with permission.

and chronic effects of psychoactive substances on the central nervous system.[1]

WHO IS AT RISK?

As discussed in the preceding chapters, knowing the pertinent risk factors can help to identify individuals who are at risk of drug abuse. However, being at risk cannot be equated with drug abuse. Conversely, being devoid of risk factors cannot be equated with immunity from drug abuse. Though risk factors per se are nothing more than statistical statements valid in large populations, they may be of considerable value when applied to the individual.

SUSPECTING THE DRUG ABUSER

The Role of the Physician

Although over 200 years ago, America's first Surgeon General, Benjamin Rush, M.D., labeled "intemperance" a disease, there has been inadequate training of health care professionals in the United States in the identification and treatment of alcohol and other drug abuse.[5] In 1971, the National Institute on Drug Abuse and the National Institute on Alcohol Abuse and Alcoholism encouraged the teaching of drug abuse education in the medical schools. The Career Teaching Training Program in the Addictions provided support for medical school faculty members.[6] It was the intent of this program to teach students to diagnose and treat patients with alcohol and drug abuse problems.[5] In 1972, the Council on Mental Health and the Committee on Alcohol and Drug Dependency, both of the American Medical Association, similarly called for the development and implementation of drug abuse curricula in medical schools.[7] By 1973, only 45 of 120 United States and Canadian medical schools offered subject matter dealing with alcoholism. By 1978, 102 of 105 medical schools reported at least some training in alcohol and drug abuse.[8]

A 1981 survey of 40 United States medical schools with drug abuse education indicated that there was a particular emphasis on end-stage alcoholism and its complications, and that the students were rarely being taught the skills necessary for the early identifica-

tion of individuals at risk of drug abuse as well as the skills necessary for early intervention.[9] A 1982 poll by the American Medical Association indicated that only 27 percent of physicians felt competent to deal with an alcoholic patient.[10] In 1986, United States medical schools devoted less than 1 percent of their required teaching hours to "an integrated approach to alcoholism and drug abuse."[11] In 1988, Davis and colleagues[11a] concluded, after surveying 98 medical schools and 1124 residency programs, that drug abuse training was moving in a positive direction. However, they noted that there was a lack of comprehensive drug abuse training across clinical specialties in both medical school and postgraduate training.

In 1986, Singer and Anglin[12] reported that in a large urban teaching hospital in 1983, health care professionals were "apt to judge far fewer adolescents as having an alcohol/drug problem than as having other problems common to this age group." Specifically, they noted that adjusted citywide (Cleveland) prevalence rates of adolescent alcohol abuse (12.7 percent) exceeded health care professionals' judgments (3 percent) by over fourfold. In this particular study, the health care professionals were primarily residents, medical students, and attending physicians.

Similar results were reported in 1987 by Coulehan and associates[13] in an 18-month study involving 3 academic primary care settings, 2 family health centers, and 1 internal medicine clinic. In this study in which the health care professionals were primarily internal medicine and family practice residents, only 40 percent (17 of 42) of drug abuse patients were recognized as such during an initial evaluation. In this particular study, physicians tended to diagnose drug abuse accurately if the patient also had an antisocial personality disorder. On the other hand, physicians failed to recognize drug abuse if the patient suffered from concomitant depression or other psychiatric disorders. Moore and Malitz[14] reported comparable findings of underdiagnosis of alcoholism by internal medicine residents in the Johns Hopkins Hospital Internal Medicine Group Practice.

Although the aforementioned studies are not directly transferable to drug abuse recognition by health care professionals in athletics, there is little doubt that there is an underrecognition of drug abuse by primary care physicians who care for individual athletes and by team or sports medicine physicians who care for athletes in organized settings.

In 1987, Lewis and co-workers[5] summarized the recent private and federal initiatives that have been undertaken to develop a core body of knowledge and skills for primary care physicians in the area of drug abuse. One such initiative led to the founding in 1976 of the Association for Medical Education and Research in Substance Abuse (AMERSA) at the Center for Alcohol and Addiction Studies at Brown University. At AMERSA's 1985 ninth annual conference entitled "Alcohol, Drugs and Primary Care Physician Education," it was the consensus of the conferees that at a minimum, "primary care physicians should demonstrate mastery of the following subject areas:

1. Epidemiology, including knowledge of the natural history of substance abuse and risk factors
2. Physiology and biochemistry of dependence and addiction
3. Pharmacology, including knowledge of effects of commonly abused drugs and drug-drug interactions
4. Diagnosis, intervention and referral
5. Case management, including short and long term consequences of abuse and dependence
6. Prevention through health promotion; early identification and patient education"[5]

Although directed primarily towards primary care physicians, these recommendations are applicable to any physician who has the responsibility for maintaining the health and well-being of athletes. It is toward this end that this text has been written.

The Role of Others

While a definitive diagnosis of drug abuse in the athlete may ultimately fall under the purview of a physician, it is far more likely that drug abuse is initially suspected by "significant others" in the athlete's life. Significant others include fellow athletes, trainers, coaches, agents, friends, relatives, and spouses. At times, however, drug abuse by the athlete may be so clandestine that it may become evident only as a result of a formalized urine drug testing program.

The sheer suspicion that an athlete is engaged in drug abuse raises many ethical and legal questions. It is clear that a team or personal physician who suspects drug abuse has a responsibility to deal directly with the athlete. Although working for "the team" or for management, the team physician is bound by the same rules of confidentiality and ethics that are extant in any other doctor-patient relationship (see Chapter 20).

However, treatment issues aside, it is a far more complicated matter if drug abuse is suspected by someone other than the team or personal physician. The athletic trainer who deals with the athlete from day to day often is the first person to recognize both the physical and behavioral changes associated with drug abuse in an athlete. In select circumstances, the trainer's engagement of the athlete about such concerns may facilitate the trainer's obtaining professional help for the athlete. On the other hand, if the trainer insensitively confronts the athlete, particularly when inadequately trained to do so, such confrontation may be counterproductive. In fact, such confrontation may adversely affect any future relationship between the athlete and the trainer. Similarly, if it is perceived that the trainer, in a "behind the back" manner, is conveying his or her concern to the team physician and/or management, there may well be a breakdown in the rapport between the trainer and the athlete, and perhaps more importantly, between the trainer and other athletes on the team. Similar scenarios can be developed for others who suspect that an athlete is abusing drugs.

THE TEAM/SPORTS MEDICINE PHYSICIAN AND THE INTERVIEW PROCESS

Unlike the physician practicing in the community who sees an individual infrequently and usually at the initiative of the individual, the team/sports medicine physician has the opportunity of observing the athlete in multiple settings under a variety of conditions over an extended period of time. These settings include the preparticipation physical examination, injury and illness examinations, and during training and actual competition. In these settings, the team/sports medicine physician may observe changes in behavior, mood, performance, appearance, and interpersonal relationships that might suggest drug abuse. Additionally, the observations of others, such as trainers, coaches, and teammates, may lead the team/sports medicine physician to suspect drug abuse.

Collectively utilizing these varied observations, as well as the results of any urine drug testing, the team/sports medicine physician is actually screening for or casefinding a substance abuser rather than actually diagnosing a drug abuse disorder. As emphasized by Babor and Kadden,[15] screening, which is a process of initial identification, is usually initiated by the health care professional, rather than by the individual seeking medical advice. While screening usually consists of only a portion of the examining or testing procedures required for a diagnosis, "diagnosis typically involves a broader evaluation of signs, symptoms, and laboratory data as these relate to the history of the patient's illness." Casefinding, as contrasted with screening and diagnosis, refers to the process of identifying a drug abuser who seeks medical care for a problem which may be unrelated to drug abuse.[16]

Once drug abuse by an athlete is suspected, the team/sports medicine physician, at an appropriate time and in an appropriate setting, should initiate the interview process in an effort to establish the diagnosis of drug abuse. "As with other medical illnesses, the earlier the physician establishes the diagnosis of substance abuse and begins treatment, the better the prognosis."[17] Numerous ways have been advanced to approach the subject of alcohol and drug abuse, and some general principles regarding the interview process will be emphasized.

1. Prior to beginning the interview process, physicians must be aware of their own personal pre-existing attitudes, prejudices, and insecurities regarding drug abuse. They must not let these attitudes, prejudices, and insecurities be a barrier to an effective assessment, which is essential to effective management. As Rohman[18] has noted: "While many . . . primary care physicians . . . were confident in treating the medical sequelae of alcoholism, comparatively few were confident about the non-biomedical or patient management aspects of treatment, such as formulating a treatment plan." Skillful physicians will demonstrate early that their questioning is an expression of concern.[19] Even the tone of the physician's voice may reflect underlying attitudes which may interfere with the effectiveness of the interview.[20] The term "interview," as used in this chapter, refers to a process and should not be construed to mean a single event.

2. Prior to the actual interview, physicians should familiarize themselves with as much information as possible regarding the reasons for suspecting that the individual is abusing drugs. However, the acquisition of such data must not jeopardize the individual's rights to privacy and confidentiality, and it should not result in any prejudgment.

3. The interview should be performed in a setting where privacy and confidentiality are absolutely assured. This takes on additional importance in organized athletics since the athlete may view any admission of drug abuse as jeopardizing his or her athletic career.

4. As an ice-breaker, the initial part of the interview should center around the use of legal substances such as cigarettes and caffeine. In addition to addressing such variables as the frequency and extent of use, there should be an assessment of the reasons for the use of these substances, as well as the setting in which the usage occurs. A discussion about the perceived effects of these substances on behavior can open the door to a future discussion about the effects of other substances on behavior. Similarly, discussions regarding the manifestations of abstinence from cigarettes and caffeine can pave the way to subsequent discussions regarding the symptoms and signs associated with abstinence from other drugs.

5. From cigarettes and caffeine, the interview can gradually shift to a discussion of alcohol (wine, beer, and liquor), which may or may not be the principal drug of abuse. Recognizing that many individuals feel uncomfortable when discussing drinking practices, it is often helpful for the physician to indicate to the athlete at the outset that many people feel uncomfortable when asked how much they drink, when they drink, or what happens when they drink. It is also frequently helpful, when discussing alcohol consumption, to emphasize the health aspects rather than any judgmental aspects. During this phase of the assessment process, terms such

as "alcoholic" should be avoided. Furthermore, the physician must avoid being pedantic and must be careful not to attack the denial mechanism.[17] In obtaining the history, appropriate attention should be directed to the risk factors and antecedents of alcoholism, such as family history of alcoholism and depression (see Chapter 2).

6. From alcohol, the interview can shift to a discussion of illicit drug use, beginning with marijuana. Since this part of the interview deals with the use of illegal drugs or illegally obtained legal drugs, it is especially important to be consistent by again emphasizing health matters. As with alcohol, the physician should avoid using labels such as "addict" and should not attack the denial mechanism. Since many athletes attempt to enhance performance by using drugs, there should be a discussion of this matter, in addition to a discussion about recreational drug abuse. However, it should be emphasized that many athletes believe physicians are poorly informed regarding drug-related performance enhancement and therefore many athletes are reluctant to discuss this subject with physicians.

7. Clues to drug abuse can be obtained by evaluating the usage patterns of legally prescribed drugs such as analgesic/narcotic combinations, anxiolytics, and hypnotics. The maintenance of a team prescription log can be very helpful in this regard.

STAGING OF "RECREATIONAL" DRUG ABUSE

Various systems have been developed to enable the physician to determine the severity and extent of an individual's drug abuse. The system utilized by MacKenzie and Jacobs,[21] which is adapted from MacDonald,[22] is representative of one such system (Table 17–3).

Stage 0 represents the phase of experimentation with a chemical substance. As discussed in Chapter 2, most youths have experimented with at least one chemical substance, be it alcohol, nicotine, or marijuana. If, after one or more times, the resultant experience is perceived as being a positive one, the individual is then poised to enter Stage 1. On the other hand, if the drug experience is not rewarding, or if it produces

Table 17–3. STAGES OF CHEMICAL DEPENDENCY IN ADOLESCENTS AND YOUNG ADULTS

Stage 0	Curiosity
Stage 1	Learns the mood swing
Stage 2	Seeks the mood swing
Stage 3	Is preoccupied with the mood swing
Stage 4	Uses substance to feel normal

From MacDonald,[22] with permission.

adverse effects, drug usage may never progress to Stage 1.

Stage 1 "is learning about the use of mood-altering chemicals."[21] Peer pressure is a principal motivating factor during this stage, and the drugs used are usually alcohol, marijuana, and occasionally cocaine. Recognition of drug abuse at this stage is difficult because there are few, if any, outward signs, though feelings of guilt may be evident.

Stage 2 "is seeking the effects of mood-altering chemicals." It is during this stage that drug abusers acquire their own drugs and paraphernalia. Drug abuse becomes a method of "relaxing." "Situational rather than social use characterizes this stage."[21] It is during this stage that personal hygiene begins to deteriorate, peer relationships become focused around drug abuse, and performance—whether academic or athletic—begins to change. Periods of increased anxiety as well as actual panic attacks may appear, which can be confused with the psychological and physical effects of stimulants (Table 17–4).

Stage 3 is characterized by a preoccupation with drugs and alcohol and by the relentless pursuit of being high. During this stage, there is a progressive deterioration in appearance, personal hygiene, behavior, and interpersonal relationships. Behavioral changes include lying, cheating, and stealing. Interpersonal relationships are often centered around the acquisition of drugs. Emotional swings are evident and reflect both underlying psychiatric disturbances as well as drug effects. Language may be increasingly pervaded by idioms of the drug culture.

Stage 4 has been referred to as the "burnout" stage of drug abuse. Drugs are no longer

Table 17–4. SYMPTOMS OF PANIC ATTACK

Apprehension
Fear
Terror
Feeling of impending doom
Shortness of breath
Dizziness
Faintness
Choking
Palpitations
Trembling/shaking
Sweating
Nausea/abdominal pain
Depersonalization
Numbness/tingling
Chest pain

used to achieve a high or a state of euphoria, but instead are used to relieve a chronic dysphoria.

FORMALIZED SCREENING INSTRUMENTS

The accuracy of the history in alcoholism and drug abuse has proven to be one of the most difficult measures in the drug abuse field. For example, with respect to alcohol, Hays and Spickard[23] note that experts cannot agree on a "safe" level of consumption, nor is the average consumption by an individual a part of the DSM-III (R) criteria for the diagnosis of alcoholism. In addition, individuals who are heavy drinkers are oftentimes inaccurate in their reporting of quantities consumed. Accordingly, various screening instruments such as questionnaires have been developed in an attempt to provide a more structured and standardized approach to the diagnosis of drug abuse, in particular, alcohol abuse and alcoholism. However, it must be emphasized that any such instrument is only adjunctive to a complete history (including a psychosocial history) physical examination, and laboratory evaluation. As Klitzner and Schonberg have emphasized: "That a screening device would be a substitute for a confidential and candid discussion between physician and young patient would seem for the moment premature."[24]

The Diagnostic Interview Schedule (DIS)[26] might be viewed as a "gold standard" diagnostic instrument for the identification of all psychiatric disorders, including alcohol abuse as well as drug abuse, and is in accordance with DSM-III criteria, the Feighner and associates criteria,[25] and the Research Diagnostic Criteria (RDC). This highly structured and comprehensive interview was designed as an epidemiologic instrument to be administered by nonclinicians. It is computer scored according to algorithms based on the DSM-III criteria for psychiatric diagnoses.[13,26]

An easily administered questionnaire that was designed in 1970 specifically for the diagnosis of alcoholism is the CAGE questionnaire[27,28] (Table 17–5). This useful, brief, and nonintimidating interviewing instrument provides a useful mnemonic device. In some studies, one "yes" response has been considered positive for alcoholism.[29] In others, a two- or three-item "yes" criterion has been used. CAGE is an insensitive indicator if a four-item "yes" is required.[28] In general, the CAGE questionnaire has been validated as both reasonably sensitive and specific in a variety of settings, including both inpatient and outpatient settings.[23] In a prospective study of over 500 medical and orthopedic inpatients, Bush has demonstrated the CAGE questionnaire to be far superior to the use of laboratory tests (MCV, GGTP, SGOT, SGPT) in identifying alcoholics.[29] However, it should be noted that the CAGE questionnaire can be administered so as to encourage negative responses and thus result in underreporting, particularly in the early stages of alcohol abuse.

Another questionnaire that has been extensively utilized is the self-reporting, Michigan Alcoholism Screening Test (MAST),[30] which was "devised to provide a consistent, quantifiable, structured interview" consisting

Table 17–5. CAGE QUESTIONNAIRE

C. Have you ever felt you ought to "C"ut down on your drinking?
A. Have people "A"nnoyed you by criticizing your drinking?
G. Have you ever felt bad or "G"uilty about your drinking?
E. Have you ever had a drink first thing in the morning to steady your nerves or to get rid of a hangover ("E"ye opener)?

From Ewing,[27] p. 1907, with permission.

Table 17–6. MAST RESPONSES OF HOSPITALIZED ALCOHOLICS AND NONALCOHOLIC CONTROLS (IN PERCENTS)

Points	Questions	Alcoholics (N = 116) Yes	No	Nonalcoholics (N = 103) Yes	No
2	*1. Do you feel you are a normal drinker?	14	86	99	1
2	2. Have you ever awakened the morning after some drinking the night before and found that you could not remember a part of the evening before?	80	20	18	82
1	3. Does your wife (or parents) ever worry or complain about your drinking?	86	12†	7	93
2	*4. Can you stop drinking without a struggle after one or two drinks?	84	66	98	2
1	5. Do you ever feel bad about your drinking?	91	9	6	94
2	*6. Do friends or relatives think you are a normal drinker?	15	82‡	99	1
0	7. Do you ever try to limit your drinking to certain times of the day or to certain places?	53	47	11	89
2	*8. Are you always able to stop drinking when you want to?	36	64	96	4
5	9. Have you ever attended a meeting of Alcoholics Anonymous (AA)?	65	35	0	100
1	10. Have you gotten into fights when drinking?	30	70	9	91
2	11. Has drinking ever created problems with you and your wife?	66	22§	7	86§
2	12. Has your wife (or other family member) ever gone to anyone for help about your drinking?	37	63	0	100
2	13. Have you ever lost friends or girlfriends/boyfriends because of drinking?	46	54	1	99
2	14. Have you ever gotten into trouble at work because of drinking?	52	48	0	100
2	15. Have you ever lost a job because of drinking?	39	61	0	100
2	16. Have you ever neglected your obligations, your family, or your work for two or more days in a row because you were drinking?	61	39	0	100
1	17. Do you ever drink before noon?	85	15	22	78
2	18. Have you ever been told you have liver trouble? Cirrhosis?	31	69	1	99
2	19. Have you ever had delirium tremens (DTs), severe shaking, heard voices, or seen things that weren't there after heavy drinking?	49	51	0	100
5	20. Have you ever gone to anyone for help about your drinking?	28	72	0	100
5	21. Have you ever been in a hospital because of drinking?	45	55	1	99
2	22. Have you ever been a patient in a psychiatric hospital or on a psychiatric ward of a general hospital where drinking was part of the problem?	21	79	0	100
2	23. Have you ever been seen at a psychiatric or mental health clinic, or gone to a doctor, social worker, or clergyman for help with an emotional problem in which drinking had played a part?	31	69	0	100
2	24. Have you ever been arrested even for a few hours because of drunk behavior?	49	51	4	96
2	25. Have you ever been arrested for drunk driving or driving after drinking?	45	55	1	99

*Negative responses are alcoholic responses; †Two (2 percent) were single with both parents out of the picture; ‡Three (3 percent) gave no response to this question; §Fourteen (12 percent) of the alcoholics and seven (7 percent) of the control group were single. From Selzer,[30] with permission.

Scoring:
≤3 points = nonalcoholic; 4 points suggests alcoholic; ≥5 points = alcoholic.

Table 17–7. THE BRIEF MAST

Points	Questions
2	*1. Do you feel you are a normal drinker?
2	*2. Do friends or relatives think you are a normal drinker?
5	3. Have you ever attended a meeting of Alcoholics Anonymous (AA)?
2	4. Have you ever lost friends or girlfriends/boyfriends because of drinking?
2	5. Have you ever gotten into trouble at work because of drinking?
2	6. Have you ever neglected your obligations, your family, or your work for two or more days in a row because you were drinking?
2	7. Have you ever had delirium tremens (DTs), severe shaking, heard voices, or seen things that weren't there after heavy drinking?
5	8. Have you ever gone to anyone for help about your drinking?
5	9. Have you ever been in a hospital because of drinking?
2	10. Have you ever been arrested for drunk driving or driving after drinking?

*Negative response = alcoholic response. Scoring same as for Table 17–6. From Pokorny, Miller, and Kaplan,[32] with permission.

of 25 yes or no questions that relate to medical, social, and behavioral events associated with excessive drinking (Table 17–6). Although there have been conflicting arguments as to the validity of self-reporting screening devices, it has been stated that a self-report device is typically faster, more efficient, and less costly than other screening devices but of comparable accuracy.[31]

Unlike the CAGE, the MAST gives more than a simple alcoholic-nonalcoholic designation. Its scoring methodology provides some indication of severity. According to Hays and Spickard,[23] the MAST and the

Table 17–8. THE ALCOHOL CLINICAL INDEX: MEDICAL HISTORY

DIRECTIONS:

The following questions are about your health. Please read each question carefully and then indicate your answer by circling either "yes" or "no."

Please answer every question. If you have difficulty understanding a question, then ask for help from your doctor or other member of the health care team.

Your medical history is a private matter. The information collected on this form will be kept strictly confidential.

	Circle your answer	
1. Do you often wake up with a headache?	yes	no
2. Do your hands shake in the morning?	yes	no
3. Do you often feel unable to concentrate (e.g. while reading or at work)?	yes	no
4. Do you find it hard to remember recent events?	yes	no
5. Have your hands been trembling a lot recently?	yes	no
6. Are you troubled by frightening dreams?	yes	no
7. Have you experienced troublesome mental confusion?	yes	no
8. Have you ever had a hallucination (experienced a sight or sound that didn't exist)?	yes	no
9. Do you often wake up feeling thirsty in the morning?	yes	no
10. Are you often troubled by a dry coated tongue?	yes	no
11. Do you cough on most days (for periods of at least 3 months)?	yes	no
12. Do you often bring up phlegm (thick mucus) from your throat or lungs?	yes	no
13. Since your 18th birthday, have you been injured in a fight or assault (exclude injuries during sports)?	yes	no

From Skinner and Holt,[34] with permission.

CAGE are equal in sensitivity and specificity. In 1972, a shortened version of the MAST was introduced and is referred to as the Brief MAST (Table 17–7), which in a VA hospital setting had correlations with the long form of the MAST ranging from 0.95 to 0.99.[32]

The Diagnostic Questions for Early or Advanced Alcoholism (DQEAA) represents

Table 17–9. THE ALCOHOL CLINICAL INDEX: CLINICAL SIGNS

	Present (check)
HAND	
1. Hand tremor (fine tremor with hands outstretched and unsupported)	_____
2. Palmar erythema (permanent red color of proximal and lateral palms)	_____
3. Nicotine stains (brown stains usually between index and middle finger)	_____
HEAD	
4. Facial erythema (persistent, red flush of the face or "whiskey nose")	_____
5. Rhinophyma (varying degrees of epithelial thickening, dilatation of sebaceous follicles and bluish-red discoloration of the distal portion of the nose)	_____
6. Coated tongue (varying degrees of fixed exudate on the surface of the tongue)	_____
7. Edema of soft palate or fauces (obvious swelling of the soft palate, tonsillar area and/or uvula, usually associated with erythema but excluding infection)	_____
ABDOMEN	
8. Collateral circulation (venous vessel enlargement in a radial distribution outward from the umbilicus or on the anterior abdominal wall, "caput medusa")	_____
9. Abdominal tenderness (tenderness elicited by normal palpation of any area of the abdomen due to any cause)	_____
BODY	
10. Cigarette burns (recent or old burn marks or scars on hands and/or body)	_____
11. Bruises/Abrasions (bruises or abrasions resulting from recent and/or past injury)	_____
12. Scars due to trauma (more than one scar due to recent and/or past injury, excluding elective surgery)	_____
13. Tattoos (subepidermal infiltration of ink or pigment for cosmetic reasons)	_____
14. Gynecomastia (male only, glandular *and* fatty tissue enlargement of *both* breasts)	_____
15. Spider nevi (>5) (greater than five vascular, spiderlike lesions with a central feeding vessel on the area of the body corresponding to the distribution of the superior vena cava)	_____
LOCOMOTOR FUNCTION	
16. Tandem gait (inability of an individual to walk in a straight line by opposing the heel of the forward foot with the toe of weight bearing foot)	_____
17. Deep knee bend (inability of a mobile subject to take up a crouching position with both knees flexed and return to an upright standing posture, excluding subjects with known musculoskeletal disease, and the frail or elderly)	_____

From Skinner and Holt,[34] with permission.

an alternative self-reporting questionnaire which may be used during the interview process. This instrument, although somewhat more subtle than the MAST, has not been subject to the same validations as the MAST.[17]

In an effort to integrate the medical history as well as clinical signs of alcohol abuse into a single diagnostic instrument, Skinner and Holt, in 1986, developed *The Alcohol Clinical Index*.[33,34] Thirteen specific questions are either asked by the examiner or are self-completed by the individual, and seventeen specified clinical signs are looked for on the physical examination. A probability of alcohol abuse exceeding 0.90 exists if 4 or more clinical signs or 4 or more medical history items in the instrument are present (Tables 17–8 and 17–9).

The aforementioned questionnaires have been directed primarily at adult populations. The recognition of the increasing problem of teenage alcoholism has prompted the development of a questionnaire geared towards this age group. The Adolescent Alcohol Involvement Scale (AAIS) (Table 17–10), primarily developed as a research tool, was not designed to diagnose alcoholism in adolescents, but rather to identify adolescents who have drinking problems.[31] In this scale, a score of less than 41 is indicative of no alcohol-related behavioral problems; a score of 42 to 57 indicates alcohol misuse; and 58 to 79 is consistent with alcoholic-like drinking patterns.

Although, as indicated above, a variety of formalized screening instruments have been developed to detect alcohol abuse, to date there has not been a parallel effort to develop similar instruments for other forms of drug abuse. The recent development of such an instrument by Klitzner and co-workers[35] for the adolescent age group awaits validation.

Table 17–10. ADOLESCENT ALCOHOL INVOLVEMENT SCALE

1. How often do you drink?
   a. never
   b. once or twice a year
   c. once or twice a month
   d. every weekend
   e. several times a week
   f. every day
2. When did you have your last drink?
   a. never drank
   b. not for over a year
   c. between 6 months and 1 year ago
   d. several weeks ago
   e. last week
   f. yesterday
   g. today
3. I usually start to drink because:
   a. I like the taste
   b. to be like my friends
   c. to feel like an adult
   d. I feel nervous, tense, full of worries or problems
   e. I feel sad, lonely, sorry for myself
4. What do you drink?
   a. wine
   b. beer
   c. mixed drinks
   d. hard liquor
   e. a substitute for alcohol—paint thinner, sterno, cough medicine, mouthwash, hair tonic, etc.

5. How do you get your drinks?
   a. supervised by parents or relatives
   b. from brothers or sisters
   c. from home without parents' knowledge
   d. from friends
   e. buy it with false identification
6. When did you take your first drink?
   a. never
   b. recently
   c. after age 15
   d. at ages 14 or 15
   e. between ages 10–13
   f. before age 10
7. What time of day do you usually drink?
   a. with meals
   b. at night
   c. afternoons
   d. mostly in the morning or when I first awake
   e. I often get up during my sleep and drink
8. Why did you take your first drink?
   a. curiosity
   b. parents or relatives offered
   c. friends encouraged me
   d. to feel more like an adult
   e. to get drunk or high
9. How much do you drink, when you do drink?
   a. 1 drink
   b. 2 drinks

Table 17–10—*Continued*

c. 3–6 drinks
d. 6 or more drinks
e. until "high" or drunk
10. Whom do you drink with?
    a. parents or relatives only
    b. with brothers or sisters only
    c. with friends own age
    d. with older friends
    e. alone
11. What is the greatest effect you have had from alcohol?
    a. loose, easy feeling
    b. moderately "high"
    c. drunk
    d. became ill
    e. passed out
    f. was drinking heavily and the next day didn't remember what happened
12. What is the greatest effect drinking has had on your life?
    a. none—no effect
    b. has interfered with talking to someone
    c. has prevented me from having a good time
    d. has interfered with my school work

e. have lost friends because of drinking
f. has gotten me into trouble at home
g. was in a fight or destroyed property
h. has resulted in an accident, an injury, arrest, or being punished at school for drinking
13. How do you feel about your drinking?
    a. no problem at all
    b. I can control it and set limits on myself
    c. I can control myself, but my friends easily influence me
    d. I often feel bad about my drinking
    e. I need help to control myself
    f. I have had professional help to control my drinking
14. How do others see you?
    a. can't say, or a normal drinker for my age
    b. when I drink I tend to neglect my family or friends
    c. my family or friends advise me to control or cut down on my drinking
    d. my family or friends tell me to get help for my drinking
    e. my family or friends have already gone for help for my drinking

Scoring Instructions: The highest total score is 79. An *a* response is scored 1 (except on questions 1, 2, 6, 12, 13 and 14, on which *a* = 0); *b* = 2; *c* = 3; and so on to *h* = 8. When more than one response is made, the one with the higher or highest score is used. An unanswered question is scored 0.

From Mayer and Filstead,[31] with permission.

FINAL NOTE

In general terms, a high index of suspicion of drug abuse should be prompted by an unexplained change in behavior, mood, performance, appearance, or concentration. Changes in interpersonal relationships may be evidenced by arguments with teammates, inappropriate challenges to authority figures, conniving, and lying. Associations may become limited to other individuals who share in their drug taking or who are involved in the procurement of drugs. Other clues include distortions of time sense, such as showing up repeatedly late or early to practice, unexplained financial difficulties, an increase in injuries, and an excessive reliance on over-the-counter and prescriptive medications for trivial illnesses and injuries.

A knowledge of the antecedents of drug abuse and the special vulnerabilities of the athlete to drug abuse as discussed in Part I of this text should be familiar to team/sports medicine physicians as well as others who render care to athletes. The physiology and pharmacology as well as the clinical characteristics of the various drugs of abuse detailed in Part II should facilitate the recognition of specific drug abuse patterns. Although formalized screening instruments are available to assist in the diagnosis of alcoholism, to date no validated comparable instruments are readily available to diagnose other forms of drug abuse. Drug tests per se must be viewed within a total clinical context and should not be the sole criterion for or against the diagnosis of a drug abuse disorder.

Once drug abuse is suspected and confirmed in an athlete, the issue of management, discussed in Chapter 19, can then be appropriately addressed.

REFERENCES

1. American Psychiatric Association: Diagnostic and Statistical Manual of Mental Disorders, ed 3, Revised. American Psychiatric Association, Washington, DC, 1987.
2. Kolb, LC: Modern Psychiatry. WB Saunders, Philadelphia, 1977, p 659.
3. Johanson, CE, Woolverton, WL and Schuster, CR: Evaluating laboratory models of drug dependence. In Meltzer, HY (ed): Psychopharmacology—The Third Generation of Progress. Raven Press, New York, 1987, p 1617.
4. Pattison, EM and Kaufman, E: Alcohol and drug dependence. In Usdin, G and Lewis, JM (eds): Psychiatry in General Medical Practice. McGraw-Hill, New York, 1984, p 305.
5. Lewis, DC, et al: A review of medical education in alcohol and other drug abuse. JAMA 257:2945, 1987.
6. Helwick, SA: Substance-abuse education in medical school: Past, present and future. J Med Ed 60:707, 1985.
7. Council on Mental Health: Medical school education on abuse of alcohol and other psychoactive drugs. JAMA 219:1746, 1972.
8. Schlesinger, SE: Substance misuse training in nursing, psychiatry, and social work. Int J Addict 21:595, 1986.
9. Coggan, P, Davis, A and Rogers, J: Teaching alcoholism to family medicine students. J Fam Pract 13:1025, 1981.
10. Holden, C: The neglected disease in medical education. Science 229:741, 1985.
11. Kamerow, DB, Pincus, HA and MacDonald, DI: Alcohol abuse, other drug abuse, and mental disorders in medical practice. JAMA 255:2054, 1986.
11a. Davis, AK, Cotter, F, and Czechowitz, O: Substance abuse units taught by four specialties in medical schools and residency programs. J Med Educ 63:739, 1988.
12. Singer, M and Anglin, T: The identification of adolescent substance abuse by health care professionals. Int J Addict 21:247, 1986.
13. Coulehan, JL, et al: Recognition of alcoholism and substance abuse in primary care patients. Arch Intern Med 147:349, 1987.
14. Moore, RD and Malitz, FE: Underdiagnosis of alcoholism by residents in an ambulatory medical practice. J Med Educ 61:46, 1986.
15. Babor, TF and Kadden, R: Screening for alcohol problems: Conceptual issues and practical considerations. In Chang, NC and Chao, HM (eds): Early Identification of Alcohol Abuse, DHHS Publication No. (ADM) 85-1258, Washington, DC, 1983, p 1.
16. Skinner, HA, Holt, S and Israel, Y: Early identification of alcohol abuse: 1. Critical issues and psychosocial indicators for a composite index. CMAJ 124:1141, 1981.
17. Gallant, DS: Alcohol and drug abuse curriculum guide for psychiatry faculty. DHHS Pub. No. (ADM) 82-1159, Washington, DC, 1982.
18. Rohman, ME, et al: The response of primary care physicians to problem drinkers. Am J Drug Alcohol Abuse 13:199, 1987.
19. Clark, WD: Alcoholism: Blocks to diagnosis and treatment. Am J Med 71:275, 1981.
20. Nace, EP: The Treatment of Alcoholism. Brunner/Mazel, New York, 1987, p. 215.
21. MacKenzie, RG and Jacobs, EA: Recognizing the adolescent drug abuser. Primary Care 14:225, 1987.
22. MacDonald, DI: Patterns of alcohol and drug use among adolescents. Pediatr Clin North Am 34:275, 1987.
23. Hays, JT and Spickard, WA, Jr: Alcoholism: Early diagnosis and intervention. J Gen Intern Med 2:420, 1987.
24. Klitzner, M and Schonberg, SK: Commentary: Concerns regarding indirect assessment for drug abuse among adolescents. J Developmental and Behavioral Peds, 1988, in press.
25. Feighner, JP, et al: Diagnostic criteria for use in psychiatric research. Arch Gen Psychiatry 26:57, 1972.
26. Robins, LN, et al: National Institute of Mental Health Diagnostic Interview Schedule. Arch Gen Psychiatry 38:381, 1981.
27. Ewing, JA: Detecting alcoholism. The CAGE Questionnaire. JAMA 252:1905, 1984.
28. Mayfield, D, McLeod, G and Hall, P: The CAGE questionnaire: Validation of a new alcohol screening instrument. Am J Psychiatry 131:1121, 1974.
29. Bush, B, et al: Screening for alcohol abuse using the CAGE questionnaire. Am J Med 82:231, 1987.
30. Selzer, ML: The Michigan Alcoholism Screening Test: The quest for a new diagnostic instrument. Am J Psychiatry 127:1653, 1971.
31. Mayer, J and Filstead, WJ: The Adolescent Alcohol Involvement Scale. J Stud Alcohol 40:291, 1979.
32. Pokorny, AD, Miller, BA and Kaplan, HB: The brief MAST: A shortened version of the Michigan Alcoholism Screening Test. Am J Psychiatry 129:342, 1972.
33. Skinner, HA, et al: Clinical versus laboratory detection of alcohol abuse: The Alcohol Clinical Index. Br Med J 292:1703, 1986.
34. Skinner, HA and Holt, S: The Alcohol Clinical Index: Strategies for identifying patients with alcohol problems. Addiction Research Foundation, Toronto, 1987.
35. Klitzner, M, et al: Screening for risk factors for adolescent alcohol and drug use. Am J Dis Child 141:45, 1987.

CHAPTER 18

Drug Testing

INTRODUCTION

Perhaps the most controversial issue of the 1980s in competitive sports is the testing of athletes for drug usage. Though testing for performance enhancing drugs in horses (saliva) dates back to 1910,[1] the testing of humans for drug use in sports is a phenomenon of only the past quarter of a century. Prompted by the amphetamine-related deaths of the Danish cyclist Kurt Enemar Knud Jensen[2] during the 1960 Olympics and the English cyclist Tommy Simpson[3] during the Tour de France in 1967, the Medical Commission of the International Olympic Committee published a list of banned drugs for the 1968 Winter Olympics.[3] There had been no official drug testing program at the 1964 Tokyo Olympics, although spot checks of cyclists at those games did indicate that some were receiving "unidentified injections" before competition.[2]

In 1965, Beckett and associates[4] were the first to apply sensitive gas chromatographic testing techniques to control drug abuse at an athletic event, the Tour of Britain Cycle Races. As a result, three individuals were disqualified. Although drug testing was first introduced at the Summer and Winter Olympic Games in 1968, it wasn't until the Munich Games, in the summer of 1972, that comprehensive drug testing was undertaken at an international event [5,7] (Table 18–1). It was during the Munich Games that Rick DeMont, an asthmatic, lost his gold medal after urine drug analysis revealed traces of ephedrine—an ingredient in one of his asthma medicines.[8]

It was not until the 1976 Montreal Olympic Games that the methodology for detecting anabolic steroids in the urine was ade-

Table 18–1. DRUG TESTING AT THE OLYMPICS[5,5a]

Site	Year	Athletes Tested	Positive
Winter			
Grenoble	1968	86	0
Sapporo	1972	211	1
Innsbruck	1976	390	2
Lake Placid	1980	426	0
Sarajevo	1984	408	1
Calgary	1988*	422	1
Summer			
Mexico City	1968	668	1
Munich	1972	2079	7
Montreal	1976†	2061	11
Moscow	1980	2200	0
Los Angeles	1984	1520	11
Seoul	1988‡	1601	10

*Personal communication (Robert Baynton, Ph.D., Calgary).[6]
†Anabolic steroid testing introduced.[7]
‡Personal communication (Prince Alexandre de Merode, Lausanne).

quately developed to be used in a drug screening program.[9,10] The disqualification of 19 athletes for using banned substances in the 1983 Pan American games in Caracas, Venezuela, heightened awareness of the potential problem of drug abuse in competitive sports.[9,11] As a consequence, in 1985 the United States Olympic Committee (USOC) implemented a comprehensive drug testing program with definitive sanctions for offenders.[12] The USOC drug testing program applies to the Olympic Games, the Olympic Trials, the World University Games, the Pan American Games, and the U.S. Olympic Festival. Additionally, any amateur sport National Governing Body (NGB) can request that the program be initiated at any of its sponsored events. Drug testing at the 1987 Pan American Games at Indianapolis resulted in disqualification of 6 athletes, as contrasted with the 19 in the 1983 Games.[13]

In 1986, the National Collegiate Athletic Association (NCAA), at a cost of approximately one million dollars in the first year, similarly implemented a drug testing program, with clear-cut sanctions for violators.[14,15] In its first year of operation, 2.5 percent of 3,500 athletes tested positive for banned drugs, the majority of which were anabolic steroids. In 1987, 12 athletes tested positive for drugs in NCAA postseason play.[16]

Both the USOC and the NCAA have pub-lished extensive lists of banned drugs (see Appendices). Drugs on these lists include psychomotor stimulants, sympathomimetic amines and other miscellaneous central nervous system stimulants, anabolic steroids, narcotic analgesics, diuretics, and in certain instances beta blockers, benzodiazepines, and alcohol.[12,13] From a national perspective, Britain has introduced perhaps the most ambitious drug testing program: amateur athletes will be subject to drug testing during practices and training sessions as well as during competitions. It is estimated that the cost of the British program will be about one million dollars per year for 4,000 tests. It was estimated that the USOC would spend about $675,000 for 2,700 tests in 1988.[17]

Drug testing in sports has frequently dominated the headlines in the mid-1980s.[11,18–22] Drug testing standards, rules, and findings have varied from sport to sport.[23–37] Drug testing has been the subject of negotiation,[38] arbitration,[39,40] legislation,[41] and litigation.[42–49] Players,[50] their associations,[39,51,52] coaches, owners, league officials,[35] legal scholars,[53,54] sociologists, ethicists,[55,56] medical historians,[57] physicians,[58] team physicians,[19] civil libertarians,[59–61] and arbitrators[62] have all voiced strong opinions regarding the intent, methodology, and implications of drug testing.[18]

The debate regarding the drug testing of athletes in the 1980s has occurred within the context of drug testing large segments of the United States work force.[63] In 1986, following 32 months of investigation, the President's Commission on Organized Crime recommended that the federal government test all federal employees and withhold federal contracts to private employers that do not begin drug testing programs.[64,64a] In 1985, 18 percent of the Fortune 500 companies had some form of employee drug testing program.[59,62] By 1986, the percentage rose to 40 percent,[65] and by 1988 more than half of the Fortune 500 companies were doing some form of drug testing,[66] with as many as two-thirds of these requiring drug testing as part of a pre-employment examination. According to preliminary findings of the 1987 American Management Association's survey of approximately 1,000 companies nationwide, 36 percent had some kind of drug testing program, as contrasted with 21 percent in 1986.[67]

INTENT OF TESTING

Historically, the principal intent of a drug testing program in sports has been to eliminate any competitive advantage that might result from ergogenic aids. However, as "recreational" drug abuse in the sports community has become increasingly apparent, the intent of drug testing in sports has been expanded to include: casefinding of individuals with a drug problem; screening teams or groups of athletes for evidence of drug abuse; protecting other athletes from injury caused by the drug-abusing athlete; enhancing the role model perceptions of athletes; deterring drug abuse by athletes; and minimizing criminality. Additionally, drug testing has been utilized to ensure compliance with drug treatment programs—a concept that gave rise to the initial drug testing protocols of the 1960s.[64a] Properly conceived, implemented, and administered, a drug testing program can also serve as an educational vehicle, and as such, it should not be adversarial.

WHO SHALL BE TESTED?

Within the context of sports, there are four options relative to selecting individuals to be drug tested. The first is not to have any drug testing whatsoever. The second is to test athletes for probable or reasonable cause. This option requires that criteria be established for determining probable or reasonable cause. It also requires that the responsibility for determining probable or reasonable cause be vested in specific individuals or categories of individuals. The third option is mandatory random testing. This methodology requires that certain predefined criteria be established for the timing of the testing as well as for the selection of individuals to be tested, for example, the first three finishers of a race are to be immediately tested after the event. The fourth option is mandatory testing of everyone. This option requires that the conditions regarding the timing of testing be pre-established, for example, mandatory testing of all participants immediately following the conclusion of a championship event, or mandatory testing of all participants in preseason training camp.

WHICH SPORTS ORGANIZATIONS DRUG TEST ATHLETES AND WHAT ARE THEIR POLICIES?

No text could possibly be current as to which sports organizations test for drugs. Similarly, drug testing policies are constantly changing as are the lists of drugs which are banned. Influenced by such factors as collective bargaining, legal challenges, and public opinion, drug testing in sports remains in a continuous state of flux. Table 18–2 summarizes the United States sports organizations that had drug testing programs in 1987. (For the details of many of these programs, see Appendices.)

While the NCAA program tests athletes for recreational and performance-enhancing drugs at its championships and football bowl games, it does not mandate its member institutions to conduct a testing program during the regular season. Nonetheless, the number of institutions conducting drug testing programs during the regular season has increased thirtyfold during the past 3 years.[68] The specifics of each of these regular season programs (intent, conditions of testing, drugs tested for, consequences of positive tests) are left to the discretion of the individual colleges and universities.[15]

The USOC drug testing program is implemented in cooperation with the National Governing Bodies of the 33 Olympic winter and summer sports. These policies must be

Table 18–2. SPORTS ORGANIZATIONS THAT TEST UNITED STATES ATHLETES FOR DRUG USE—1987

Organization	Testing Policy	Banned Drugs	Who Gets Tested	When Tests Are Done	Penalty for Positive Test
Amateur Level US Olympic Committee (USOC) 1750 E Boulder St Colorado Springs, CO 80909-5760	Provides a list of banned drugs to National Governing Bodies (NGBs); administers tests at Olympic and Pan Am trials, USOC-sponsored competitions, and, when requested, at NGB events	Stimulants, narcotic analgesics, anabolic-androgenic steroids, systemic corticosteroids, diuretics, and in some sports, beta-blockers, sedatives, hypnotics, tranquilizers, depressants, anticonvulsants, and alcohol	Most top finishers at NGB- and USOC-sponsored competitions; a random sampling of other finishers and participants at training camps; all prospective team members at Olympic trials	Within 1 hr after event; frequency of tests varies with each NGB; alcohol may be tested before event	Athlete is suspended 6 mo from USOC and NGB activities; repeat offenders suspended for 4 yr; some NGBs have stiffer penalties
National Collegiate Athletic Association (NCAA) Box 1906 Mission, KS 66201	Provides a list of banned drugs to member institutions; administers tests at NCAA championships and football bowl games	Psychomotor and CNS stimulants, sympathomimetic amines, anabolic steroids, "street drugs," diuretics, and in some sports, alcohol and beta-blockers	Procedures to choose athletes to be tested are sport specific but may include random selection, position of finish, suspicion of use, playing time, and position	Before, during, or after events, depending on institution and event; usually within 1 hr after an event	Athlete is deemed ineligible for postseason championships for minimum of 90 days; if retested positive, athlete will lose postseason eligibility for the current season and succeeding season
US Powerlifting Federation (USPF) Box 18485 Pensacola, FL 32523	Provides a list of banned drugs; follows testing procedures similar to those of the USOC	Psychomotor stimulants, anabolic steroids	Top two finishers in each weight class; all record holders at various national championships	Immediately after last lift at major championships	Athlete is suspended 3 yr from USPF and International Powerlifting Federation events
Amateur and Professional Level US Tennis Association (USTA) 1212 Avenue of the Americas New York, NY 10036	Follows USOC policy for junior level; follows Men's Tennis Council (MTC, see below) policy for professional level	USOC list for juniors; MTC for pros	Follows USOC guidelines for juniors; requires mandatory testing of all professional members, including athletes, staff officials, and committee members	At all tennis championships; time of testing depends on specific championship but usually occurs right after event	Enforces USOC rules for juniors; enforces MTC rules for pros

Professional Level

Organization	Function	Drugs Tested	Who Is Tested	Schedule	Penalties
Major League Baseball (MLB) Office of the Commissioner 350 Park Ave New York, NY 10022	Conducts centralized, regular, random testing of certain MLB and minor league employees; program includes evaluation, education, and rehabilitation	Cocaine, marijuana, heroin, morphine	MLB ownership, executives, field managers, umpires, and players with guaranteed contracts containing drug testing clauses or who have known drug involvement	No regular schedule; tests randomly	Differs for specific cases
Men's Tennis Council (MTC) Fourth Floor 437 Madison Ave New York, NY 10022	Provides a list of banned drugs and outlines testing procedures for MTC championships	Cocaine, heroin, amphetamines	MTC members, including athletes, staff, officials, and committee members	Starting on first day of tournament until all members are tested; tests occur annually at no more than two MTC-sanctioned tournaments	Athlete must undergo treatment program; failure to comply or three positive tests result in disqualification and suspension; reinstatement considered after 1 yr
National Basketball Association (NBA) 645 Fifth Ave New York, NY 10022	Follows the collective bargaining agreement between the NBA and the National Basketball Players Association on drug testing	Cocaine, heroin	Individual players, only if confronted with "reasonable cause," ie, the belief that an athlete is engaged in use, possession, or distribution of prohibited substances	No regular screening; tests only in cases of "reasonable cause"; tests may be conducted without prior notice	Disqualification from NBA; reinstatement considered after 2 yr
National Football League (NFL) 419 Park Ave New York, NY 10022	Provides a list of banned drugs and administers drug tests to NFL employees	"Street drugs," anabolic steroids, and amphetamines and similar substances found in decongestants	All payroll players on both active and reserve teams; draft-eligible players at scouting sessions; may also include nonplaying NFL employees	All preseason camps, at scouting sessions, and in cases of "reasonable cause"	Depending on extent of abuse, outpatient counseling, which results in 30-day probation, or 30-day inpatient treatment, off payroll; after three positive tests, athlete is banned from NFL
World Boxing Council (WBC) Calle Geneva, No. 33 Room 503 Mexico City, D.F. 06600 Mexico	Provides a list of banned drugs and instructions for testing procedures	Similar to USOC list with certain modifications	All contenders for WBC world title	Immediately after bout at WBC championships	Athlete is suspended for 2 yr from WBC-recognized fights; any boxing title nullified

(Adapted from Gall, SL, et al.[68])

rigorously adhered to in USOC-sponsored events. However, in NGB-sponsored events, the NGB may modify the drug testing program.[68]

Some sports organizations and associations, such as the Professional Golf Association (PGA), have drug testing policies, but the details are kept confidential. Some sports organizations, such as the National Hockey League, have articulated firm anti-drug positions, but have no formal drug testing program (see Appendices). Other sports organizations and associations have elected to emphasize drug prevention education in lieu of having a drug testing policy. Drug prevention education is the principal approach currently utilized at the level of high school athletics.[68]

LEGAL ISSUES

The drug testing of athletes raises numerous legal issues (see Chapter 20), including, but not limited to, informed consent, confidentiality, internal and external chain of custody or evidence (to assure that the urine samples are not adulterated or exchanged during transport), chain of communication, due process, the appeal process, the right of privacy and medical privilege (which vary from state to state), job security, rights of those refusing to be tested, and the testing of minors. Civil libertarians have been particularly outspoken regarding their concern that drug testing represents an invasion of an individual's civil rights.[15,44−46,48,59−61] In the fall of 1986, the American Civil Liberties Union filed a potentially precedent-setting court challenge to the University of Colorado's random drug testing program for athletes. The Union claimed: "It's an issue of invasion of privacy, freedom from unreasonable search and seizure and due process."[42] However, it was also in the fall of 1986, in a precedent-setting case, that the U.S. Supreme Court allowed states to require drug and alcohol tests for people involved in thoroughbred horse racing.[43] Parenthetically, in the first 2 years of random drug testing of jockeys and harness racers in New Jersey, there were 13 positive results from 2,343 samples in 1985, and 14 positive results (primarily cocaine) from 2,416 samples in 1986.[69]

In December of 1986, a federal judge upheld an NCAA ruling forbidding a Louisiana State football player from playing in the Sugar Bowl because of a positive urine test for anabolic steroids.[47] In the fall of 1987, on the other hand, a Superior Court judge ruled that the NCAA drug testing program violated student-athletes' right to privacy as guaranteed by the California constitution.[70] Stating that the mandatory drug program was "overbroad," he ruled that all Stanford athletes except football and male basketball players were exempt from urine drug testing, and that the testing would be limited to cocaine, anabolic steroids, and amphetamines.[15] He further ruled that testing would not be accompanied by visual monitoring.[70]

In 1988, the legality of drug testing in the workplace was brought for the first time to the United States Supreme Court.[66] The Supreme Court agreed to hear a case brought by agents of the U.S. Customs Service (*National Treasury Employees Union vs. William Von Raab*), in which it is argued that urine testing of public employees violates the Fourth Amendment to the Constitution, which prohibits unwarranted search and seizure.[64a] It is anticipated that the decision in this case will have a considerable impact on drug testing activities in the workplace. It should be emphasized that in those cases in which drug testing was not ordered by the government, such as in sports, the Fourth Amendment does not necessarily apply.[64a] However, as noted in Chapter 20, drug testing in the sports setting has been challenged, at least in part, on the basis of invasion of privacy.[42] Sports such as professional tennis, which are played by non-U.S. citizens and which are played internationally, present additional legal considerations.

WRITTEN POLICY

The implementation of an effective drug testing program requires that a written policy be developed, distributed, and publicized to all those potentially affected by the program[12,13] (see Appendices). Included in the written policy should be the purpose of testing, the criteria for testing, the conditions of testing, the drugs to be tested for, the actions to be taken if drugs are detected, and a description of the appeal process.

LOGISTICS

In recent years the myriad logistical problems—particularly resulting from human error—in the collection, securing, and transporting of specimens for the most part have been solved, especially when relatively small groups of individuals are tested, as in organized sports.[13,71,72] However, mistakes such as transcription errors and the misspelling of names, and even the confusion of specimens, can occur in the processing of specimens. As recently as 1983, the U.S. Army admitted to large-scale mishandling and mix-ups in the urine testing of 60,000 soldiers.[63] Observed specimens have minimized the risks of cheating by such methods as switching urines, scooping from the toilet bowl, or adding salt, vinegar, bleach, or detergents to the urine.[73-75] Measuring peak urine temperatures has been suggested as a way of discriminating fresh from previously voided urines, thereby eliminating the problem of urine switching and as an alternative to witnessed collections.[76] The above techniques notwithstanding, there are those who will continually try to outwit the drug testing system. During the 1987 Pan American Games, the uricosuric drug, probenecid, which was not on the banned list, was found in an undisclosed number of athletes' urine specimens. Because of its ability to delay the excretion of some drugs, it was alleged that probenecid was used in an attempt to mask anabolic steroid usage.[17,77] In the fall of 1987, the International Olympic Committee officially banned probenecid and related compounds.[15]

SELECTION OF BODY FLUID OR TISSUE

Urine has been chosen as the body fluid most frequently analyzed for evidence of drug abuse. The American Medical Association (AMA) Council on Scientific Affairs has enumerated the following reasons for this selection:[78]

1. The collection of urine is not invasive.
2. Large volumes can be collected easily.
3. Drugs and their metabolites are generally present in higher concentrations in urine than in other tissues or fluids because of the concentrating function of the kidneys.
4. Urine is easier to analyze than blood and other tissues because of the usual absence of protein and cellular constituents.
5. Drugs and their metabolites are usually very stable in frozen urine, allowing long-term storage of positive samples.

There are a number of disadvantages of using urine to screen for drug abuse. Providing an observed urine is difficult for many, and some perceive it to be a humiliating experience. Ingenious techniques of urine specimen tampering have been developed which include substituting and adulterating the specimens so as to interfere with the testing procedure.

The use of blood or plasma to measure the concentration of a drug may permit better correlations with the effects of that drug or its active metabolites on athletic performance. For some substances, such as growth hormone, a blood assay is the only method available to detect its abuse. Current methods of detecting autologous blood transfusions (blood doping) similarly require blood specimens.[79] However, the use of blood or plasma presents a number of limitations. As an invasive technique, technical proficiency is required in the securing of the specimen, though this would reduce the risk of specimen tampering. It is likely that an invasive technique would result in even greater resistance to any form of drug testing than exists for urine drug testing. From a laboratory perspective, "the analyses of the specimens are more expensive, and more complex; the amount of specimen is smaller; and the concentrations of drugs and metabolites are lower."[80]

One of the more recent developments in the field of drug testing involves the analysis of human hair for the presence of drugs by means of radioimmunoassay (RIA). Although in its infancy, this inexpensive technique can be used to detect cocaine, marijuana, barbiturates, morphine, phencyclidine (PCP), methaqualone, amphetamines, and LSD. Currently an enzyme-linked immunoabsorbent assay (ELISA) variation of the RIA methodology, described later in this chapter, is under development.[81] When hair is so analyzed it reveals not only what drugs have been taken, but when. In fact hair from long-dead famous individuals has revealed evidence of drug usage.[63] In 1988, the New York State appeals court ruled that hair analysis for cocaine use (RIA) could be used as legitimate evidence to determine whether a woman seeking custody of her children had stopped using cocaine.[81a]

Salivary analysis has also been investigated as a body fluid which could be utilized for detecting and measuring drug use. One of its major advantages resides in the fact that it is easy to obtain. Salivary analysis has been utilized to better ascertain the last usage of marijuana. Though tetrahydrocannabinol (THC)—the active ingredient of marijuana—is not secreted into saliva, it does attach to the oral mucosa during smoking and can be detected in the saliva for as long as 6 hours after smoking. Whereas urine testing can be positive for THC for up to 4 weeks after smoking, saliva which tests positive for THC suggests marijuana smoking within a time frame of hours.[82]

In 1987, Thompson and associates[83] reported that cocaine can be reliably detected in human saliva following intravenous administration. Analysis of saliva by gas chromatography–mass spectrometry (GC/MS), described later in this chapter, confirmed that cocaine is excreted in saliva and that the saliva and blood levels parallel each other. This observation leaves open the possibility that saliva screening tests may be possible in the future. Problems with salivary analysis include limited knowledge of the salivary clearance of various drugs, small sample size, variability in saliva flow rates and pH, variability in duration of positive results, and difficulties with quantification and confirmation.[80,84,85]

THE LABORATORY

Aside from the legal issues, the accuracy of testing remains one of the most questioned and controversial aspects of drug testing.[21,59] The discovery of commercial laboratory errors through proficiency testing has given credence to reports of laboratory errors that have appeared in the lay press.[86] These reports, together with the many ramifications of drug testing, have prompted the Department of Health and Human Services to es-

tablish a National Accreditation Program for Urinalysis Testing which will develop standards to certify the analytic capability of laboratories which perform drug testing.[87] These standards were to be put into effect in 1988. To ensure adherence to professional standards, laboratories performing drug tests should maintain "records of procedures and worksheets regarding instrument operation, maintenance and quality control, and records of personnel training and experience,"[62] as well as participate in accreditation and proficiency testing programs. In 1988, the National Institute on Drug Abuse reported that 100 laboratories were seeking federal certification, twice as many as was expected.[64a]

An understanding of the concepts of sensitivity and specificity is critical to the interpretation of data received from the drug testing laboratory. *Sensitivity* refers to the smallest quantity of a substance that can be detected by a given drug testing method. Techniques are currently available that can detect one part in a billion of a forbidden substance.[8] *Specificity* relates to the ability to exclude false positives.[88] A *false positive* means that a positive result is produced when the substance being sought is not present, is not confirmable as present, or is present at a concentration below the cut-off value.[80]

There are two general methodologic categories for evaluating urine for drugs of abuse: immunologic assays and chromatographic assays. The former includes radioimmunoassays (RIA) and enzyme immunoassays (EIA). The latter includes thin-layer chromatography (TLC), gas-liquid chromatography (GLC), high-pressure liquid chromatography (HPLC), and combined gas chromatography–mass spectrometry (GC/MS).[88–90]

Thin-Layer Chromatography

Chromatography is a technique which is used to separate a mixture of substances by taking advantage of the specific physicochemical characteristics of each of the components in the mixture.[91] The principle that is common to all forms of chromatography is that the separation of the substances in the mixture is achieved by virtue of differences in each substance's migration rate on or

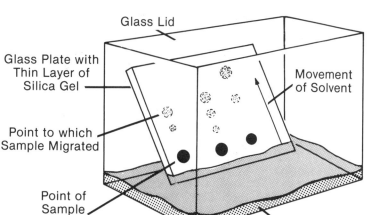

Glass Lid

Glass Plate with
Thin Layer of
Silica Gel

Movement
of Solvent

Point to which
Sample Migrated

Point of
Sample
Application

Solvent

Figure 18–1. Principle of thin-layer chromatography.

through a porous supporting medium called an "adsorbent."[92] Thin-layer chromatography (TLC)[88–92] is an inexpensive, relatively crude chromatographic technique which primarily has been used in the emergency room setting to qualitatively detect high-dose drug abuse or toxic levels of drugs in the comatose patient.[93] In the context of screening for drugs of abuse, TLC is considered "inadequate and obsolete."[94]

TLC is a time-consuming, relatively nonspecific, and insensitive technique that separates different molecules in a mixture. Results are only reported in the qualitative terms of positive or negative. A technician subjectively reads the results by comparing the presence of spots, usually the color of spots, on a chromatographic plate to known standards (Fig. 18–1). High concentration of a drug or its metabolites must be present in the urine to be detected. The drug concentration must be in the range of 1000 to 2000 ng per ml, as contrasted with the concentrations of 10 to 20 ng per ml which can be detected by other chromatographic and certain immunologic techniques.

Because of its relative insensitivity, TLC can only detect a limited number of substances 12 to 24 hours after ingestion, and false negative reports are common.[92] A *false-negative* report refers to a negative report when a sought-after substance is actually present in a concentration greater than a cutoff value. For example, one may falsely conclude that cocaine was not used 24 hours previously when examining urine with TLC as contrasted to more sensitive methods.

Immunoassay

Radioimmunoassay and enzyme immunoassay[75,88–90] are immunologic techniques based on the principles of antigen-antibody interaction. Both are useful for screening large numbers of specimens rapidly and inexpensively.[7] In both, the test is only as good as the sensitivity and the specificity of the antibody being used. Though the antibodies used in these immunoassays are highly selective, they are not absolutely specific for their respective drug.[94] Neither procedure utilizes monoclonal antibodies. The RIA technique utilizes known amounts of I-125 tagged antigen in the determination, whereas the EIA technique utilizes the enzyme glucose-6-phosphate dehydrogenase as the active tag. With EIA, technicians are not exposed to radioactive substances. Both procedures are generally used for screening urine specimens, and both are more sensitive and specific than TLC.

EIA is generally less sensitive than RIA, the former detecting levels in the 150 to 300 ng per ml range (except for cannabinoids, which can be detected in the 20 ng range), whereas RIA can detect most compounds at levels in the 10 to 20 ng per ml range. Both procedures produce automated semi-quantitative results. These techniques may not differentiate between specific drugs within a class of drugs since immunologic assays are known to be less specific for a single molecule and may cross-react with molecules similar in structure to the desired substance.[94] The Enzyme Multiplied Immunoassay Technique (EMIT, trademark of Syva Co., a subsidiary of Syntex Corp. of Palo Alto, CA) was introduced in the early 1970s and is perhaps the best known and the most frequently used of the EIA procedures.[21,64a,80] It has become the standard approach for screening large numbers of urine samples, and is the most widely employed methodology for the detection of marijuana.[64a,93] The system referred to as EMIT-dau is designed to detect marijuana metabolites at concentrations of 20 ng/ml or greater.[75] The principle of EMIT as applied to the detection of marijuana is shown in Figure 18–2.

Both EIA and RIA have been known to yield false-positive results with decongestants such as pseudoephedrine, anorectants such as phenylpropanolamine, and nonsteroidal anti-inflammatory drugs such as ibuprofen and naproxen.[78,80] The latter drugs are especially important to athletes given their high usage rate of nonsteroidal anti-inflammatory drugs. Consequently, positive drug screens with EIA or RIA should only be considered presumptive, since other substances may interfere with any assay, thereby producing erroneous results. Thus, before a preliminary result leads to an action that could be deleterious to an individual, confirmatory testing with a more specific assay such as GC/MS is essential.[21,90,95] Urine specimens, whether positive or negative, should be stored for an appropriate period of time so as to enable further testing if necessary. An algorithm demonstrating the concept of confirmatory testing appears in Figure 18–3.

Gas-Liquid Chromatography

Gas-liquid chromatography (GLC) is a process by which a mixture of compounds in a volatized form is separated into its component parts by moving a mobile (gas) phase over a stationary (absorbent or liquid) phase.[88,91,93,94,96,97] Therefore, this technique requires that the substance of interest be put into a gaseous (volatile) state. If the substance is not particularly volatile in its native state, then a new compound (a derivative compound) that is volatile needs to be formed from the compound of interest.[7,91] Once separated by this chromatographic technique, the individual drugs or their metabolites can be individually identified and

quantitated by a variety of analytic techniques. In routine gas-liquid chromatography, compounds are identified by their rate of speed traveling through the chromatographic column. This rate is referred to as the retention time and is unique and reproducible for each drug in a given type of chromatographic column. Chromatographic columns are available which are packed with different types of material. While substance A may have a retention time of 5 minutes in a chromatographic column packed with material X, it may have a retention time of 3 minutes in a chromatographic column packed with material Y. In the field of drug testing, GLC is primarily used as a screening technique.

High-Performance Liquid Chromatography (HPLC)

Another form of chromatography which is similar to gas chromatography is high-performance liquid chromatography, or high-pressure liquid chromatography (HPLC).[91] HPLC is easily automated and is both sensitive and specific. Unlike GLC, HPLC does not require the preparation of a gaseous or volatile derivative of the substance being studied, and its use is usually somewhat simpler and more rapid than GLC.[97] At present, HPLC is primarily used in sports as a screening technique, particularly for substances such as the psychomotor stimulant pemoline (Cylert), which has poor GLC properties. It has also been used to quantitate urinary caffeine levels.[10] In some settings HPLC has been used to confirm the positive results obtained from other screening techniques; however, its acceptability in forensic settings has not been firmly established.[78,80]

Gas Chromatography–Mass Spectrometry (GC/MS)

The most precise way of accomplishing drug identification is to combine the chemical separating power of gas chromatography with the molecular identifying power of mass spectrometry, a procedure referred to commonly as GC/MS.[78] As each separated compound leaves the chromatographic column, it is introduced, one compound at a time, into a mass spectrometer. The mass spectrometer, under high vacuum, then

Normal Urine

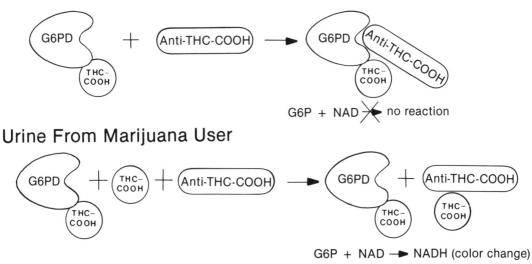

G6P + NAD ⟶✕ no reaction

Urine From Marijuana User

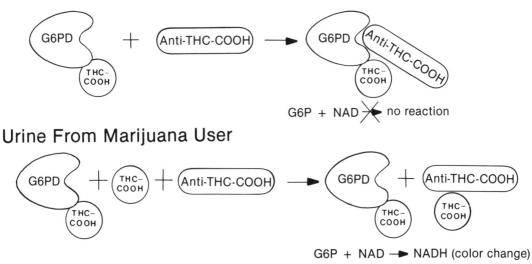

G6P + NAD ⟶ NADH (color change)

Figure 18–2. Principle of enzyme-mediated immunotechnique (EMIT) for detection of marijuana in a urine specimen. Enzyme activity of glucose-6-phosphate dehydrogenase (G6PD) serves as a marker for presence or absence of marijuana metabolites (tetrahydrocannabinol-11-carboxylic acid [THC-COOH]). The G6PD used in the assay has been chemically modified to incorporate THC-COOH covalently. In the absence of free metabolite in the urine specimen, an antibody that recognizes THC-COOH binds to G6PD at the site where THC-COOH is covalently bound. Antibody binding distorts the tertiary structure of G6PD and causes it to lose activity. Enzyme substrates, glucose-6-phosphate (G6P), and nicotinamide-adenine dinucleotide (NAD) are present in the assay system, but because the enzyme is inactive, no colored reaction product (reduced form of NAD, NADH) is formed. When unbound THC-COOH is presented to the assay system in the specimen, the anti-THC-COOH preferentially binds to it rather than to G6PD. In this case, the enzyme remains active and catalyzes the reaction to form NADH. In the presence of marijuana metabolites, color is detected, and intensity of color is proportional to metabolite concentration. (From Moyer,[75] with permission.)

Figure 18–3. Algorithm for testing for use of marijuana. The type of report issued is dictated by the clinical situation. In cases in which the preponderance of evidence points to drug use, a presumptive result is adequate. If the test result is the primary evidence that will be used in making the decision to take major action, such as expulsion from a treatment program, job probation or loss, or other major societal effect, confirmation of the positive result is imperative. EMIT-dau = enzyme-mediated immunotechnique; GC/MS = gas chromatography/mass spectrometry. (From Moyer,[75] with permission.)

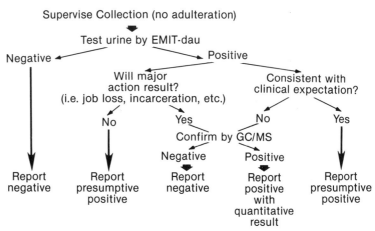

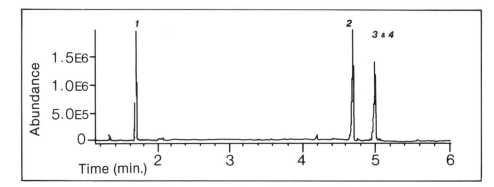

NAME	RELATIVE RETENTION TIME	MASS
(1) Ecgonine Methyl Ester	0.338	182
(2) Cocaine	0.938	182
(3) Benzoylecgonine	1.00	240
(4) Benzoylecgonine 2H3	1.00	243

Figure 18–4. Gas chromatography/mass spectrometry for cocaine and its metabolites. (Courtesy of Psychiatric Diagnostic Laboratories of America, Inc.)

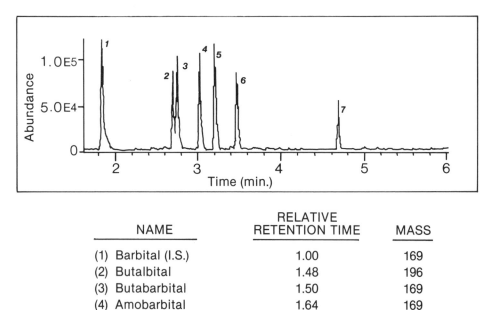

NAME	RELATIVE RETENTION TIME	MASS
(1) Barbital (I.S.)	1.00	169
(2) Butalbital	1.48	196
(3) Butabarbital	1.50	169
(4) Amobarbital	1.64	169
(5) Pentobarbital	1.74	169
(6) Secobarbital	1.88	196
(7) Phenobarbital	2.46	232

Figure 18–5. Gas chromatography/mass spectrometry for barbiturates. (Courtesy of Psychiatric Diagnostic Laboratories of America, Inc.)

bombards the separated compound with high-energy electrons. Because not all bonds in a drug molecule are of equal strength, the bombardment of the molecule by the high-energy electrons is more likely to break the weaker bonds than the stronger ones, thereby producing ionized fragments or breakage products. The fragmentation ions or patterns, the so-called "molecular finger-prints" which are produced by this proce-dure, are unique for each compound (Figs. 18–4 and 18–5). Like fingerprints, these frag-mentation patterns are matched against known patterns in a computer library, thereby permitting precise identification.

GC/MS is available in two modes: full scan and selected ion (SIM). The full-scan mode provides a unique pattern of ions which describes the complete mass spectrum of the drug or the metabolite. However, it is less sensitive than the selected ion mode. In the selected ion mode only a few preselected masses of fragments characteristic of the drug are measured. While this provides greater sensitivity, it is less specific than the full-scan mode.[95]

GC/MS, which in most cases is about 100 to 1,000 times more sensitive than TLC, is the most sensitive and accurate technique currently available in the field of drug test-ing, but it is also the most expensive.[21,54,90,93] GC/MS requires expertise and experience by the technician. Because of its sensitivity, it can detect very low levels of drugs and their metabolites in the urine (nanogram range for most drugs, and picogram range for some drugs when special detectors are used) (Table 18–3); therefore, it can detect evi-dence of drug usage by an individual many days after the fact.

GC/MS is regularly used to confirm pre-sumptively positive urines as determined by the aforementioned screening techniques. In fact, the IOC and essentially all of the inter-national sports federations have required GC/MS identification of the drugs or their metabolites for all positive screening tests.[7] Because of its extreme accuracy, GC/MS, as a forensic procedure, is accepted by the courts as being the gold standard. McBay[80] notes: "The combination of a positive im-munoassay and a GC/MS result with the proper retention times and three mass ions of the proper intensities should distinguish the compound of interest from more than 10^6 other organic compounds. Two mass ions of the proper intensities will distinguish the compound from about 10^4 compounds."

As Vereby has emphasized: "When confir-mation of positive samples is required, this should be performed by a method for which the scientific principle differs from that of the screening method. This means that a positive sample by an immunologic method (EMIT, RIA) must be confirmed by a chromato-graphic method (GLC, GC/MS) and vice versa."[95] However, even this approach does not completely eliminate the problem of drug misidentification. For example, as McBay[80] has reported, although the skeletal muscle relaxant cyclobenzaprine (Flexeril) differs structurally from the antidepressant amitriptyline (Elavil), they give "identical responses to three different TLC procedures, have the same retention times to GC and HPLC procedures, give positive EMIT res-ponses, and produce a GC/MS ion of m/e 275." However, a GC/MS method of iden-tification is available that produces different mass ions that can distinguish between the two compounds.[80]

LEGAL DEFENSIBILITY

Legal defensibility is of utmost importance in the selection of a specific drug testing pro-tocol for the detection of prohibited sub-stances in situations where an individual's freedom, reputation, and career are in jeop-ardy (see Chapter 20). In addressing this issue, Hoyt and associates[62] sought the opin-ion of experts in the drug testing field as to the most defensible methods for a variety of abused drugs. The results are detailed in Table 18–4.

Table 18–3. EQUIVALENT UNITS OF MEASURE

1 g = 1 gram = $\frac{1}{28}$ ounce
1 mg = 1 milligram = one thousandth of a gram
1 μg = 1 microgram = one millionth of a gram
1 ng = 1 nanogram = one billionth of a gram
1 pg = 1 picogram = 1 trillionth of a gram

Table 18–4. LEGAL DEFENSIBILITY OF METHODS AS DETERMINED BY EXPERTS (96% RESPONSE)*

| | Single-Procedure Methods† | | | | | Multiple-Procedure Methods† | | | | | | | | | | |
	EMIT	RIA	TLC	GC	GC/MS	EMIT, RIA	EMIT, TLC	EMIT, GC	EMIT, GC/MS	RIA, TLC	RIA, GC	RIA, GC/MS	TLC, EMIT	TLC, RIA	TLC, GC	TLC, GC/MS
Amphetamines	3.9	3.9	3.8	3.4	1.7	3.7	2.6	2.2	1.0	2.7	2.2	1.0	2.8	2.8	2.3	1.2
Barbiturates	4.0	4.0	3.8	3.4	1.7	3.7	2.5	2.1	1.0	2.6	2.1	1.1	2.7	2.7	2.3	1.2
Benzodiazepines	4.0	4.0	3.8	3.5	1.7	3.8	2.5	2.1	1.0	2.6	2.2	1.1	2.7	2.7	2.4	1.2
Cannabinoids	3.9	3.9	3.7	3.6	1.7	3.7	2.6	2.3	1.0	2.7	2.3	1.0	2.7	2.7	2.5	1.2
Cocaine	3.9	3.9	3.7	3.4	1.7	3.6	2.5	2.1	1.0	2.5	2.1	1.0	2.5	2.5	2.3	1.2
Methaqualone	3.9	3.9	3.8	3.4	1.7	3.7	2.5	2.1	1.0	2.5	2.1	1.0	2.5	2.5	2.3	1.2
Opiates	4.0	4.0	3.7	3.5	1.7	3.6	2.5	2.1	1.0	2.6	2.1	1.0	2.7	2.7	2.3	1.2
Phencyclidine	3.9	3.9	3.8	3.4	1.7	3.6	2.5	2.1	1.0	2.6	2.1	1.0	2.6	2.6	2.4	1.2

*Scale: 1, fully defensible against legal challenge; 2, somewhat defensible; 3, difficult to defend in legal challenges; 4, unacceptable for legal defense.

†EMIT indicates enzyme-multiplied immunoassay technique; RIA, radioimmunoassay; TLC, thin-layer chromatography; GC, gas chromatography; and GC/MS, gas chromatography/mass spectrometry. First procedure is a "screen"; second procedure is a "confirmation."

From Hoyt, et al,[62] with permission.

OTHER CONSIDERATIONS

Confounding the already complex issues of drug testing has been the observation that passive inhalation of large quantities of marijuana smoke can result in the appearance of marijuana metabolites in the urine. In 1986, Cone and associates[98] studied five volunteers who were exposed to the smoke of 16 marijuana cigarettes for an hour a day for 6 consecutive days while in a small, unventilated room. When their urine specimens were tested for total cannabinoids (EMIT), the specimens were positive at concentrations of 20 ng per ml as well as 100 ng per ml of urine. By contrast, when subjects were exposed to the smoke of only 4 marijuana cigarettes in a similar setting, their urines tested positive for total cannabinoids only at the 20 ng per ml level.

In 1987, Cone and associates[99] essentially repeated the study. However, this time they measured not only total cannabinoids (EMIT) but also the urine concentration of the acid metabolite of marijuana, THC-carboxylic acid (THC-COOH), by RIA and by GC/MS. Using these methods, they demonstrated that for individuals exposed to the smoke of 16 marijuana cigarettes, urine THC-COOH levels of 100 ng per ml could be achieved. However, it must be emphasized that the concentration of marijuana smoke was so great in the enclosed room that eye irritation alone prevented most subjects from tolerating this level of smoke for extended periods of time. Thus, it is unlikely that subjects would unknowingly passively inhale sufficient quantities of marijuana smoke so as to have urine THC-COOH levels of 100 ng per ml. In 1988, Mule and colleagues[99a] concluded from their studies of passive inhalation that cannabinoid levels in the urine (RIA) are consistently below 10 ng per ml in conditions where passive inhalation is likely to reflect realistic exposure to marijuana smoke.

In 1981, when the U.S. Navy first initiated large-scale urine drug testing for marijuana, a cut-off level of 100 ng per ml (total cannabinoids, RIA) was used.[98,100] Confirmation by GC/MS required a concentration of 50 ng per ml of THC-COOH. Since October 1986, the initial RIA screen cut-off remains at 100 ng per ml, but confirmation by GC/MS requires THC-COOH to be present at a concentration of at least 15 ng per ml.[101]

Because of their high degree of sensitivity, techniques such as GC/MS might, on occasion, lead one to wrongly conclude that an individual intentionally used illicit drugs. As Imwinkelried[54] commented: "Even poppy seeds and some herbal teas can leave signs of morphine or cocaine in the urine of innocent people."[54] Beginning in 1983, coca leaf tea was imported into the United States and was commercially available. Two such products which were exported from Peru were sold as Health Inca Tea and Mate de Coca, and it has been estimated that 1.5 million tea bags have been sold in the United States.[102] Analysis of Health Inca Tea bags showed an average cocaine content of 4.8 mg per bag.[102a] Within weeks of an article appearing in the medical literature describing the presence of cocaine in these teas, these products essentially disappeared from the shelves of health-food stores.[85]

New technology is being directed at enhancing the sensitivity and accuracy of screening procedures. These in turn can be confirmed by tests which have great specificity, such as GC/MS. In addition to identifying drugs by their fragmentation patterns, other methods are currently being developed, such as identifying drugs by their unique electrochemical patterns.

Specific application of the various aforementioned laboratory techniques to the XXIII Olympiad in Los Angeles have been detailed by Catlin and associates.[10]

DRUG TESTING METHODOLOGY AND IMPLICATIONS FOR THE ATHLETE

From the above discussion, it is apparent that the selection of the initial drug screening methodology, that is, TLC, immunoassay, or GC/MS, will have a significant bearing on the results (Table 18–5). This in turn relates to the intent of a given drug testing program. If an athlete uses cocaine even in moderate amounts on a Wednesday, and his or her urine is screened by TLC on Sunday, it will most likely test negative. If, on the other hand, his or her urine is tested by GC/MS, it may well test positive, depending on the detection limits or cut-offs that are used. Although there are sociologic and medical implications to Wednesday's drug usage, there will probably be no performance enhancement from that usage. Put differently, the most sensitive method of drug screening,

Table 18–5. DRUG TESTING METHODOLOGY AND DRUG DETECTABILITY

Drug	Detection Limits (ng/ml)			Detection Windows (days)		
	TLC	EIA	GC/MS	TLC	EIA	GC/MS
Amphetamines	1000–2000	300	100	1	2	2–4
Barbiturates	1000–2000	300	100	1	2–3+	7†
Benzodiazepines	1000–2000	300	100	18 hr	3	7†
Cocaine**	1000–2000	300	50	12 hr	2	5–6
Opiates	1000	300	100	1–2	2–3	5–6
Marijuana (Cannabinoids)	—	20	10	—	10*	10*
Alcohol‡						
Anabolic Steroids§			10¶			

*As long as 30 days in chronic users.

†As long as 2–3 weeks with long-acting sedatives.

‡Sensitivity is 10 mg/dl in blood, 20 mg/dl in urine; blood level decrement is 15 mg/dl/hour; urine/blood ratio approximately 1:3.

§A 6:1 testosterone/epitestosterone ratio is considered as evidence of exogenous testosterone usage. The normal ratio is 1:1. Exogenous steroids can be detected from 2–3 weeks (all) to as long as 12 months (parenteral).

¶May be as low as 1 ng/ml in the near future (David Black, personal communication).

**Measured as benzoylecgonine.

GC/MS, performed at the time of an athletic event, may reveal the presence of drugs at concentrations that likely have nothing to do with performance enhancement.[44]

Implicit in any urine drug testing program aimed at the detection of drugs that might affect performance is the notion that there is a predictable relationship between the presence of a banned substance in the urine and a quantifiable effect of that substance on performance. Correlating degrees of driving impairment with alcohol levels as measured in blood and breath, and rarely in urine, has served as the prototypic model for assessing the effects of drugs on performance. However, alcohol has several pharmacodynamic properties which make such correlations meaningful: it is both water and lipid soluble, it is distributed in the body water, it is not bound to plasma proteins, it produces no long-lived active metabolites, and it equilibrates rapidly between blood and brain.[103] Additionally, there are a variety of accepted cognitive and motor simulators to measure driving performance.

Using urine drug testing to evaluate the effect of drugs on athletic performance is far more complicated. Even ignoring the lack of uniform standards to measure performance, there are pharmacodynamic reasons which make the correlation between the urine concentration of a drug and its pharmacologically active metabolites and their effect on performance extremely difficult. Urine concentrations of a drug are influenced by too many variables. These include, but are not limited to: route of administration, dose and dosing patterns (single, multiple, or chronic), peak absorption times, diurnal variations, lipid and water solubility, degree of hydration and urine flow, the presence of active metabolites, protein binding, body habitus, and disposition kinetics. The complexity of trying to correlate drug effect with urine screening is exemplified by the study of Vereby and associates,[104] in which the detectability of diazepam (Valium) depended on the build of the subject and the sensitivity cut-off of the assay that was used. Detection windows are only intended as general guidelines. They indicate the length of time a drug can be detected by a given method and, as noted, can change as a function of such variables as weight, frequency and extent of drug use, and individual pharmacokinetics.

DRUG TESTING AND THERAPEUTIC DRUGS

Both the NCAA and the USOC have published extensive lists of drugs "banned" because of their theoretical potential for enhancing performance.[12,13] Such widely used drugs as pseudoephedrine, hydrochlorothiazide, atenolol, and isoetharine are included in one list or the other, or in both. In each category of banned drugs, the USOC includes the phrase "and Related Substances."[12] Similarly, the NCAA includes the phrase "and Related Compounds."[13] Such phrases can lead to uncertainty for the athlete and physician alike.

Extensive lists of banned drugs pose a particular problem to those athletes who travel frequently as individuals rather than as part of a team. These athletes are frequently treated by local physicians in accordance with accepted community medical standards. Yet they may be inadvertently treated with medications which are on a "banned" list despite the fact that these medications are being prescribed appropriately. This problem may be compounded further by the different medications and languages an athlete encounters in international travel. To help obviate these and other problems, the USOC has a "Drug Control Hot Line" (1-800-233-0393).[12]

REFERENCES

1. Dyment, PG: Drugs and the adolescent athlete. Ped Ann 13:602, 1984.
2. Puffer, J: The use of drugs in swimming. Clin Sports Med 5:77, 1986.
3. Hanley, DF: Drug and sex testing: Regulations for international competition. Clin Sports Med 2:13, 1986.
4. Beckett, AH and Cowan, DA: Misuse of drugs in sport. Br J Sports Med 12:185, 1979.
5. Blakeslee, S: Drug cheaters are growing smarter. The New York Times, July 13, 1988.
5a. Janofsky, M: Drug-free games expected. The New York Times, February 5, 1988.
6. Personal Communication, Robert Baynton, Ph.D., Calgary.
7. Catlin, DH: Detection of drug use by athletes. In Strauss, RH (ed): Drugs and Performance in Sports. WB Saunders, Philadelphia, 1987, p. 103.
8. Cowart, V: State-of-art drug identification laboratories play increasing role in major athletic events. JAMA 256:3068, 1986.
9. Perlmutter, G and Lowenthal, DT: Use of anabolic steroids by athletes. Am Fam Physician 32:208, 1985.

10. Catlin, DH, et al: Analytic chemistry at the games of the XXIIIrd Olympiad in Los Angeles, 1984. Clin Chem 33:319, 1987.

11. Wolff, C: Bosworth barred from bowl for steroids. The New York Times, December 26, 1986.

12. US Olympic Committee, Division of Sports Medicine and Science: Drug Education & Control Policy. Colorado Springs, 1988.

13. The 1988–89 NCAA Drug Testing Program. NCAA Publishing, Mission, Kansas, September, 1988.

14. Dodds, T: NCAA believes its drug test passed. Los Angeles Times, January 6, 1987.

15. Cowart, VS: Drug testing programs face snags and legal challenges. Phys Sportsmed 16(2):165, 1988.

16. Cowart, V: On to 1988 Olympics . . . with lessons learned. JAMA 256:2649, 1986.

17. Janofsky, M: British expand drug testing. The New York Times, November 11, 1987.

18. Lamar, JV, Jr: Scoring off the field. Time, August 25, 1986, p 52.

19. Breo, DL: Team MDs call for mandatory drug tests. Am Med News, March 14, 1986, p 25.

20. Topol, M: Drug testing gaining foothold. Newsday, July 9, 1985.

21. Rust, M: Drug deaths heat up testing debate. Am Med News, July 18, 1986, p 1.

22. Drug deaths revive test issue. Newsday, July 1, 1986.

23. Duda, M: Drug testing in professional sports. Phys Sportsmed 13:46, 1985.

24. Duda, M: Drug testing challenges colleges and pro athletes. Phys Sportsmed 12:109, 1984.

25. Drug testing for tennis pros. The New York Times, November 7, 1985.

26. Vecsey, G: After race, testing starts. The New York Times, November 3, 1986.

27. OK of riders' drug tests in New Jersey may set precedent. Newsday, July 14, 1986.

28. Pricci, J: Drug issue still cloudy. Newsday, December 14, 1986.

29. Monahan, P: Golden gloves—drug testing now required. The New York Daily News, December 30, 1986.

30. Marathon drug test. Newsday, October 17, 1986.

31. Marathoner's drug test positive, friends say. Newsday, July 14, 1986.

32. A matter of policy. Newsday, July 11, 1986.

33. Drug ban for 15 pentathletes. Newsday, November 25, 1986.

34. Cowart, V: Road back from substance abuse especially long, hard for athletes. JAMA 256:2645, 1986.

35. King, P: The NFL drug plan. Newsday, July 8, 1986.

36. Goodwin, M: Should baseball have mandatory drug testing? The New York Times, November 13, 1985.

37. IAAF to expand drug-testing rules. The New York Times, August 25, 1987.

38. Time right to resolve plan for drug testing. Newsday, June 22, 1986.

39. Noble, M: Drug tests are in violation. Newsday, July 31, 1986.

40. Rozelle's plan for unscheduled drug testing overturned. The New York Times, October 26, 1986.

41. Rust, M: County may bar most drug testing. Am Med News, Septermber 12, 1986.

42. Drug plan challenged. The New York Times, October 22, 1986.

43. Drug test lost by jockeys. Newsday, December 2, 1986.

44. Pickett, AD: Drug testing: What are the rules? Athletic Training 211:331, 1986.

45. Kerr, P: Drug tests losing most court cases. The New York Times, December 11, 1986.

46. Gianelli, DM: Drug testing programs face legal challenge. Am Med News, December 12, 1986.

47. Steroid ruling upheld. The New York Times, January 1, 1987.

48. ACLU files lawsuit on drug testing. Newsday, January 7, 1987.

49. Curran, WJ: Compulsory drug testing: The legal barriers. N Engl J Med 316:318, 1987.

50. Gaskins, SE and DeShazo, WF, III: Attitudes toward drug abuse and screening for an intercollegiate program. Phys Sportsmed 13(9):93, 1985.

51. King, P: Laying down the law—tougher drug plan has NFLPA unhappy. Newsday, July 8, 1986.

52. Berkowitz, H: Drug tests—harder union look. Newsday, October 19, 1986.

53. Imwinkelried, EJ: Some preliminary thoughts on the wisdom of governmental prohibition or regulation of private employee urinalysis testing. Clin Chem 33/11B(Suppl):19B, 1987.

54. Imwinkelried, EJ: False positive = shoddy drug testing is jeopardizing the jobs of millions. The Sciences, September/October, 1987, p 23.

55. Murray, TH: Drug testing and moral responsibility. Phys Sportsmed 114:47, 1986.

56. Cowart, V: Drug use, no matter why, raises ethical issues. JAMA 256:2649, 1986.

57. Swick, T: War on drugs: Taking the longer view. Am Coll Phys Observer 6:120, 1986.

58. Ryan, AJ: Drug abuse in sports—A physician's view. Postgrad Med 80:213, 1986.

59. Chapman, FS: The ruckus over medical testing. Fortune, August 19, 1985, p 57.

60. Glasser, I: Drug tests and searches violate workers' rights (Letter). The New York Times, March 25, 1986.

61. Siegel, N: Should pro contracts include drug-test clauses? (Letter). The New York Times, September 28, 1986.

62. Hoyt, DW, et al: Drug testing in the workplace—Are methods legally defensible? JAMA 258:504, 1987.

63. Castro, J: Battling the enemy within. Time, March 17, 1986, p 52.

64. Brinkley, J: U.S. panel urges testing workers for use of drugs. The New York Times, March 3, 1986.

64a. Marshall, E: Testing urine for drugs. Science 241:150, 1988.

65. Drug testing methods vary in defensibility—study. Am Med News, August 7, 1987.

66. Tyler, A: Value of drug screening in workplace questioned. Am Med News, March 11, 1988.

67. Roel, RE: Drug test at work. Newsday, December 7, 1987.

68. Gall, SL, et al: Who tests which athletes for what drugs? Phys Sportsmed 16(2):155, 1988.

69. Moran, P: Drug-testing talk eclipses awards. Newsday, February 7, 1987.
70. Vecsey, G: A gain for civil rights. The New York Times, December 6, 1987.
71. Blanke, RV: Quality assurance in drug-use testing. Clin Chem 33/11(b):41B, 1987.
72. Catlin, DH, et al: Chemistry at the Games of the XXIIIrd Olympiad in Los Angeles, 1984. Clin Chem 33:319, 1987.
73. Legwood, G: Have we learned a lesson about drugs in sports? Phys Sportsmed 12(3):175, 1985.
74. Clarke, KS: The United States Olympic Committee drug control program. In Butts, NK, Gushiken, TT and Zarins, B (eds): The Elite Athlete. SP Medical and Scientific Books, New York, 1985, p 27.
75. Moyer, TP, et al: Marijuana testing—How good is it? Mayo Clin Proc 62:413, 1987.
76. Person, NB and Ehrenkranz, JRL: Fake urine samples for drug analysis: Hot, but not hot enough (Letter). JAMA 259:841, 1988.
77. Cowart, V: On to 1988 Olympics . . . with lessons learned. JAMA 258:2485, 1987.
78. Council on Scientific Affairs, The American Medical Association: Scientific issues in drug testing. JAMA 257:1310, 1985.
79. Berglund, B, Hemmingsson, P and Birgegard, G: Detection of autologous blood transfusions in cross-country skiers. Int J Sports Med 8:66, 1987.
80. McBay, AJ: Drug-analysis technology—Pitfalls and problems of drug testing. Clin Chem 33/11(B):33B, 1987.
81. Bullock, C: Cocaine: Use now revealed by RIA of hair. Medical Tribune, December 17, 1986.
81a. Buder, L: Court allows testing of hair for cocaine. The New York Times, October 28, 1988.
82. Vereby, K, Gold, MS and Mule, J: Laboratory testing in the diagnosis of marijuana intoxication and withdrawal. Psychiat Ann 16:235, 1986.
83. Thompson, LK, et al: Confirmation of cocaine in human saliva after intravenous use. J Analyt Toxicol 11:36, 1987.
84. Mucklow, JC, et al: Drug concentrations in saliva. Clin Pharmacol Ther 24:563, 1978.
85. Jatlow, PI, et al: Panel discussion: The major drugs of abuse. Clin Chem 33/11(B):87B, 1987.
86. Hansen, HJ, Caudill, SP and Boone, J: Crisis in drug testing. Results of CDC blind study. JAMA 253:2382, 1985.
87. Walsh, JM: Reliability of urine drug testing (Letter). JAMA 258:2587, 1987.
88. Sandler, KR: The role of the clinical laboratory in diagnosing and treating substance abuse. In Biopsychiatric Insights on Substance Abuse (A Symposium). Psychiatric Diagnostic Laboratories, Inc., Princeton, 1986, p 68.
89. Gold, MS and Dackis, CA: Role of the laboratory in the evaluation of suspected drug abuse. J Clin Psychiat 47:1(Suppl):17, 1986.
90. Ehrlich, NEP: The athletic trainer's role in drug testing. Athletic Training 21:225, 1986.
91. Evenson, MA: Principles of instrumentation. In Henry, JB (ed): Todd-Sanford-Davidson Clinical Diagnosis and Management by Laboratory Methods, ed 17. WB Saunders, Philadelphia, 1984, p 24.
92. Spitzer, RH: Chromatography. In Tietz, NW (ed): Fundamentals of Clinical Chemistry. WB Saunders, Philadelphia, 1976, p 157.
93. Gold, MS, Vereby, K and Dackis, CA: Diagnosis of drug abuse, drug intoxication and withdrawal states. Fair Oaks Hospital Psychiatric Letter 3:23, 1985.
94. Finkle, BS: Drug-analysis technology: Overview and state of the art. Clin Chem 33/11(B):13B, 1987.
95. Vereby, K: Cocaine abuse detection by laboratory methods. In Washton, AM and Gold, MS (eds): Cocaine. The Guilford Press, New York, 1987, p 214.
96. Chattoraj, SC: Gas chromatography. In Tietz, NW (ed): Fundamentals of Clinical Chemistry. WB Saunders, Philadelphia, 1976, p 167.
97. Bauer, JD: Clinical Laboratory Methods, ed 9. The CV Mosby Company, St. Louis, 1982, p 441.
98. Cone, EJ and Johnson, RE: Contact highs and urinary cannabinoid excretion after passive exposure to marijuana smoke. Clin Pharmacol Ther 40:247, 1986.
99. Cone EJ, et al: Passive inhalation of marijuana smoke: Urinalysis and room air levels of delta-9-tetrahydrocannabinol. J Analyt Toxicol 11:89, 1987.
99a. Mule, SJ, Lomax, P and Gross, SJ: Active and realistic passive marijuana exposure tested by three immunoassays and GC/MS in urine. J Analyt Toxicol 12:113, 1988.
100. Dougherty, RJ: Controversies regarding urine testing. J Subst Abuse Treatment 4:115, 1987.
101. Personal communication, Commander John Irving, U.S. Naval Military Command, 1988.
102. Siegel, RK, et al: Cocaine in herbal tea (Letter). JAMA 225, 1986.
102a. El Sohly, MA and El Sohly, HN: Coca tea and urinalysis for cocaine metabolites. J Analyt Toxicol 10:256, 1986.
103. Consensus Development Panel: Drug concentration and driving impairment. JAMA 254:2618, 1985.
104. Vereby, K, Jukofsky, J and Jule, SJ: Confirming of EMIT benzodiazepine assay with GLC/NPD. J Analyt Toxicol 6:305, 1982.

CHAPTER 19

Management

INTRODUCTION

Beginning in the 1960s, a variety of treatment approaches were developed in response to the burgeoning problem of drug abuse. Most of these approaches have been predicated on the medical model in which drug abuse is considered primarily to be an illness or a disease.[1,2] Since alcoholism was the first form of drug abuse to be considered as a disease, it follows that the treatment of alcoholism has served as a prototype for the treatment of other forms of drug abuse. The escalation in the abuse of narcotics, specifically heroin, in the 1960s and early 1970s led to the development of additional methods for the treatment of drug abuse, such as methadone maintenance and therapeutic communities. In response to the rapid escalation in cocaine abuse, the most recent major development in the field of drug abuse treatment relates to the development of strategies for the treatment of this disorder.[3]

It is not the intent of this chapter to delineate the treatment details for each of the drugs discussed in the preceding chapters. Rather, it intends to familiarize the reader with both the language and the concepts associated with drug abuse treatment. The management approaches of two of the more common drug abuse disorders, alcohol abuse (and alcoholism) and cocaine abuse, will be emphasized. It is particularly noteworthy that the frequently observed coexistence of cocaine abuse and alcohol abuse[4] has necessitated the breaking down of barriers between drug abuse and alcoholism treatment. As Zweben has noted, "These endeavors have remained separate for numerous historical reasons, partly because of stereotypes held by one group about the other, and very

213

much perpetuated by the division of the two funding empires on the federal and state level."[5]

WHO SHOULD BE TREATED?

In addressing the question "Who should be treated?" a frame of reference such as Resnick and Resnick's classification of the patterns of cocaine use is useful:[6]

1. Experimental—This term is self-explanatory. It is particularly applicable to the adolescent, who, in the process of psychoactive drug experimentation, tries cocaine. Given the increased availability of cocaine, the young athlete, like other youths, may experiment with cocaine as he or she might experiment with alcohol and marijuana.

2. Recreational—This pattern of cocaine abuse is the most common. Its use is usually limited to social settings and is generally intended to facilitate social interaction. The recreational user, who usually does not buy cocaine, but accepts it when offered, rarely escalates the amount or frequency of cocaine used. The successful athlete, like the successful businessperson, may find himself or herself in social settings in which this type of usage is commonplace.

3. Circumstantial—This type of cocaine use, which is sizable but not nearly that of recreational use, pertains to the use of the drug under very specific circumstances. Musicians have been purported to use cocaine in this manner, that is, cocaine use is limited to musical performances. Similarly, stimulant drugs such as cocaine have been used by athletes circumstantially to enhance athletic performance.

4. Intensified—As contrasted with the above categories, this group is relatively small. Cocaine is "snorted" daily at a frequency which does not interfere with daily functioning. "These individuals usually do not experience 'crashing' and they maintain their jobs and usual level of psychosocial functioning without disruption."[5]

5. Compulsive—At this stage, cocaine use dominates the individual's life. It becomes his or her raison d'être. This stage of drug use is manifested by disintegration at the psychosocial, physical, and vocational levels. The use of cocaine progresses to a point beyond which the individual can control it.

From this classification, it is evident that the finding of cocaine in the urine, as part of a drug testing protocol, does not differentiate between the experimental cocaine user, on the one hand, and the compulsive cocaine user or "addict," on the other. Accordingly, it would not be appropriate for sports organizations, associations, and governing bodies to mandate "treatment" merely on the basis of a positive urine test. Rather, it would be more appropriate to mandate an "evaluation" by a qualified health care professional. The finding of an unequivocally positive urine test should not be ignored. However, as with all laboratory tests in clinical medicine, a positive urine for illicit drugs must be viewed within a specific clinical context. The finding of a positive urine, when taken *together* with the concepts and principles outlined in Chapter 17, will enable the qualified health professional to determine and establish the necessity, if any, and type of treatment.

Conversely, the absence of a positive drug test does not obviate the diagnosis of drug abuse. The casefinding of drug abuse in sports should not be limited to positive urine tests. If a positive drug test were the sine qua non of casefinding, many alcohol abusers and alcoholics, as well as other drug abusers, would go undetected depending on the specifics of a drug testing protocol. Here too, the principles and concepts outlined in Chapter 17 should enable the identification of the athlete in need of treatment in the absence of a positive drug test.

In this regard, it must be emphasized that regardless of any drug testing result, if it is determined on clinical grounds that a drug abuse disorder is present, it is preferable that treatment efforts should be initiated early. Valuable time can be wasted if one arbitrarily waits first to fulfill the minimal DSM-III (R) criteria of a Psychoactive Substance Abuse Disorder,[7] which stipulate a "maladaptive pattern" of psychoactive substance use must be present for at least 1 month.

Employee Assistance Programs

In recent years, the consequences of alcoholism and drug abuse have stimulated the development of employee assistance programs (EAPs) in industry. Since employers or other supervisory personnel are usually in a good position to recognize drug abuse at an early stage, EAPs were designed to facilitate the identification, treatment, and rehabilitation of drug abusers. A well-designed EAP should have a clear statement of policy, ensure confidentiality, provide health insurance for drug abuse treatment, ensure that the employee gets appropriate treatment, and, whenever possible, allow the employee to continue working while in treatment.[8] Building on this concept, EAPs have been recently integrated into university health programs. Troubled university faculty and staff can be identified by trained supervisory staff and can be referred for treatment with the assurance that once treatment is completed, they may return to work and remain, provided their job performance is acceptable. As has been stated by Spickard and Tucker,[9] "The denial of the existence of alcoholism in colleagues, the 'conspiracy of silence,' enables the obviously ill faculty member to deteriorate without proper treatment."

The concept of employee assistance programs can also be applied to the athletic community and to all forms of drug abuse. In sports, the "conspiracy of silence" must also be overcome. A sympathetic, compassionate, but firm confrontation of the troubled athlete need not await a positive urine screening test, clinical deterioration ("hitting the bottom"), or impaired athletic performance.[10] In 1981, the San Diego Padres baseball team established one of the first EAPs in professional sports. In this program, any player with a drug problem can, without penalty or cost, refer himself for professional treatment and counseling services which have been put in place by the team.[11] Since then, the Commissioner of Major League Baseball has mandated an EAP for all 26 major league organizations.[12]

OBJECTIVES AND GOALS OF TREATMENT

As Blum[13] has emphasized, the drug abuse literature is consistently inconsistent in defining "success" in the drug abuse treatment field, at least in part because of inconsistencies in defining outcome goals and objectives. Is total abstinence from one or more specific drugs as defined by negative urine tests the criterion of success? Is improvement in social functioning a criterion? If yes, to what degree? Is improved psychological functioning a criterion, and how is it to be measured? Does the remediation of a drug abuse–related medical problem constitute a successful outcome? The reality is that the objective of drug abuse treatment is directed not only at these criteria but to many more not enumerated here. Assuming agreement is achieved as to the requisite elements of treatment success, the question then arises, for how long? 6 months, 1 year, 2 years?

Inherent in defining the goals and objectives of any specific drug abuse treatment program or approach is the philosophical orientation of the program. What does the program see as the etiologic factors in the development of a drug abuse disorder? The program goals and objectives are further influenced by the case mix of patients it treats—demographic and socioeconomic factors, psychopathology, specific substances abused, age of patients, educational level, and severity of abuse, just to name some.

In general terms, the objective of treatment of the athlete with a drug abuse disorder is the same as that for any other individual with a drug abuse disorder. It is to have him or her become and remain abstinent from psychoactive substances while defining and dealing with the specific etiologic factors that were contributory to the development of his or her drug abuse disorder. The contributory factors which relate to the athlete's sport-focused lifestyle have been detailed in Chapter 3. From a more specific and limited perspective, it may be argued that the principal objective of a drug abuse treatment program in sports is to have the athlete become drug-free while participating more effectively in his or her sport. Where there had been impairment of performance, performance should improve. Where there had been dysfunctional relationships with teammates, coaches, management, and others, relationships should improve. Where there had been problems with meeting obligations, such as attending practice on time, these problems should resolve. Where injuries had become commonplace, these should diminish.

Although complete abstinence from psychoactive drugs has been a stated objective of most drug abuse treatment efforts, there have been efforts to assess the possibility of achieving what has been called stable "moderate drinking" or "normal drinking" in treated alcoholics. Interest in this question was stimulated by the report of Davies in 1962, in which he reported that 7 of 93 alcoholic patients were able to return to "normal drinking" for 7 to 11 years after treatment for alcoholism.[14] However, recent reports have indicated that when the follow-up period is longer than 1 to 2 years, the number of moderate drinkers falls off substantially. Specifically, by the end of 3 years, less than 3 percent could still be categorized as moderate drinkers.[15] The only predictors that appeared to correlate with the potential of an alcoholic subsequently becoming a stable, moderate drinker were being a less severe alcoholic initially and being female.[16]

PREDICTORS OF TREATMENT SUCCESS

While there exists no consensus on what constitutes a treatment success, Blum has outlined those variables that apparently predict an improved treatment outcome in drug abusing adolescents:[13]

1. Demographic
   a. Residential stability
   b. Higher educational attainment
   c. Fewer arrests
   d. Higher social class
2. Attitudinal
   a. Self-referral, more motivated for treatment, and having less denial of symptoms.
   b. More active participation in therapy (as assessed by treatment team)
3. Psychological
   a. Fewer psychoneurotic and psychopathologic symptoms
   b. Higher degree of distress
   c. More stable social relationships

In Gibbs and Flanagan's review[17] of 45 studies to assess those personal characteristics of alcoholics which might correlate with treatment outcome, they concluded: (1) there is a great diversity of opinion among various researchers about those personal characteristics of alcoholics which correlate with an improvement from treatment; and (2) highly stable, general predictors of treatment success are quite elusive. More recently, Neuberger and associates[18] have highlighted the fact that when two specific demographic indicators coexist, namely, marriage and employment, there is a 73 percent probability of achieving 12 months of sobriety.

Predicting treatment success not only requires an assessment of patient characteristics but also an assessment of the treatment methodology. Assessing treatment success is confounded by the observation that many drug abusers recover "spontaneously." As Moos and Finney[19] have pointed out in their discussion of alcoholism treatment evaluation, 10 to 20 percent of problem drinkers may recover without therapy, depending on the criteria that are used, and 32 to 53 percent of problem drinkers improve with minimal treatment. Nonetheless, they concluded, as have others, that since many studies indicate treated individuals show a higher rate of improvement than do minimally treated or untreated individuals, treatment may "facilitate" the recovery process or at least "reduce" the drinking problem.[20]

SELECTING TREATMENT APPROACHES

In response to the escalation of drug abuse over the past 3 decades, numerous treatment approaches have been advocated. While some, such as Alcoholics Anonymous (AA), date back to 1935,[21] others are of much more recent vintage. While each has its proponents, many substance abusers will require a mix of treatment approaches. For some, treatment strategies will have to be changed or modified during the course of therapy.

The effectiveness of treatment of drug abuse has been viewed by some as being of limited value, with some workers in the field suggesting that the outcome is the same regardless of the treatment approach.[22] As underscored by Rounsaville,[23] "Carefully designed, controlled studies, with randomized assignment evaluating efficacy of different approaches to treatment of substance abusers are comparatively rare." For any analysis of treatment efficacy, there must exist: (1) specificity relative to the patients treated; (2) specificity relative to the treatment approaches used; and (3) a clear delineation of the treatment goals and objectives. As McLellan[22] has noted:

> Given a large population of substance abuse patients with a wide range of treatment needs, it seems likely that any single therapeutic program will be successful

with only the small sample of patients whose particular treatment needs correspond with the specific treatment approach of the program. Thus, while a program may be only 35–40 percent effective with the total patient population, each individual program may be much more effective in treating the particular sample of patients for which it is best suited. By determining the specific treatment needs most successfully addressed by a therapeutic program, and then assigning patients with those needs to that program, it seems possible to improve the overall level of treatment success.

Accordingly, as in other branches of medicine, the selection of a treatment approach or approaches should be predicated on a careful and specific assessment of the patient. Factors which can be helpful in the selection process include: medical problems (drug abuse related and others); drug abuse pattern (type or types, severity); economics (employment, financial background); legal status (arrests, court-ordered treatment); family status (marital status, functional or dysfunctional relationships); education (level attained, aspirations); social issues (peer group, stability of relationships); residence (living arrangements, stability); and psychological considerations (psychopathology).

Additional factors come into play in selecting a treatment plan for the drug-abusing athlete. These include, but are not limited to, athletic status (amateur or professional), nature of sport (team or individual), rules of governance with respect to drug abuse (mandatory "treatment," suspension, no rules), policies regarding alcohol, regulations regarding follow-up drug testing (frequency, conditions, which substances), living arrangements (home, dorms, hotels, roommates), travel (extensive, minimal), available sports medicine services (comprehensive, nominal), and available psychological services (readily available, consultation only, none). Whereas the vast majority of drug abusers are unknown to the public, the athlete, and particularly the successful athlete, is frequently well known. Entering treatment under the scrutiny of the media and being periodically monitored by the media (and thus the public) throughout the treatment process might well impact on the treatment approach chosen and, in particular, the selection of an aftercare approach.

TREATMENT APPROACHES

Since most athletes are either teenagers or young adults, any approach to the treatment of an athlete's drug abuse disorder must be tailored to meet the needs of adolescents and young adults. Accordingly, some treatment approaches which had been designed for the older "hard-core" addict are not suitable for the competitive athlete who is more likely to be either a youthful circumstantial drug abuser or, perhaps, an intensified alcohol or cocaine abuser. Regardless of the specifics of any given approach, Wheeler and Malmquist[24] have noted that most programs directed at youthful drug abusers "share a belief that treatment begins with the *interruption of use*, requires a stable *maintenance of sobriety*, and has as its goal the development of a *chemical-free life-style*."

In addition to the requirement of abstinence, Semlitz and Gold[25] have emphasized that all drug abuse treatment programs geared towards youth should share the following characteristics:

1. The program should provide accurate and current information on the health hazards of drug abuse.
2. The program should actively help users overcome their dependence rather than rely on lectures and harangues.
3. The program should be directed to the age, interests, and special problems of the participants.
4. The program should include family involvement.
5. The program should emphasize the present "so that those in treatment understand the immediate damage they experience from their drug use and, just as important, realize that they will be held accountable for their actions and suffer the consequence of their destructive behavior."

Representative Approaches

Inpatient, Short Term

Most programs that offer short-term inpatient care do so in a hospital setting. The judgment to hospitalize a drug abuser depends on many factors. Included in these are the extent, compulsivity, and progression of drug abuse, the need for detoxification, the presence of polysubstance abuse, prior out-patient treatment failures, concurrent medical problems, medical complications, severe psychiatric symptoms, severe impairment of social or vocational functioning, and inadequate mobilization of outpatient and community resources. The athlete may enter an inpatient treatment program in order to facilitate treatment so that he or she may return to athletic competition in as short a time as possible. It has become an increasingly common phenomenon that athletes are so hospitalized for the treatment of one or more addictions. The involvement of team management or a sport's governing body is often crucial in motivating the athlete to seek and accept such treatment. As Kaufman[26] has stated: "The employer who clearly makes treatment a precondition of continued employment, who supports time for treatment and who guarantees a job on completion of the initial treatment course is a valuable ally."

The period of hospitalization allows for intensive program planning, as well as the actual initiation of the treatment program. Aside from detoxification, the elements that might be implemented in the short-term hospital setting include individual and group psychotherapy, family therapy, and introduction to self-help groups such as Alcoholics Anonymous, Narcotics Anonymous, and Cocaine Anonymous. Counseling, frequently by recovering alcoholics and drug abusers, offers insights from their own experiences. It is during the period of hospitalization that a detailed plan of aftercare, incorporating these elements, is orchestrated so that there is no break in the continuity of care following discharge.

The length of stay in the hospital usually approximates 28 days, although this varies according to patient needs, insurance policies, and program design.

Pharmacologic Approaches

Pharmacologic strategies have been employed in the management of alcohol and drug withdrawal and in the maintenance of abstinence. Sustained use of psychoactive drugs such as alcohol, narcotics, and barbiturates produces a physical dependency on these drugs, whereas sustained use of drugs such as cocaine produces a psychophysio-logic dependency with symptoms of intense craving. Cessation of their use results in a withdrawal syndrome, the manifestations of which depend on the drug, the dose, the duration of abuse (may be as short as weeks or months), and the frequency of use.[27,28] If withdrawal is anticipated, the patient should be admitted to the hospital for observation and treatment or should be closely supervised in an ambulatory setting.[29]

Once abstinence has been achieved, three pharmacologic approaches have been utilized to maintain abstinence from alcohol and other abused substances—agonist drugs, antagonist drugs, and negative reinforcing drugs. Agonist drugs, such as methadone, have similar effects to the abused drugs, as in the case of heroin. The objective in this case is to provide replacement therapy and reduce the self-destruction and the destruction to society caused by continued heroin use, notably increasing crime rates in order to sustain ever-increasing drug habits, and the spread of infections such as acquired immunodeficiency syndrome (AIDS). This approach is based on the phenomenon of cross-tolerance between the different opiate drugs. Antagonist drugs, such as naltrexone, reduce the positive reinforcing properties of heroin by blocking its subjective effects.[30] A third category of drugs that have been employed to maintain abstinence is negative reinforcing drugs. Agents such as disulfiram produce profound negative reinforcement if the abused substance (alcohol) is used after a period of abstinence.[23]

Alcohol withdrawal. The alcohol withdrawal syndrome occurs when an individual abruptly stops drinking alcohol following prolonged consumption. The symptoms of withdrawal, which are frequently overlooked, can begin within 6 to 8 hours after cessation. Clinical features include anxiety, agitation, irritability, tremor, hyperreflexia, hallucinations, insomnia, and a reduction of the individual's seizure threshold. Systemic symptoms can include nausea, vomiting, tachycardia, sweating, agitation, systolic and diastolic hypertension, and cardiac arrhythmias (see Chapter 11). Only a small percentage of individuals will progress to the extreme form of withdrawal, delirium tremens (DTs). This latter disorder, which can occur 3 to 4 days after the cessation of alcohol consumption, is characterized by marked disorientation, fever, vivid hallucinations, tachycardia, hypertension, and profuse sweating. In its extreme form, cardiovascular collapse and death can occur.[31]

If the symptoms are mild, no pharmacologic treatment may be required. If sedation is required, generally the benzodiazepines have been utilized.[32] Because the alcohol withdrawal syndrome, in part, is mediated through the autonomic nervous system, autonomic blocking agents such as clonidine and atenolol have been used to block the sympathetic response.[31,33]

Cocaine withdrawal and craving. Although chronic cocaine use can lead to an extreme degree of psychophysiologic dependence, true tolerance is equivocal and an "opiate" type of dependence does not develop (see Chapter 7).[34] It is noteworthy that the DSM-III (R) requires neither tolerance nor withdrawal for the diagnosis of cocaine dependence.[7] Over time, the use of cocaine leads to brain neurochemical changes which manifest themselves by an intense craving for increasing amounts of cocaine. The symptoms of craving are most evident following the smoking of cocaine in the form of "crack." Crack smoking produces a euphoria referred to as a "rush," which is followed by a dysphoric withdrawal referred to as a "crash." With increased usage, the craving increases and results in behaviors which are singularly directed at obtaining more and more crack. This severe psychophysiologic dependence can occur in a matter of days to weeks.[35]

The abstinence syndrome is considered to be more complex than merely experiencing a "crash" after the cessation of cocaine usage. It has been described as a three-phase syndrome.[36] The first phase, a dysphoric withdrawal commonly referred to as the "crash," can last from approximately 9 hours to as long as 4 days. Early agitation, anorexia, and intense craving for cocaine are followed shortly by symptoms of tiredness, depression, oversleeping, increased dreaming, overeating, irritability, and a loss of craving for cocaine.[37] As the second phase, which can last from 1 to 10 weeks, is entered, there is an improvement in mood and a normalization of sleeping and eating patterns. However, the craving for cocaine returns, and it is in this phase that the risk of relapse is particularly high. During the third phase, "where

mood and hedonic responses are generally normal for patients without additional psychiatric diagnoses," craving for cocaine still may result from environmental stimuli many months to years, and perhaps indefinitely, after the last use of cocaine[32] (Fig. 19–1).

Additionally, many crack users, as well as heavy users of intranasal cocaine, are polysubstance abusers. These other substances, including alcohol, barbiturates, and opiates, are used to relieve the agitation, dysphoria, and insomnia commonly associated with cocaine use, and may produce dependency in their own right. Therefore, the management of withdrawal from these drugs may also be required.

A number of pharmacologic approaches have been employed to diminish the craving for cocaine.[38-42] These include a dopamine receptor agonist (bromocriptine [Parlodel]), tricyclic antidepressants (e.g., desipramine [Norpramin], imipramine [Tofranil]), lithium (Lithobid), and methylphenidate (Ritalin). The latter has been used in patients whose cocaine use is thought to be associated with an attention deficit disorder of the residual type.[28,37] Both lithium and methylphenidate act rapidly to curb withdrawal symptoms but appear to lose their efficacy with time. On the other hand, tricyclic antidepressants require weeks before their actions become evident. Recent efforts are being directed at using drug combinations such as lithium and desipramine, and amantadine (Symmetral) and imipramine.[43] Both tyrosine—the precursor of dopamine and norepinephrine—and tryptophan—the precursor of serotonin—have also been used to diminish the withdrawal symptoms and craving for cocaine.[35,40,44] When psychopharmacologic approaches are added to psychotherapeutic interventions, Kleber and Gawin[38] observed that the patient retention rate approached twice the retention rate for psychotherapeutic intervention alone.

Disulfiram. Disulfiram (Antabuse) has been used for the pharmacologic treatment of alcoholism over the past 3 decades. Its effect on alcohol metabolism was found quite by accident by two Danish physicians who had taken disulfiram as part of a study to evaluate this drug as a treatment for parasitic diseases. They became ill when drinking alcohol after having taken disulfiram. As a result, they initiated the studies that became the

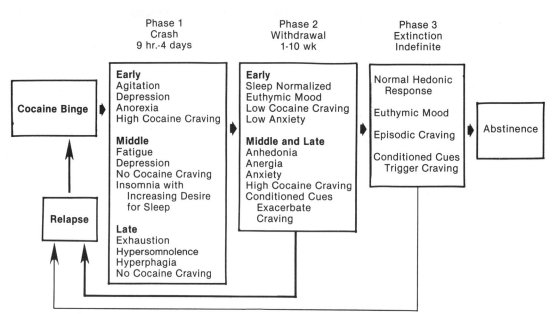

Figure 19–1. Post-cocaine withdrawal symptoms. Duration and intensity of symptoms vary based on binge characteristics and diagnosis. Binges range from under 4 hours duration to 6 or more days. High cocaine craving early in phase 1 continues for up to 20 hours, but usually lasts less than 6 and is followed by a period of noncraving with similar duration in the next subphase (middle-phase 1). Substantial craving then returns only after a lag of up to 5 or more days, during phase 2. (From Gawin and Kleber,[36] with permission.)

basis for the use of disulfiram as an adjunct in the treatment of alcoholism.[45]

Disulfiram is referred to as an alcohol-sensitizing drug which produces an aversive reaction when it is taken shortly before the ingestion of alcohol. Disulfiram is the only alcohol-sensitizing drug that is used for this purpose in the United States. Calcium carbimide, another alcohol-sensitizing drug, is not available in the United States. Disulfiram inhibits the enzyme aldehyde dehydrogenase, which is responsible for the metabolism of acetaldehyde to acetate, an important step in the metabolism of alcohol (see Chapter 11). Consequently, alcohol consumed after the ingestion of these drugs results in a rapid rise in the blood acetaldehyde level. The more alcohol, the higher the acetaldehyde level. High levels of acetaldehyde are in turn associated with intensely distressing symptoms which collectively have been referred to as the disulfiram-alcohol reaction. The symptoms, which begin within 5 to 10 minutes after ingesting alcohol and can last from 30 minutes to hours, include: facial flushing, a rapid heart rate, decreased blood pressure, nausea and copious vomiting, chest pain, and shortness of breath.[45,46] In severe cases, myocardial infarction, seizures, cerebrovascular hemorrhages, congestive heart failure, and cardiovascular collapse have been reported.[32] In most fatal cases, excessive doses of disulfiram in conjunction with 2 or more alcoholic drinks were consumed.[46] Sensitization to alcohol may last 6 to 14 days after the last ingestion of disulfiram.[45]

In the early days of its usage, when doses were 1 to 2 grams per day, disulfiram was reported to have produced psychiatric disturbances in up to 20 percent of patients. However, with currently used doses, the incidence of psychiatric disturbances is extremely low.[47] With the low doses that are currently used—250 mg per day—the side effects of disulfiram are minimal and do not exceed those reported with placebos. Disulfiram can impair the metabolism of certain drugs such as diazepam (Valium), chlordiazepoxide (Librium), and warfarin (Coumadin).[46]

Disulfiram has been used in alcoholics who are seeking abstinence, who are willing to take the drug, and who have no medical contraindications such as heart disease, pulmonary insufficiency, neuropathy, organic mental syndromes, and psychoses. Since disulfiram is not a cure but an adjunct for alcoholism treatment, the patient must be participating in other forms of therapy, for instance, psychotherapy and/or self-help groups. Continuous medical monitoring during therapy is necessary.

Despite the fact that disulfiram has been used for more than 35 years, there is still uncertainty regarding its efficacy. Schuckit has suggested those men who may do better with disulfiram are individuals who are married, are affluent, drink less often, and have greater degrees of social stability.[48] A 1986 study has concluded that disulfiram did not enhance the attainment of continuous abstinence, time to relapse, or employment status any more than counseling alone. However, in those patients taking disulfiram who did relapse, a statistically significant reduction in the extent of alcohol use relative to non-disulfiram-treated individuals occurred.[49] Any reduction in intake is important, since an increased number of "dry days" may reduce the medical complications associated with alcoholism.[50]

Methadone maintenance. Although methadone maintenance has little applicability to the treatment of drug abuse in sports, it is briefly discussed in this chapter because of its historic significance in the pharmacologic management of drug abuse. Methadone is a synthetic narcotic which was developed by the Germans during World War II. In 1964, Dole and Nyswander[51] of Rockefeller University introduced the concept of methadone maintenance for the treatment of heroin addiction. They observed that the regular oral administration of methadone to heroin-addicted patients reduced the patients' craving for heroin. Additionally, methadone appeared to block the "rush" and the euphoric effect associated with heroin use. Consequently, these patients were not only able to resist their desire to use heroin, but they were able to function within society as evidenced by their ability to resume their education and/or to hold jobs.

Much of the early success reported by Dole and Nyswander has been attributed to careful patient selection as well as the provision of supportive services. As the number of methadone maintenance programs grew (well over 100,000 patients worldwide) and the patient selection process became less discriminating (less motivated patients), and as the supportive services became less available, successful treatment outcomes were often less dramatic.[32] Nonetheless, methadone maintenance, a treatment approach in which opiate addicts receive a daily oral dose of methadone, remains a major approach to the treatment of heroin addiction.[52]

As a treatment for opiate addiction, methadone maintenance is not without its detractors. Some feel "it is merely a replacement of one addiction for another" and that success "can only be measured by abstinence, not substitution."[53] Others have voiced concern that methadone programs, while concentrating on opiate addiction, have ignored or neglected dealing with the problem of associated chronic dependencies, such as alcohol, cocaine, and tobacco. For example, it has been estimated that heavy alcohol consumption in methadone treatment populations ranges from 20 to 50 percent.[8]

Psychotherapy

As Khantzian[54] has noted:

> Substance abusers suffer because they are unable to manage their feelings, self-esteem, relationships and behavior. It is for these reasons that they need treatment in general, and psychotherapy in particular. They have substituted extraordinary chemical solutions for more ordinary human ones and as a consequence they need to discover in the context of a human relationship with another individual or a group of individuals that their problems can be identified, understood and treated in more ordinary ways.

Psychotherapy has been particularly effective in drug abusers with psychiatric problems of "comparatively high severity."[23,55] There exists an abundant literature on the philosophies, approaches, and techniques of psychotherapy for the management of drug abuse disorders.[56] These run the gamut from traditional psychoanalytically oriented psychotherapy, to gestalt therapy, to cognitive-behavioral therapy. Requisite to any discussion of psychotherapy for drug abuse is an understanding of the interrelationship of psychiatric disorders and drug abuse disorders. Psychiatric disorders which may be antecedent to, or coincident with, the development of a drug abuse disorder are discussed in Chapter 2. Additionally, psychopathology may occur as a consequence of drug abuse. Accordingly, in assessing the potential role of psychotherapy in a drug abuse disorder, it is important to distinguish which is primary, the drug abuse disorder or the psychiatric disorder. In making this assessment, obtaining a past psychiatric history is very helpful. This may be available from the patient or from significant others in the patient's life. Since it may be difficult to distinguish which is primary, the determination may have to be deferred until the patient is drug or alcohol free for a period of 3 to 4 weeks.[56-58]

Although specifically addressing the psychotherapeutic treatment of cocaine abuse, the treatment objectives of Kleber and Gawin[28] can be adapted to other primary drug abuse disorders:

> 1) To help the abuser recognize deleterious effects of cocaine use and accept the need to stop it. . . .
> 2) To help the abuser manage impulsive behavior in general, and cocaine in particular; for example, exploring ways to dissociate the abuser from cocaine use situations and cocaine sources. . . .
> 3) To bring the abuser to an understanding of the functions that cocaine has played in his life and to help him serve these functions without drugs.

In addition to being used to treat primary drug abuse disorders, psychotherapy has been utilized for the treatment of frequently associated affective disorders such as depression and bipolar affective disorder. From his review of the literature, Nace[58] concluded, with respect to alcohol, that "the coexistence of alcoholism and depression is common . . . that depression in alcoholics often remits with brief treatment, and that alcoholics remaining depressed are likely to need specific treatment for depression if abstinence is to be gained."

Individual therapy. Many drug abusers, particularly younger ones, enter individual psychotherapy at the behest of others. Accordingly, they may enter therapy begrudgingly and without a commitment. It is imperative that the therapist be aware of this and that at the outset he or she establish ground rules that will permit the development of a rapport and trust. During the treatment process, Nace highlighted four treatment phases.[59] The *recognition phase* is directed at having the patient recognize and admit that a substance abuse problem exists. It is characterized by confrontation and education. During the *compliance phase*, the patient superficially participates in therapy although not convinced it is needed. However, it is in the third phase, the *acceptance phase*, that the patient begins to recognize his or her inability to use psychoactive substances. Denial, defensiveness, and manipulation are stripped away. It is not until the fourth phase, the *integration phase*, that the drug abuser is fully accepting of the fact that he or she cannot use psychoactive substances. It is during this phase of psychotherapy that issues not directly related to drug abuse come into focus.

By definition, all drug abuse disorders have the self-administration of a drug as a central objective. Thus, a specific goal of drug abuse treatment is to eliminate drug self-administration.[60] One specific form of behavioral psychotherapy that has been utilized to accomplish this objective is referred to as contingency contracting or contingency management.[61-63] This technique, which has primarily been used in the management of cocaine abuse, is predicated on the fact that some drugs are biologically reinforcing. The drug itself serves to reinforce the continued use of the drug, leading to its sustained use. Contingency contracting is a behavioral technique designed to competitively promote or develop more desirable behaviors than that of drug self-administration. Contingency contracting utilizes a system of severe, individualized penalties mutually agreed upon by the patient and the therapist. Penalties are selected in such a manner that negative consequences will accrue to the patient if he or she uses the drug as evidenced by positive urine tests. This technique has been used to treat a variety of professionals.[63] Early in therapy, a letter or "contract" is drawn up by the patient detailing his or her drug abuse which is addressed, for example, to an employer or a licensing agency such as a state education or health department. Such letters or contracts are written for a specified period of time, frequently several months. Patients could choose to include other drugs in the contract. The letter would only be sent contingent upon the patient reinitiating his or her drug use. This in turn would trigger some official action by the licensing agency. In sports, a similar approach could be undertaken with a contingency letter directed to team management or to the governing body of the sport. The contingency contracting technique relies on the notion that the aversive effects associated with drug use can be powerful determinants in creating new drug-free behaviors.[62]

Group therapy. Whereas individual psychotherapy provides the drug abuser with a confidential, one-on-one, ongoing relationship, group psychotherapy provides the individual with a setting in which his or her concerns and problems crucial to abstinence and recovery can be expressed, challenged, and validated among his or her peers.[64,65] It is a process in which the patient not only receives support and guidance from others with similar problems, but he or she is also able to help others as well. Group psychotherapy has had wide application in the treatment of both youthful drug abuse and alcoholism.[59,62,64]

Although the composition of the group may be homogeneous with respect to the substance or substances abused, it is likely to be heterogeneous with respect to socioeconomics, sex, age, occupation, and religion, as well as to prior and concurrent psychotherapeutic experience. It is imperative for the group to be homogeneous in terms of its objective to achieve total abstinence from the use of psychoactive drugs. Accepting "controlled" or "moderate" use of these substances by some members of the group, while demanding total abstinence by others, will become a focus of divisiveness within the group. In group psychotherapy, as contrasted with self-help groups, the therapist is a professional who may be a psychiatrist, a psychologist, a psychiatric social worker, or a nurse trained as mental health worker. The specific training and orientation of the therapist will determine the actual approach and techniques to be used in the group process. As with individual therapy, these might include behavioral, gestalt, and psychoanalytically oriented approaches. Groups usually consist of 6 to 15 persons, they usually meet once or twice a week, and sessions last from 1½ to 2 hours.[60,66] The length of time a group exists is a function of its objective. If the group process is used merely to get the abuser through a period of detoxification, then its life will be short. On the other hand, if the objective is to have the individual develop insight into the psychodynamics of his or her drug abuse, then the life of the group may be years. As Smith and associates[64] have noted: "Modern group therapy tends to focus on 'here and now' in interpersonal interactions and communication, while they are occurring within the group therapy sessions, and on the relationships, feelings, and problems between group members." Table 19–1 is illustrative of ground rules that have been established for participation by cocaine abusers in group psychotherapy.

Family therapy. According to Kaufman, family therapy is the most promising, nonpharmacologic intervention for the treatment of drug abusers to have evolved in the past decade.[26] It is predicated on the following notions: (1) the family is a distinct behavioral entity with unique characteristics rather than merely being the sum of the characteristics of the individual members of the family; and (2) a close interrelationship exists between the psychosocial functioning of the family as a distinct unit or group and the emotional adaptation of each individual member of the group.[67] It follows that family therapy involves the treatment of more than one family member simultaneously.

The familial genetic and environmental contributions to drug abuse are discussed in Chapter 2. A variety of dynamics can be at play in the family of the drug abuser. Oftentimes, the family will unwittingly deny the existence of drug abuse in a family member. By accepting rationalizations for the family member's drug-related behavior, the family may actually be in collusion with the patient's use of drugs and alcohol, thereby forestalling treatment.[5] In other situations, more than one family member may be a drug abuser, particularly given the contribution of genetics to alcoholism. Still other families are dysfunctional or severely dysfunctional, independent of drug abuse, and if abstinence is achieved in one family member, such families may actually break up. The relatively high incidence of other psychiatric diagnoses, such as depression, bipolar disorders, and antisocial personality disorders in the families of drug abusers cannot be overlooked. It was originally thought that there were sharp lines of distinction between the

Table 19–1. COCAINE TREATMENT PROGRAM GROUP THERAPY
GROUND RULES

Purpose: To support and assist self and other members in abstaining from cocaine.

Rules:
1. Absolute commitment to never use cocaine.
2. Absolute honesty about drug use.
3. Regular attendance: you may not continue in the group if you have more than the occasional absence (e.g., once per 2 months).
4. No coming to group under the influence of any drug.
5. "Slips" will be looked on as potential learning experiences. However, you cannot continue in the group if you have a regular pattern of slips (e.g., every week). This is destructive for everyone.
6. Random urine tests for all group members.
7. Group therapists will be in regular contact with individual therapists.
8. No socializing outside of the group.
9. Fee will be on a monthly basis, due at the first session each month.
10. *Confidentiality:* Anything said in the group must be respected and not used for "gossip" or other purposes outside the group. Serious breaches of confidentiality are grounds for dismissal from the group.

From Spitz,[66] with permission.

families of heroin addicts, alcoholics, and cocaine abusers. However, as these substances have crossed socioeconomic lines, and as polysubstance abuse has increased, it has become clear that there are large areas of overlap.[68]

There are many schools of family therapy, a discussion of which is beyond the scope of this book. Some approaches to family therapy include conjoint therapy, couples group therapy, and spouse (or parent or child) group therapy.[58] The most common, conjoint therapy, involves the drug abuser and his or her spouse, and it may include their children. In the case of minors, conjoint therapy may involve siblings as well as the parents. In their discussion of the role of family therapy in cocaine abuse, Spitz and Spitz[68] have detailed a step-by-step approach to this form of therapy. While the specific goals of family therapy in the treatment of drug abuse will necessarily depend on the specifics of each case, in general the goal of family therapy is to develop a plan of abstinence that the family can consistently maintain. Educationally, family members are taught to recognize the signs and symptoms of drug abuse in order to reduce the likelihood of manipulation and lying about alcohol and drug usage by the patient. Family members learn to modify their own behaviors which may have contributed to the drug abuse by a family member.

Although not a family in the traditional sense of the word, the relationships that an athlete has with his or her team are often akin to those seen in families. Traveling together, living together, and competing together for months at a time creates interpersonal dynamics and tensions that are not experienced in most professions. Although the concepts of "family therapy" have not been generally applied to athletic teams when a team member is treated for drug abuse, the potential exists for this type of approach when specific members of the team are committed to helping a drug-abusing teammate. Such an approach could enable problems of communication to be addressed. Specifically, a therapist could encourage teammates to talk and listen to each other, could correct distorted communications, and could help teammates to find other ways of communicating.[69]

One example of a team "family" approach to drug abuse can be found in the program established in 1982 by the Cleveland Browns football team. This program revolves around a group of current and former players with drug-related problems. Members of the group, referred to as the Inner Circle, meet weekly in an encounter format and are available to meet with other players. Supportive services for the group are provided by a psychiatrist with expertise in chemical dependency, the coach, the team administrative assistant, the employee assistant consultant, and a spiritual counselor. Collectively, this support group is called the Outer Circle. Both the Inner Circle and the Outer Circle are but parts of a *"total organizational commitment* aimed at prevention, identification, and treatment, not only for the drug abuse itself, but also for the problem of the 'whole person'."[70a] The Cleveland Browns' program, which was developed jointly by the Cleveland Browns and the Cleveland Clinic Foundation, reports a substantial improvement, as measured by drug free status and other psychosocial and biologic parameters, in 75 percent of the cases.[70,70a]

Some individual athletes relocate during their teenage years to train with world-class coaches. They live with surrogate families, and much of their time is devoted to the development of athletic skills. Here too, the concept of family therapy has applicability.

Whether in the sports setting or the traditional family setting, the principles of confidentiality and privacy must be adhered to, particularly when discussing the use of illicit drugs. Violations of confidentiality only serve to subvert the therapeutic process. Traditional concepts of confidentiality associated with individual psychotherapy must be expanded when working with familities.[71]

Self-Help Groups

Alcoholics Anonymous (AA) is considered by many to be the mainstay of alcoholism treatment and has become a prototype for self-help groups dealing with other compulsive and addictive disorders. However, some feel that because of its emphasis on "spiritual" recovery, it is out of the mainstream of alcoholism treatment.[72] Officially dating its beginning to June 10, 1935, its membership in the United States and Canada was reported to approximate 653,000 by 1984.[73] Whereas historically AA primarily serviced older adults, by 1983 20 percent of its members were under the age of 31, as contrasted with only 6 percent in 1971.

The AA Preamble succinctly describes its mission.[73]

> Alcoholics Anonymous is a fellowship of men and women who share their experience, strength, and hope with each other that they may solve their common problem and help others to recover from alcoholism.
>
> The only requirement for membership is a desire to stop drinking. There are no dues or fees to AA membership; we are self-supporting through our own contributions. AA is not allied with any sect, denomination, politics, organizations, or institution; does not wish to engage in any controversy, neither endorses nor opposes any causes. Our primary purpose is to stay sober and help other alcoholics achieve sobriety.

At the heart of AA are the Twelve Steps of Alcoholics Anonymous (Table 19–2) and the Twelve Traditions of Alcoholics Anonymous (Table 19–3). In his book *The Treatment of*

Table 19–2. THE TWELVE STEPS OF ALCOHOLICS ANONYMOUS

1. We admitted we were powerless over alcohol—that our lives had become unmanageable.
2. Came to believe that a Power greater than ourselves could restore us to sanity.
3. Made a decision to turn our will and our lives over to the care of God as we understood Him.
4. Made a searching and fearless moral inventory of ourselves.
5. Admitted to God, to ourselves, and to another human being the exact nature of our wrongs.
6. Were entirely ready to have God remove all these defects of character.
7. Humbly asked Him to remove our shortcomings.
8. Made a list of all persons we had harmed, and became willing to make amends to them all.
9. Made direct amends to such people wherever possible, except when to do so would injure them or others.
10. Continued to take personal inventory and when we were wrong promptly admitted it.
11. Sought through prayer and meditation to improve our conscious contact with God as we understood Him, praying only for knowledge of His will for us and the power to carry that out.
12. Having had a spiritual awakening as the result of these steps, we tried to carry this message to alcoholics, and to practice these principles in all our affairs.

Reprinted with permission of Alcoholics Anonymous World Services, Inc.

Table 19–3. THE TWELVE TRADITIONS OF ALCOHOLICS ANONYMOUS

1. Our common welfare should come first; personal recovery depends upon AA unity.
2. For our group purpose there is but one ultimate authority—a loving God as He may express Himself in our group conscience. Our leaders are but trusted servants; they do not govern.
3. The only requirement for AA membership is a desire to stop drinking.
4. Each group should be autonomous except in matters affecting other groups or AA as a whole.
5. Each group has but one primary purpose—to carry its message to the alcoholic who still suffers.
6. An AA group ought never endorse, finance, or lend the AA name to any related facility or outside enterprise, lest problems of money, property, and prestige divert us from our primary purpose.
7. Every AA group ought to be fully self-supporting, declining outside contributions.
8. Alcoholics Anonymous should remain forever nonprofessional, but our service centers may employ special workers.
9. AA, as such, ought never be organized; but we may create service boards or committees directly responsible to those they serve.
10. Alcoholics Anonymous has no opinion on outside issues; hence the AA name ought never be drawn into public controversy.
11. Our public relations policy is based on attraction rather than promotion; we need always maintain personal anonymity at the level of press, radio, and films.
12. Anonymity is the spiritual foundation of all our Traditions, ever reminding us to place principles before personalities.

Reprinted with permission of Alcoholics Anonymous World Services, Inc.

Alcoholism, Nace has offered four reasons why AA has worked.[73]

1. Unconditional Acceptance—Regardless of any prior experience with treatment, the alcoholic is always welcome. The only requirement for participation is "a desire to stop drinking."
2. Overcomes Denial—At the outset, Step 1 states: "We admitted we were powerless over alcohol—that our lives had become unmanageable." This is continuously reinforced by the tradition of adding the phrase "I'm an alcoholic," when an individual introduces himself or herself to the group.
3. Group Process—Many of the elements inherent in group therapy are incorporated into AA. The importance of the group process is evidenced by the use of the pronoun "we" 7 times in the Twelve Steps and "our" 7 times. "Us" is used twice, as is "ourselves." New members have the opportunity of identifying with the experiences of older members. Recognizing the diversity of the alcoholic population, AA has adapted to this by establishing groups centered around special subgroups and special needs, such as women, professionals, day groups, night groups.
4. Deflation of Pathological Narcissism— Nace has suggested that Steps 1, 2, and 11

serve to undermine the alcoholic's defenses of grandiosity and self-sufficiency. This is evident, for example, in Step 1's "our lives had become unmanageable."

Alcoholics Anonymous has been viewed by some as a religious organization because of its emphasis on "spiritual" recovery[72] and because many of its members are committed to it with a religious fervor. However, AA is not affiliated with any religious denomination and the "concept of 'Higher Power' is allowed wide conceptual latitude ranging from the organized religious concept of God to the AA group itself."[73]

In years past, physicians viewed AA with skepticism, in part because of physicians' reliance on the scientific method and their demand for documentation, uniform criteria, and controls. However, more recently the health care community has increasingly recognized and accepted Alcoholics Anonymous as a valuable component of the armamentarium in the treatment of alcoholism. Oftentimes, involvement with AA is initiated during periods of hospitalization for alcoholism. By 1977, it was estimated that about 10 percent of alcoholics entering AA were referred by physicians.[73]

As with other treatment approaches, there have been attempts to assess statistically the efficacy of Alcoholics Anonymous. Success has been variously defined in terms such as days of total abstinence, decrease in the amount or frequency of drinking, and attendance at AA meetings. In 1976, Bebbington underscored the difficulty in obtaining the hard data upon which to draw efficacy conclusions.[74] Anonymity in AA means no names, no addresses, and no case histories. Even the definition of membership is arbitrarily defined as attendance at 10 or more meetings. Nonetheless, some observations are noteworthy. In 1983, Hoffman and associates[75] reported that follow-up data on 900 inpatients revealed a high correlation between total abstinence 6 months after discharge and weekly attendance at AA meetings during this period. Seventy-three percent of regular attendees remained chemically free, compared with 33 percent of the nonattendees. Put differently, alcoholics who attend AA meetings regularly may be more than twice as likely to be abstinent as the alcoholic who does not.[75]

The 1983 data from the General Services Office of Alcoholics Anonymous indicated that 60 percent were still attending meetings 3 months after starting.[73] Data from 1968 and 1971 surveys indicated that 60 percent of AA members had been abstinent for 1 year, and other programs utilizing the steps of AA in the treatment process had 2-year abstinence rates of approximately 60 percent.[72] Data also suggest that the longer the period of sobriety, the greater the likelihood that sobriety will continue. Thus, in a 7-year follow-up of 393 members of AA, 70 percent of those who were sober for 1 year were likely to be sober for 2 years, and of those who were sober after 2 years 90 percent were likely to be sober at the end of 3 years.[73]

The concepts and principles that have been applied to the treatment of alcohol abuse have more recently been applied to the treatment of other drug abuse disorders. Examples of these are Cocaine Anonymous (CA), Drugs Anonymous (DA), and Narcotics Anonymous (NA).[76] Support groups have been developed for significant others, for example, spouses, children, and friends, who are intimately involved with the drug-dependent individual. Groups such as Al-Anon and Narc-Anon allow members to share experiences and to assist each other in coping with the stresses engendered by substance abuse.

Self-help groups such as AA can be especially valuable to the athlete. Anonymity is at the heart of the program. This can be particularly important to the athlete whose name might well be a household word. Importantly, AA groups are present all over the country so that the athlete can attend meetings irrespective of travel commitments attendant to his or her sport. Accordingly, participation can continue year round, in-season and off-season. Finances are not a consideration, as there are no fees associated with self-help groups such as Alcoholics Anonymous.

Therapeutic Community

Originally developed in 1959 to serve the needs of the urban street heroin addict, the "therapeutic community" has developed into a treatment modality in which more than 100,000 individuals participate. As originally conceived, the therapeutic community (TC) primarily catered to male heroin addicts in their thirties who had spent time in prison, lived in the ghetto, and had a long history of treatment failures.[64]

Predicated on the concept that drug abuse and addiction is a complex psychosocial problem, TCs have utilized the techniques of confrontation and challenge to foster maturity and responsibility. Although not denying the contribution of physiologic influences, the TC's emphasis has traditionally been on the behavioral and social aspects of substance abuse.[77] In the early years of their existence, TCs were characterized by rigidity and by a system of social rewards and harsh punishments. The latter often took the form of "humiliating and degrading rites such as shaved heads, the wearing of signs and costumes and verbal reprimands."[64] By removing the abuser or addict from his or her dysfunctional environment and by using "older" members of the TC as role models, it is the goal of the TC to have the individual return to the outside community as a more mature, independent, drug-free, and functioning member of society.[77]

The very harsh methods utilized by the TCs in their early years were associated with high dropout rates. Since then, the programs have been modified and the clientele have changed. Participants are younger, often in their teens (adolescents), and the principal drugs of abuse have changed. In the mid-1980s, the CODAP (Client-Oriented Data Acquisitions Process) indicated that only 40 percent of the individuals seeking treatment in TCs had heroin as their principal drug of abuse, whereas 88 percent had heroin as their principal drug of abuse in 1969.[77] As the heroin population in the TCs has declined, the cocaine population has increased. With this change, the population of the TC has shifted from the urban poor to the middle class. Zweben has suggested that because many of these middle-class cocaine addicts may still be working, and they may be unable or unwilling to make a commitment to a 1-year residential program, it may be necessary to modify the traditional TC approach by combining a shortened stay in the TC with a very structured, intensive, outpatient program.[4] Although traditionally TCs have primarily utilized paraprofessionals and ex-addicts, they do utilize professional disciplines and they generally incorporate self-help groups, such as AA, CA, and NA. As with other therapeutic approaches such as methadone maintenance or outpatient drug-free treatment, there is a positive relationship between the length of a treatment episode (tenure) and the favorableness of post-treatment outcome with respect to drug abuse, employment, and crime. According to the Drug Abuse Reporting Program (DARP), individuals in treatment for less than 3 months exhibited outcomes that were not significantly different from that of persons in short-term outpatient detoxification programs or in no treatment program at all.[78]

Zweben has observed one philosophic change in TCs that has resulted from the shift from heroin to cocaine as the primary drug of abuse. She notes: "Historically, TC staff have viewed drinking privileges as a reward for successful progress, mirroring the societal attitude that drinking is what successful people do to celebrate."[4] However, she has emphasized that because alcohol (and marijuana) are major factors in the relapse of the cocaine abuser, complete abstinence from alcohol and other drugs is necessary. Following discharge from TCs, and on occasion from inpatient facilities, many individuals are referred to halfway houses.

These are structured settings which enable the abstinent individual to return to the community without returning home.

RELAPSE AND RECOVERY

The concept of a "cure" in the drug abuse field remains both enigmatic and elusive. High rates of relapse are commonplace, leading to the notion that addiction is a "chronic relapsing disease."[79] That the process of recovery in alcoholism and drug addiction is lifelong is reflected in the first steps of Alcoholics Anonymous and Narcotics Anonymous, respectively: "We admitted we are powerless over alcohol . . ." or "We admitted we are powerless over our addiction. . . ." Or as stated in Narcotics Anonymous, Third Edition, Revised: "We suffered from a disease from which there is no known cure. It can, however, be arrested at some point, and recovery is then possible."[76]

Relapse can be defined variously. While the return to pretreatment drug abuse patterns would be universally accepted as a definition of relapse, how might occasional use be classified? How would the occasional or regular use of a "lesser" drug be classified? Nonetheless, whereas relapse, whatever the operational definition, is usually readily observable, recovery is a "complex, long-term phenomenon."[80] As Leukefeld and Tims have stated:[79] "Recovery is a desired end in which drug abuse and related behavior are no longer problematic in the individual's life."

Wesson and associates[81] have reviewed various considerations underlying relapse, which include genetic influences, metabolic explanations, learning theories (both conditioning theory and social learning theory), psychopathology, stress, and social support factors. The specific mechanisms of relapse notwithstanding, diverse intervention strategies, enumerated below, have been formulated in order to minimize the likelihood of relapse, an event which Rounsaville has stated: "is the rule and not the exception in substance abusers entering or completing treatment."[23]

1. **Formalizing discharge procedures.** A special vulnerability to relapse exists in the days immediately following discharge from intensive treatment, such as short-term in-

patient treatment. Accordingly, specific treatment contracts, such as contingency contracts, can be of value during this period of high vulnerability. Such contingency contracting may be of particular value in the sports setting.

2. **Anticipating relapse.** Since the likelihood of relapse is high, there should be explicit policies and procedures for re-entry into the treatment program should relapse occur. Family members and, where appropriate, teammates and team officials should be made aware of the potential for relapse, and they should be encouraged to facilitate the re-entry of the relapsed individual into treatment.

Education during abstinence can dispel or diminish the guilt and self-loathing associated with relapse while focusing attention on issues of compulsive behavior and loss of control.[67]

3. **Assessing commitment to abstinence.** Although achieving abstinence is of paramount importance in initiating treatment for the drug abuser, an assessment of the motivation for, and commitment to, long-term abstinence is essential to the formulation of a plan of treatment and aftercare.

4. **Establishing a program of aftercare.** As previously noted, the initial approach to the drug abuser and addict is multidimensional. It is essential that the appropriate elements of that multidimensional approach be incorporated into a program of aftercare, and that program should be formulated sufficiently early in treatment so that there is no lapse in treatment which could lead to a relapse by the abuser or addict.

5. **Assessing stressors.** In recognition that stress is a significant contributor to drug abuse relapse, specific stressors need to be identified during the period of abstinence, and plans must be formulated to cope with those stressors. Towards that end, the abstinent patient should avoid those environments and individuals that contributed to their drug abuse and addiction. To the extent that participation in organized athletics is a contributory stressor, specific therapeutic interventions should be designed to deal with this stress.

6. **Recognizing and managing "craving."** During abstinence, the patient should be helped to identify those specific thoughts and emotions that typically appear immediately preceding their drinking an alcoholic beverage or using a drug. Building on this recognition, the patient can be taught in behavioral terms how to obviate the use of alcohol and drugs during craving periods. Specifically, with respect to cocaine, Gawin and Ellinwood note that such craving can be "evoked by circumstances (moods, people, locations, other intoxicants) and objects (money, white powders, pipes, mirrors, syringes) that cue conditioned associations to memories of euphoria."[82] They further state that "if conditioned cues repeatedly fail to be followed by the reward that established them, their potency diminishes,"[82] a process referred to as extinction.

7. **Drug testing.** As noted in Chapter 18, drug testing was initiated in the 1960s as a way of ensuring compliance with drug treatment protocols. As an extension of that concept, drug testing has been utilized as a deterrent to relapse as well as a method for objectively assessing relapse. As discussed previously, contingency contracting with respect to cocaine abuse has been shown to be an effective method of relapse deterrence. Examples of the powerful significance of drug testing[83] in terms of relapse are highlighted in Table 19–4.

Table 19–4. PENALTIES IMPOSED BY MAJOR SPORTS ORGANIZATIONS FOR POSITIVE DRUG TEST FOLLOWING TREATMENT

Organization	Penalty for Positive Test after Treatment
USOC	Repeat offender suspended for 4 years
NCAA	If retested positive, loss of eligibility for the current season and the succeeding season
NFL	After three positive tests, banned from NFL
Men's Tennis Council (MTC)	Three positive tests result in disqualification and suspension; reinstatement considered after 1 year

Table 19–5. TIME UNTIL FIRST USE IN THE FIRST YEAR AFTER
TREATMENT AMONG CLIENTS WHO REPORTED
POSTTREATMENT USE OF EACH OF FOUR DRUG TYPES

| | Drug Used Posttreatment | | | |
Weeks after Termination	Heroin (%)	Other Narcotics (%)	Cocaine (%)	Other Nonnarcotics (%)
Used at termination	15.3	14.4	10.7	15.2
Within 1 week	28.9	22.8	21.6	24.3
2–4 weeks	21.4	24.1	24.6	24.5
5–13 weeks	15.8	13.9	17.6	16.0
14 or more weeks	18.6	24.8	25.5	20.0
Total	100.0	100.0	100.0	100.0
Number of Posttreatment Users	720	626	984	1026
Mean Days to Relapse Among Those Who Used Drugs Posttreatment	55.0	68.3	71.9	58.8

From Hubbard and Marsden,[84] with permission.

8. **Time frames of maximal risk.** It is during the first 3 months of treatment that the risk of relapse is greatest in the short term,[78] and during the first year in the long term.[23] Thus, Leukefeld and Tims[79] have emphasized the need for periodic clinical assessment, at least at the following intervals: first week after treatment, the first month, the third month, and the first year. Table 19–5 is illustrative of the time sequence from treatment to relapse for various drugs of abuse.

In 1986, Gold and associates[65] reported on preliminary treatment outcomes of 63 middle- and upper-class chronic cocaine users ranging in age between 25 and 40 years. They similarly noted that the treatment success rates were directly related to the amount of time spent in treatment. "Among patients completing at least six months of treatment, 95% were still drug-free at follow-up. For those completing either three to five months of treatment or less than three months of treatment, the percentage remaining drug-free at follow-up were 65% and 0%, respectively."

In alcoholics, Pickens and co-workers[85] note that 44 percent of treated patients relapsed in the first year, and of those that relapsed, about half subsequently stopped drinking and returned to abstinence. Thus, after one year, 74 percent were abstinent from alcohol.

THE ATHLETE

The athlete entering a drug abuse treatment program frequently has a self-image of being quite different from other drug abusers. The successful amateur athlete grows up very much the center of attention—at home, at school, and in the community, often with a sense of invincibility.[70a] While success in the amateur ranks brings fame and stature, success in the professional ranks may bring fortune as well. As a consequence, the successful athlete's expectations, upon entering treatment, are that of being treated as someone special. Their physical stature and strength often set them apart from other patients. Because of the pampering and adulation they have become accustomed to, athletes may believe themselves to be invulnerable. Star status frequently produces a resistance to treatment which compounds the denial so common in drug abuse patients.[86] As Washton has commented, athletes "live in an ultrapermissive environment and they think they're exempt from normal consequences."[57]

Once in treatment, other factors come into

play which set the athlete apart from other patients. Those who are providing direct treatment services may themselves, either consciously or unconsciously, be perpetuating the special status that the athlete had grown accustomed to prior to treatment. The therapist may be under pressure from the team to get the athlete back to the field of play as soon as possible. Complete anonymity, so important in self-help groups, may not be possible with a public figure.

The provision of aftercare services, particularly in the early stages when individual, group, and family therapy in one combination or another may be required, is difficult to implement because of the frequent travel necessitated by the sport. "An athlete is on the road all the time. Most of the time, he can't obtain what he needs to stay clean."[88] A network of aftercare services, in various cities, may have to be established, particularly with respect to participation in self-help groups such as AA, NA, and CA. As Gross has commented: "It's hard enough to find a meeting where you feel comfortable. Imagine trying to find it in every city you go to."[87] In addition to specific aftercare services, a program of random testing is required to ensure continued abstinence from drugs.

Although rehabilitation of the athlete is the objective of management, the pressures to get the athlete back to the playing field cannot be ignored or denied. However, given the time frame of relapse, particularly in the first 3 months following discharge from inpatient care, it is important to assess the relapse potential on a patient-by-patient basis. For some, early return to competition may even be therapeutic. For others, it may be preferable to bring the athlete back more slowly. Skills may be honed in the "minor leagues," that is, at lower levels of competition, away from the scrutiny of teammates, the public, and the media. Thus, as skills are refined, there is an opportunity to ensure that the aftercare program is in place and is working. As more time has elapsed, there is a statistically decreased risk of relapse, so that the athlete can then return more safely to regular competition in an environment which previously had been associated with his or her drug abuse. For some, contingency contracts may further increase the likelihood of continued abstinence. In the final analysis,

it is in the best interest of the athlete, management, and the sports community that the athlete not return to competition prematurely.

REFERENCES

1. Wadler, GI: Hospital role called vital in treatment of drug addicts. The New York Law Journal, December 6, 1971.
2. Wadler, GI, McCartney, JR and Buckley, DF: Health-hospital approach to drug abuse. New York State J Med 72:1194, 1972.
3. Gawin, FH and Kleber, HD: Cocaine abuse treatment. Arch Gen Psychiat 41:903, 1984.
4. Smith, DE: Cocaine-alcohol abuse: Epidemiological, diagnostic and treatment considerations. J Psychoactiv Drugs 18:117, 1986.
5. Zweben, JE: Treating cocaine dependence: New challenges for the therapeutic community. J Psychoactiv Drugs 18:239, 1986.
6. Resnick, RB and Resnick, EB: Cocaine abuse and its treatment. Psychiatr Clin North Am 7:713, 1984.
7. American Psychiatric Association: Diagnostic and Statistical Manual of Mental Disorders, ed 3, Revised. American Psychiatric Association, Washington, DC, 1987.
8. Goldstein, PJ, Hunt, D and Des Jarlais, DC: Drug dependence and abuse. In Almer, RW and Dull, HB (eds): Closing the Gap: The Burden of Unnecessary Illness. Oxford University Press, New York, 1987, p 89.
9. Spickard, WA and Tucker, PJ: An approach to alcoholism in a university medical center complex. JAMA 252:1894, 1984.
10. Spickard, WA and Billings, FT: Alcoholism in a university faculty. Trans Am Clin Climatological Assn 27:191, 1985.
11. Meer, J: Drugs and sports. In Snyder, SH (ed): The Encyclopedia of Psychoactive Drugs. Chelsea House Publishers, New York, 1987, p 107.
12. Jacobs, B: Cheers! Here's to the players who have bid farewell to booze and drugs. Family Weekly, August 7, 1983.
13. Blum, RW: Adolescent substance abuse: Diagnostic and treatment issues. Pediatr Clin North Am 34:523, 1987.
14. Davies, DL: Normal drinking in recovered alcoholics. Quart J Stud Alcohol 23:94, 1962.
15. Taylor, JR, Helzer, JE and Robins, LN: Moderate drinking in ex-alcoholics: Recent studies. J Study Alcohol 47:115, 1986.
16. Helzer, JE, et al: The extent of long-term moderate drinking among alcoholics discharged from medical and psychiatric treatment facilities. N Engl J Med 312:678, 1985.
17. Gibbs, L and Flanagan, J: Prognostic indicators of alcoholism treatment outcome. Int J Addict 12:1097, 1977.
18. Neuberger, OW, et al: Replicable abstinence rates in an alcoholism treatment program. JAMA 248:960, 1982.
19. Moos, RH and Finney, J: The expanding scope of

alcoholism treatment evaluation. Amer Psychol 38:1036, 1985.

20. Emrick, CD: A review of psychologically oriented treatment of alcoholism. II. The relative effectiveness of different treatment approaches and the effectiveness of treatment versus no treatment. J Stud Alcohol 36:88, 1975.

21. Leach, B and Norris, JL: Factors in the development of Alcoholics Anonymous (A.A.). In Kissin, B and Beigleiter, LH (eds): Treatment and Rehabilitation of the Chronic Alcoholic. Plenum Press, New York, 1977, p 441.

22. McLellan, AT, et al: Matching substance abuse patients to appropriate treatments: A conceptual and methodological approach. Drug and Alcohol Dependence 5:189, 1980.

23. Rounsaville, BJ: Clinical implications of relapse research. In Tims, FM and Leukefeld, CG (eds): Relapse and Recovery in Drug Abuse. NIDA Research Monograph No. 72, NIDA, Rockville, Maryland, Publication No. (ADM) 86-1473, 1986, p 172.

24. Wheeler, K and Malmquist, J: Treatment approaches in adolescent chemical dependency. Pediatr Clin North Am 34:437, 1987.

25. Semlitz, L and Gold, MS: Adolescent drug abuse—Diagnosis, treatment, and prevention. Psychiatr Clin North Am 9:455, 1986.

26. Kaufman, E: The workable system of family therapy for drug dependence. J Psychoactiv Drugs 18:43, 1986.

27. Acute drug abuse reactions. The Medical Letter 27:77, 1985.

28. Kleber, HD and Gawin, FH: Cocaine abuse: A review of current and experimental treatments. In Grabowski, J (ed): Cocaine: Pharmacology, Effects, and Treatment of Abuse. NIDA Research Monograph 50, NIDA, Rockville, Maryland, DHHS Publication No. (ADM) 84-1326, 1984, p 111.

29. Clark, WDF: Alcoholism: Blocks to diagnosis and treatment. Am J Med 71:275, 1981.

30. Kleber, H: Naltrexone. J Subst Abuse Treatment 2:117, 1985.

31. Treatment of alcohol withdrawal. The Medical Letter 28:75, 1986.

32. Jaffe, J: Pharmacologic agents in treatment of drug dependence. In Meltzer, HY (ed): Psychopharmacology: The Third Generation of Progress. Raven Press, New York, 1987, p 1605.

33. Kraus, ML, et al: Randomized clinical trial of atenolol in patients with alcohol withdrawal. N Engl J Med 313:905, 1985.

34. Gay, GR: Clinical management of acute and chronic cocaine poisoning. Ann Emerg Med 11:562, 1982.

35. Rosecan, JS, Spitz, HI and Gross, B: Contemporary issues in the treatment of cocaine abuse. In Spitz, HI and Rosecan, JS (eds): Cocaine Abuse—New Directions in Treatment and Research. Brunner/Mazel, New York, 1987, p 299.

36. Gawin, FH and Kleber, HD: Abstinence symptomatology and psychiatric diagnosis in cocaine abusers—Clinical observations. Arch Gen Psychiatry 43:107, 1986.

37. Dackis, CA and Gold, MS: Bromocriptine as treatment of cocaine abuse (letter). Lancet 1:1151, 1985.

38. Kleber, H and Gawin, F: Psychopharmacological

trials in cocaine abuse treatment. Am J Drug Alcohol Abuse 12:235, 1986.

39. Rosecan, JS and Nunes, EV: Pharmacological management of cocaine abuse. In Spitz, HI and Rosecan, JS (eds): Cocaine Abuse—New Directions in Treatment and Research. Brunner/Mazel, New York, 1987, p 255.

40. Gawin, F and Kleber, H: Pharmacologic treatments of cocaine abuse. Psychiatr Clin North Am 9:573, 1986.

41. Dackis, CA and Gold, MS: Pharmacological approaches to cocaine addiction. J Subst Abuse Treatment 2:139, 1985.

42. Giannini, AJ and Billett, W: Bromocriptine—desipramine protocol in treatment of cocaine addiction. J Clin Pharmacol 27:549, 1987.

43. Tricyclic antidepressants curbing cocaine use. Med World News, October 12, 1987, p 12.

44. Cocaine withdrawal step by step. Emerg Med, April 30, 1987, p 65.

45. Ritchie, JM: The aliphatic alcohols. In Gilman, AG, et al (eds): Goodman and Gilman's The Pharmacological Basis of Therapeutics, ed 7. Macmillan, New York, 1985, p 372.

46. Peachey, JE and Annis, H: Pharmacologic treatment of chronic alcoholism. Psychiatr Clin North Am 7:745, 1984.

47. Branchey, L, et al: Psychiatric complications of disulfiram treatment. Am J Psychiatry 144:1310, 1987.

48. Schuckit, MA: A one-year follow-up of men alcoholics given disulfiram. J Stud Alcohol 46:191, 1985.

49. Fuller, RK, et al: Disulfiram treatment of alcoholism. A Veterans Administration cooperative study. JAMA 256:1449, 1986.

50. Tennant, FS, Jr: Disulfiram will reduce medical complications but not cure alcoholism (Editorial). JAMA 256:1489, 1986.

51. Dole, VP and Nyswander, ME: Heroin addiction—A metabolic disease. Ann Intern Med 120:19, 1967.

52. Newman, RG: Methadone treatment: Defining and evaluating success. N Engl J Med 317:447, 1987.

53. M.F., R.Ph.: Methadone treatment (Letter). N Engl J Med 318:385, 1988.

54. Khantzian, EJ: Psychotherapeutic interventions with substance abusers—The clinical context. J Subst Abuse Treatment 2:83, 1985.

55. McLellan, AT, et al: Predicting response to alcohol and drug abuse treatment. Role of psychiatric severity. Arch Gen Psychiatry 40:620, 1983.

56. Woody, GE, et al: Psychotherapy for substance abuse. Psychiatr Clin North Am 9:547, 1986.

57. Washton, AM: Nonpharmacologic treatment of cocaine abuse. Psychiatr Clin North Am 9:563, 1986.

58. Nace, EP: The Treatment of Alcoholism. Brunner/Mazel, New York, 1987, p 201.

59. Nace, EP: The Treatment of Alcoholism. Brunner/Mazel, New York, 1987, p 162.

60. Bigelow, GE, Stitzer, MOL and Liebsdon, IA: The role of behavioral contingency management in drug abuse treatment. In Grabowski, J, Stitzer, ML and Henningfield, JE (eds): Behavioral Intervention Techniques in Drug Abuse Treatment. NIDA Research Monograph 46, NIDA, Rockville, Maryland, DHHS Publication No. (ADM) 86-1282, 1984, p 36.

61. Pickens, RW and Thomson, T: Behavioral treatment of drug dependence. In Grabowski, J, Stitzer, ML and Henningfield, JE (eds): Behavioral Intervention Techniques in Drug Abuse Treatment. NIDA Research Monograph 46, NIDA, Rockville, Maryland, DHHS Publication No. (ADM) 86-1282, 1984, p 53.

62. Spitz, HI and Rosecan, JS: Overview of cocaine abuse treatment. In Spitz, HI and Rosecan, JS (eds): Cocaine Abuse—New Directions in Treatment. Brunner/Mazel, New York, 1987, p 97.

63. Anker, AL and Crowley, TJ: Use of contingency contracts in specialty clinics for cocaine abuse. In Harris, LS (ed): Problems of Drug Dependence, 1981. NIDA Research Monograph 41, Rockville, Maryland, 1982, p 452.

64. Smith, D, Levy, SJ and Striar, DE: Treatment services for youthful drug abusers. In Beschner, GM and Friedmans, AS (eds): Youth Drug Abuse. DC Heath, Lexington, MA, 1979, p 537.

65. Gold, MS, et al: New treatment for opiate and cocaine abusers: But what about marijuana. Psychiatr Ann 16:206, 1986.

66. Spitz, HI: Cocaine abuse: Therapeutic group approaches. In Spitz, HI and Rosecan, JS (eds): Cocaine abuse—New directions in treatment. Brunner/Mazel, New York, 1987, p 156.

67. Ackerman, NW and Kempster, SW: Family therapy. In Freeman, AM and Kaplan, HI (eds): Comprehensive Textbook of Psychiatry. Williams & Wilkins, Baltimore, 1967, p 1244.

68. Spitz, HI and Spitz, ST: Family therapy of cocaine abuse. In Spitz, HI and Rosecan, JS (eds): Cocaine abuse—New directions in treatment and research. Brunner/Mazel, New York, 1987, p 202.

69. Lask, B: Family therapy. Br Med J 294:203, 1987.

70. Hill, C: Are the teams doing enough in N.F.L. drug cases? Browns, says Calvin Hill, are facing the problem. The New York Times, July 31, 1983.

70a. Collins, GB, et al: Recreational drug use in sports. In Grana, WA, et al (eds): Advances in Sports Medicine and Fitness, Vol 1. Year Book Medical Publishers, Chicago, 1988, p 97.

71. Rinella, VJ and Goldstein, MR: Family therapy with substance abusers: Legal considerations regarding confidentiality. J Marital Fam Ther 6:319, 1980.

72. Hays, JT and Spickard, WA, Jr: Alcoholism: Early diagnosis and intervention. J Gen Intern Med 2:420, 1987.

73. Nace, EP: The Treatment of Alcoholism. Brunner/Mazel, New York, 1987, p 236.

74. Bebbington, PE: The efficacy of Alcoholics Anonymous: The elusive hard data. Br J Psychiat 128:572, 1976.

75. Hoffman, NG, Harrison, PA and Belille, CA: Alcoholics Anonymous after treatment: Attendance and abstinence. Int J Addict 18:311, 1983.

76. Narcotics Anonymous, ed 3, revised. World Service Office, Van Nuys, CA, 1986.

77. O'Brien, WB and Biase, DV: Therapeutic community: A current perspective. J Psychoactiv Drugs 16(1):9, 1984.

78. Simpson, DD: Treatment for drug abuse. Arch Gen Psychiat 38:875, 1981.

79. Leukefeld, CG and Tims, FM: Relapse and recovery: Some directions for research and practice. In Tims, FM and Leukefeld, CG (eds): Relapse and Recovery in Drug Abuse. Research Monograph No. 72, NIDA Publication No. (ADM) 86-1473, NIDA, Rockville, MD, 1986, p 185.

80. Tims, FM and Leukefeld, CG: Relapse and recovery in drug abuse: An introduction. In Tims, FM and Leukefeld, CB (eds): Relapse and Recovery in Drug Abuse. Research Monograph No. 72, NIDA Publication No. (ADM) 86-1473, NIDA, Rockville, MD, 1986, p 1.

81. Wesson, DR, Havassy, BE and Smith, DE: Theories of relapse and recovery and their implications for drug abuse treatment. In Tims, FM and Leukefeld, CG (eds): Relapse and Recovery in Drug Abuse. NIDA Research Monograph 72. NIDA, Rockville, MD, Publication No. (ADM) 86-1473, 1986, p 5.

82. Gawin, FH and Ellinwood, EH: Cocaine and other stimulants: Actions, abuse, and treatment. N Engl J Med 318:1173, 1988.

83. Gall, SL, et al: Who tests which athletes for what drugs? Phys Sportsmed 16(2):155, 1988.

84. Hubbard, RL and Marsden, ME: Relapse to use of heroin, cocaine, and other drugs in the first year after treatment. In Tims, FM and Leukefeld, CG (eds): Relapse and Recovery in Drug Abuse. NIDA Research Monograph No. 72, NIDA, Rockville, MD, DHSS Publication No. (ADM) 86-1473, 1986, p 157.

85. Pickens, RW, et al: Relapse by alcohol abusers. Alcoholism: Clin and Exper Res 9:244, 1985.

86. Bunn, CG: Drugs, the toughest rebound in sports. Newsday, July 19, 1987.

87. Gross, J: A permanent cure is difficult for athlete-addicts. The New York Times, December 17, 1984.

88. Cowart, V: Road back from substance abuse especially long, hard for athletes. JAMA 256:2645, 1986.

CHAPTER 20

Legal Considerations

H. RICHARD BERESFORD, M.D., J.D.

PROLOGUE

In November 1987, a California superior court barred the National Collegiate Athletic Association (NCAA) from conducting a drug testing program for college athletes.[1] Two athletes from Stanford, one a member of the women's track team and the other a football player, had sued the NCAA on the grounds that its testing program unlawfully invaded their privacy, including their right to receive care from team physicians. Stanford joined the students in their suit, asserting that the hearing process for those who tested positive for any of a large number of prohibited drugs was inadequate to protect the interests of student-athletes. The NCAA defended its program as necessary to promote "integrity" of sporting competition and to protect athletes from the adverse effects of "performance-enhancing" drugs. Invoking constitutional doctrines that bar invasions of personal privacy for all but "compelling" reasons and that require justifiable invasions to be narrowly tailored, the court concluded the NCAA had failed to demonstrate a sufficiently compelling need for its program and that, in any event, its testing program was too broad to satisfy constitutional norms. The court excepted football and male basketball players from its prohibition on testing because of evidence these athletes used banned drugs (especially anabolic steroids).

This case is but one facet of the continuing debate about what latitude social institutions should have when it comes to restricting usage of drugs that may be harmful to users or that are seen by these institutions as threats to important social values. Here the court agreed with the Stanford athletes that the NCAA had gone too far, despite the NCAA's assertion of altruistic goals. It noted that in 1986 and 1987 the NCAA had tested 3,511 athletes and had declared only 34 ineligible for competition, including 26 who tested positive for anabolic steroids and 7 for cocaine. Of the 34 made ineligible, 31 were football players and none was a woman. In 11 of the 14 sports surveyed, no athlete tested positive. Against this factual background, the court thought it inappropriate for the NCAA to treat athletes as if they were suspected criminals, especially since use of the major offending drugs, anabolic steroids, was not in itself unlawful. It gave little weight to the NCAA's argument that its program was a justifiable means of promoting fair competition.

Whatever the long-range impact of this decision, it highlights particular themes that will emerge in future legal disputes over drug use by athletes. These include (1) the extent to which privacy rights can be used to defeat attempts to identify users of unlawful or putatively harmful drugs; (2) the degree of justification that private agencies (such as the NCAA or other sports associations) and employers of athletes must demonstrate before acting to identify or sanction users of drugs; (3) the potential for conflicts of interest when sports team physicians prescribe drugs primarily to allow athletes to compete or to enhance their performance; and (4) the extent to which athletes, as public figures, have an obligation to moderate their usage of drugs beyond the ordinary dictates of law. These themes will be explored in the following sections.

THE PRIVACY RIGHTS OF ATHLETES

Privacy as a Protected Legal Interest

The notion that persons enjoy a right of privacy that is separate and distinguishable from other fundamental rights (such as freedom of speech or an entitlement to due process of law) is a relatively recent legal development. Perhaps the best-known expression of the doctrine is the Supreme Court decision

in *Roe* v *Wade*[2] where it was held that the federal constitution protects the right of a woman to abort a nonviable fetus. Even though the Constitution does not codify a right of privacy or say anything about reproductive freedom, the Court regarded decisions of this nature as of such fundamental personal importance as to be immune from state intrusion. It interpreted the Constitution as creating a penumbra of derivative rights, including reproductive freedom, and this penumbral concept has served to bring other decisions of uniquely personal significance (such as the right to refuse life-sustaining medical treatment) into the zone of constitutional protection.[3,4] The outer limits of the right of privacy are ill-defined, however, and a major area of controversy among legal scholars is the proper scope of the privacy doctrine. The recent Supreme Court decision in *Bowers* v *Hardwick*[5] exemplifies problems of line-drawing in this area. Here the Court held that the federal constitution does not bar a state from prosecuting a person for homosexual acts performed in the privacy of the home. In so doing, it signaled that certain concededly intimate, cloistered, and personal actions are not protected against state intervention if they offend against social norms as expressed in statutes criminalizing these actions. Strong dissenting opinions characterized the majority's opinion as a retreat from previous decisions of the Court with respect to privacy, and it seems likely the Court will soon have other opportunities to refine its views about the scope of the right of privacy under the federal constitution.

Regardless of developments under federal constitutional law, there will remain a variety of protections for privacy under state constitutions and legislation. Several state constitutions expressly recognize a right of privacy,[4,6] and courts in other states have read a right of privacy into state constitutions that are not explicit about it.[4] Moreover, many states have laws protecting confidentiality of communications between physicians and patients and of records containing medically significant or other highly personalized data.[7,8] Thus, highly intrusive efforts by state governments and private organizations to deal with drug use may also encounter legal barriers erected by state legislators and judges.

Drug Use and Privacy

In their suit against the NCAA, the Stanford athletes characterized the NCAA testing program as infringing upon their privacy by its potential for interfering with the ability of team physicians to treat them, by enabling a "searching review" of their personal lifestyles, and by its requirement of monitored urination to assure proper collection of test samples.[1] They did not assert an unfettered right to take drugs. Instead they emphasized those features of the NCAA program that reflected a disregard for individual sensitivities or well-being. In this way, they centered the case on whether the NCAA's rather abstract interest in protecting the "integrity" of sport outweighed their quite personal interests in receiving appropriate medical care and avoiding potentially humiliating or stigmatizing intrusions into their lives. Had they only asserted a general interest in personal autonomy, they might have been less successful in convincing the court that the NCAA was overreaching.

As the Supreme Court decision in *Bowers* v *Hardwick*[5] indicates, the constitutional right of privacy does not encompass conduct society has expressly condemned. Thus, users of illicit drugs will not be heard to say that the Constitution protects their right to do as they please, even though it does protect against unreasonable searches and seizures and provides a privilege against self-incrimination and rights to due process of law. The assertions that only users are harmed by taking unlawful drugs or that they take such drugs only in private lack constitutional weight, even though they may be relevant to the issue of the social utility of criminalizing drug use by individuals. On the other hand, if persons take drugs they have lawfully obtained (such as those prescribed by a physician), a claim that law bars coercive attempts to discover this fact merits more attention. On the NCAA's list of banned drugs were several lawful agents (e.g., diuretics, anabolic steroids, some sympathomimetic amines) that were included only because of the suspicion that athletes were using them to try to better their performance. It was this effort to restrain use of lawful drugs that evoked the concern of the California court about overinclusiveness in the testing program. The court was satisfied that amphetamines and anabolic steroids deserved inclusion on the list and accepted in principle the NCAA's plan to test football and male basketball players, among whom there was evidence of more than trivial use of anabolic steroids. But it was unwilling to approve a wide-ranging effort to identify users of other lawfully obtainable drugs.

Implementing any program to identify users of drugs is inevitably intrusive. Either a blood sample must be withdrawn or a urine sample collected. In the latter situation, monitoring of urination is seen as essential to assuring that the sample is what and whose it purports to be. As a matter of constitutional law, governmental agencies or officers must justify such intrusions as reasonable in light of the particular goal of testing.[9-12] This entails demonstrating that the sample is required in order to serve an important governmental interest, such as protecting public safety.[13-15] But where private organizations seek to impose testing, constitutional constraints may not be applicable.[16,17] Federal constitutional doctrines formally apply only to actions by governments or their officials and do not explicitly cover nongovernmental efforts to identify drug users. However, in contexts other than drug testing, actions by the NCAA have been classified as the equivalent of governmental actions where it was argued either that the NCAA was serving a public function or that its activities were so entangled with state funding or programs as to blur the distinction between state and private actions.[18-20] Moreover, several state constitutions (including that of California) codify a right of privacy with respect to intrusions by both state or private agencies and persons.[4,21,22] Thus, the Stanford athletes were able to invoke the California constitution[6] in support of their suit against the NCAA. Also, where private agencies receive governmental funding or purport to act under the authority of state law, conduct that violates constitutional norms may subject them to liability under civil rights legislation.[4,17]

Even if it is conceded that privacy doctrines apply to efforts by teams or other organizations to identify drug use by athletes, athletes who resist testing may not benefit. A team may simply refuse to employ athletes without pre-employment testing or require that an agreement to undergo testing be included in the employment contract. Or an organization (e.g., International Olympic Committee, NCAA) may bar participation in its events without such testing. In these circumstances, athletes may avoid testing if willing to pay the price of unemployment or nonparticipation, and the team or organization can plausibly argue that the athletes' choice is a voluntary one, however dire the consequences for them. Still, the case of the Stanford athletes and some other authorities[20,23-25] suggest that confronting athletes with such a harsh choice may be seen as violating protected economic or property interests.

Athletes may find themselves covered by agreements negotiated by their agents or players' unions under which management is permitted to test for drugs under specified circumstances. Athletes are bound by these provisions unless they are misapplied or it can be shown that the agreements themselves are invalid, and teams can lawfully fire or suspend them if they refuse to undergo testing. Bargaining over drug testing clauses is of growing importance in negotiations concerning both individual and standard player contracts. As part of these negotiations, teams may ask athletes to waive whatever rights they have to refuse testing and agree to testing under procedures developed by the teams. Once an agreement is reached, later disputes about testing become resolvable under the contract rather than under more general principles of law.

Whether or not law recognizes that a right of privacy generally includes a right to refuse testing for drugs, the entitlement of athletes, as public figures, to claim privacy protection may be questioned. Some judicial decisions have emphasized that a person's reasonable expectation of privacy with respect to a particular activity or choice is an important factor in determining whether government or others may intrude.[10,26,27] In this context, it is proper to ask if athletes can reasonably expect the legal system to bar inquiries about drugs that may affect their performance in competitions open to the public. Athletes may of course prefer to shield their drug use from public view and avoid the stigma or legal complications disclosure of drug use might bring. But it does not follow that the legal system will operate to impede efforts of those who can show good and sufficient reasons for trying to identify drug use by athletes.

JUSTIFYING INVASIONS OF ATHLETES' PRIVACY

Rationale for Drug Testing

There are sports-specific and more general reasons why teams or other sports organizations may wish to test athletes for drug use. Sports-specific reasons include preventing drug users from taking unfair advantage of competitors and protecting athletes from drugs that may impair their ability to perform. General reasons may include protecting the long-term physical and mental health of athletes, identifying athletes who may pose disciplinary problems or who are risking compensable permanent disability, and participating in societal efforts to control drug abuse.

When these considerations are invoked in support of testing, the central legal inquiry is whether they justify intruding on the person of another. This inquiry has two parts, one factual and the other doctrinal. For example, if a sports association asserts testing for drug X is needed because X is a "performance enhancer," the first step is to ascertain what evidence exists that X indeed enables an athlete to perform more skillfully than otherwise (see individual drug chapters in Part II). Only if there is credible evidence that X has this potential is it proper to address the doctrinal question of whether the interest of the sports association in drug-free competition is weighty enough to allow coercive testing. Moreover, the fact that X may enhance certain types of performance does not provide a scientific basis for testing athletes unlikely to benefit from using it. Anabolic steroids may help some football players or weight lifters to excel in their respective sports, but the relevance of steroid usage to performance in basketball, tennis, or skiing, for example, is less apparent (see Chapter 4). Testing competitors in these latter sports for anabolic steroids seems irrelevant to the goal of preventing use of drugs that may generate a competitive edge.

Identifying an empirical basis for a testing program is an essential step in providing a legal justification for testing that involves coercion.[17,28] Where disputes have arisen over the power of governmental agencies to mandate testing of individuals, courts have sought to balance personal interests in privacy against governmental interests in data that testing may reveal.[4,10–12,17] Even if a privacy claim is regarded as weak as a matter of law, the governmental tester must at least offer some rational basis for intrusive testing. The court that heard the suit of the Stanford athletes against the NCAA was unimpressed by the need for comprehensive testing of athletes, given the NCAA's own findings that only a few football and male basketball players had used suspect drugs.[1] If a privacy claim is viewed as stronger, as where privacy is expressly recognized as a protected right under a state constitution, the governmental tester may be required to show a compelling interest in the results of testing.[4,6,21] What is a sufficiently compelling interest in this circumstance is not obvious. But the least a governmental tester should be required to demonstrate is that the data are needed to deal with an important societal problem and cannot be obtained by less intrusive means. In other words, where a strong claim of privacy exists, a potential governmental intruder must offer a highly persuasive justification for the intrusion.

While private organizations may succeed in avoiding the full force of constitutional doctrines, it nevertheless seems useful to scrutinize testing by private organizations in the same light as if it were being proposed by public agencies. Constitutional norms have evolved out of judicial and legislative efforts to protect vulnerable individuals from those more powerful than they, and the fairness of a particular testing scheme can profitably be evaluated in this context.[25,28] Also, as has been stressed, some state constitutions and other legislation may apply to activities of private organizations that offend against constitutional norms.[4,21] **Thus, where teams or players' associations propose testing of athletes for drugs, one criterion of the legal sufficiency of testing programs should be that there is an empirically demonstrable relationship between use of target drugs and their adverse effects on performance, health, or the quality of competition. If this criterion is not met, it would seem that athletes' interests in freedom from intrusion should outweigh testers' interests in trying to identify users of the drugs.**

Conduct of Testing

Identifying Subjects of Testing

A threshold inquiry for any testing program is determining who should be tested for what drugs. One of the asserted defects of the NCAA program was that it tested athletes in sports in which there was little or no empirical evidence of drug use, and the California court agreed that this sort of blanket testing was a matter of special legal concern.[1] To avoid invalidation on the grounds that it is overinclusive, a testing program should therefore be selective in its determinations about whom to test.

Implementing a principle of selectivity may prove troublesome in practice. Options include testing all athletes in sports where use of particular drugs is thought to be significant (e.g., anabolic steroids in football and weight lifting), or limiting testing to athletes in whom there is specific reason to suspect drug use (e.g., dramatic gain in weight or muscle mass as might occur with anabolic steroids, unexpectedly fast time in a cycling race possibly attributable to amphetamines). The first option is obviously easier to implement since it involves no individualized judgments and avoids disputes over the validity of suspicions of drug use. The second has the advantage of restricting intrusions on privacy to those for whom there are nontrivial reasons to believe they are using drugs. On the other hand, it may entail a degree of snooping or informing that is uncomfortable for all concerned. In this respect, across-the-board testing of all competitors may be more palatable, even though this implicitly assumes that *any* competitor may be using an offending drug.

Those who seek to test nonprofessional athletes for drugs may reduce the chances of later legal disputes by clearly informing competitors in advance that testing is being contemplated and why. Information about testing can be circulated among coaches or team managers, team physicians, and local sports associations, and entry blanks for specific events can refer to planned testing and include a waiver of rights to object to such testing. These measures should help defeat later assertions by athletes that they expected to be free from drug-related investigations when they chose to participate in a particular sport. Such measures would also convey the message that testing is a routine procedure designed to protect the quality of competition and is not a device for stigmatizing individual competitors. In the case of professional athletes, procedures for determining who can be tested and when will ordinarily be spelled out in written contracts with teams or other organizations. If these contracts are carefully drawn, prospects for later legal controversy over testing will be diminished.

The Testing Process

The act of providing a sample of bodily fluid for testing may be distressing, particularly if it involves venipuncture or monitored urination. Routine though these procedures may seem to health care workers, athletes may view the yielding up of samples as assaults or humiliations, especially where they feel they have been coerced. While individual sensitivities about modes of sample collection are not in themselves a basis for invalidating testing, they bear directly on the legal issue of whether the potential testers have chosen the least intrusive means of obtaining the data they seek. For example, if analysis of hair samples or saliva provides the same information as obtainable from a blood or urine sample, then it might be appropriate to require the tester to utilize hair or saliva for testing, even though these analyses are more complex or expensive (see Chapter 18). Similarly, if comparable data about a drug can be derived from analyses of either blood or urine, subjects of testing might be given the option as to which sample to provide. Some might even prefer venipuncture to monitored urination, but offering a choice would show that testers recognize the need to minimize intrusiveness by accommodating sensitivities of those providing samples for testing.

Once samples have been collected and analyzed, questions may arise about reliability of the analyses. These may relate to the skill with which analysis was performed or the quantitative capacities of the chosen analytic method (see Table 18–4).[29] While such questions are technical or scientific in nature, they have important legal implications. If scientific consensus about reliability of a particular method is lacking, the method yields more than a tiny number of false positives, or the method cannot distinguish metabo-

lites of banned drugs from those of acceptable drugs, the legal balance shifts in favor of the opponents of testing.[17,28,29] The potential adverse consequences of wrongly labeling athletes as users of prohibited drugs seem to outweigh almost any interest a team or sports association may have in identifying true users.[28] However, if questions about accuracy of a given result can be resolved by additional more reliable tests, the fact that an ultra-sensitive screening method yields false-positives should not be grounds for invalidating an otherwise lawful testing program.

Merely because athletes submit to testing and accept that positive results may bar competing should not entitle testers to publicize positive results. Publication may serve the testers' goal of deterring use of particular drugs by other athletes and respond to public curiosity about why certain athletes are not competing, but it may disproportionately stigmatize or embarrass the athletes. This would be especially true for athletes who are banned because prescription drugs they were taking contain prohibited agents (e.g., sympathomimetic amines). While athletes in this predicament have no obvious legal remedy against testers who choose to publicize positive test results, the testers' conduct may be taken as evidence that they are not particularly concerned about the interests of individual athletes. This might become relevant where, in response to a legal challenge to a testing program, a tester asserts that a fundamental goal of testing is to protect the welfare of the athletes themselves.

Due Process in Testing

Stanford supported its athletes in their suit against the NCAA because it believed the NCAA's testing program did not afford adequate protection for athletes who tested positive for banned drugs. The university particularly objected to the hearing process for the athletes because of its asserted failure to assure a neutral hearing officer, its not giving athletes a right to be present at any hearing, its failure to provide adequate notice to affected athletes, and the lack of a written procedure for appeals from an adverse finding. These objections underscore the principle that even justifiable invasions of privacy should be coupled to procedures observing basic principles of fairness. These procedures include timely notification, a hearing in which affected persons have an opportunity to appear and refute adverse findings, and an appeals process that permits correction of major errors.[28] Of particular importance with respect to testing athletes for drugs is that there be a chance to explain adverse findings and to request confirmatory testing or retesting if there is any reason to believe test results are inaccurate or represent false-positives. Providing this sort of procedural due process will increase the cost of testing programs, but it accommodates concerns that athletes not be denied a livelihood or much-desired participation without an opportunity to correct technical errors or present evidence of mitigating factors.

TEAM PHYSICIANS AND DRUG USE BY ATHLETES

Physicians and Access to Drugs

Athletes may obtain drugs from various sources, including physicians, trainers, fellow athletes, or dealers. Of these sources, physicians are the only ones who can lawfully authorize use of scheduled or prescription drugs. If a physician is an athlete's personal physician, the assumption is that prescription of a particular drug derives from a medical judgment about what will benefit the patient, irrespective of the patient's status as an athlete. This does not imply that a physician will necessarily refuse to respond to an athlete's desire for medication that will, for example, permit competition before optimal recovery from injury. In this situation, doctor and patient negotiate based on their mutual definition of what best suits the patient. But if the physician is employed by a team or other organization, the possibility exists he or she will be influenced by goals of the employer in decisions about treating players. Thus, the physician may be tempted to prescribe drugs perceived as ergogenic or that will permit athletes to play with pain, even if this puts them at risk for temporary or permanent harm. In a less direct way, the team physician may give priority to interests of his employer by collaborating or acquiescing in provision of drugs by team trainers or simply choose to ignore evidence that athletes for whom he or she is responsible are using ergogenic, analgesic, or "recreational" drugs obtained from other sources.

Some athletes will recognize the possibility that a team physician may be a "double agent" and thereby protect themselves against inappropriate prescriptions. Moreover, ethically sensitive team physicians will appreciate the potential for conflict of interest in their role and will achieve a reasonable balance in their prescribing practices, which might include seeking a second opinion. But despite these constraints on harmful prescribing, the combination of an intense desire among athletes to gain a competitive edge and organizational or other collective pressures to win at all costs creates an atmosphere in which athletes and physicians collaborate in using drugs as vehicles for winning. The question then arises about the extent to which legal duties of team physicians to their athlete-patients differ from those of other physicians whose patients happen to be athletes. As will be seen, existing legal doctrines support the conclusion that team physicians owe the same legal duties to their patients as do other physicians, and must observe reasonable or accepted standards of medical practice in their relationship with athletes for whom they are responsible.

Legal Duties of Team Physicians

Before a physician can be held legally responsible for harm to a patient, the patient must prove a doctor-patient relationship existed at the time the harm occurred.[30] In the case of the team physician, it might be argued that neither physician nor athlete view their relationship as a professional one because both parties know (or should know) that the physician may have divided loyalties. Judicial decisions in nonathletic contexts indicate that a corporate physician must exercise reasonable care in treating other employees of the company, even though the physician is being paid primarily to protect the employer's interest in a healthy workforce.[30-32] While it doesn't necessarily follow that physicians have the same duty to employees who are quite willing to risk their health to serve goals of the organization, as in the case of professional athletes, policies underlying the existing medical liability system support holding team physicians to the same duty as other employee physicians. These policies emphasize compensating persons who are wrongfully harmed and deterring conduct that threatens harm. Applying these policies to athletic injuries, the objectives would be to assure legal remedies for athletes harmed by physicians who wrongfully prescribe drugs and to discourage other physicians from similar prescribing practices. For example, a California court found a professional football team liable for a linebacker's knee injury upon proof that the team physician instructed a trainer to give the player amphetamines so that he would play with more abandon.[33] This ruling thus provided both a monetary award to an injured athlete and a warning to those who would prescribe or counsel use of amphetamines as means of maximizing competitive effort. It is also consistent with established principles of medical ethics that exhort physicians to give priority to the best interests of their patients.[34]

Liabilities of Team Physicians

Assuming a doctor-patient relationship exists between athletes and team physicians, the physicians may be found liable for negligence if harm results from failure to observe reasonable or accepted professional standards.[30] To prove negligence, claimants must show what the appropriate professional standards are and establish that physicians did not meet these standards. In practical terms, this means injured athletes must find other physicians willing to testify that a team physician's conduct in prescribing drugs was unreasonable or unacceptable.

Before opinions of other physicians are admissible as evidence against a team physician, their qualifications as experts on the subject of the claim must be established. Since sports medicine is a new and ill-defined area of specialization, it is probably unnecessary for testifying physicians to be specialists in sports medicine before their opinions are allowed as evidence. Rather they must show they are knowledgeable about the potentially harmful effects of the drugs involved.[30,35] For example, a specialist in clinical pharmacology could qualify as an expert on the long-term adverse effects of anabolic steroids even if his own clinical practice does not include athletes, provided he shows reasonable familiarity with properties of these agents. By the same token, testimony of a specialist in sports medicine might not be admissible if his or her expertise was in musculoskeletal injuries. It should be noted, however, that rules regarding use of expert testimony have undergone progressive liberalization and courts tend to allow considerable latitude in admitting scientific evidence.[30,36] This leaves it to opposing lawyers to show lack of relevant expertise through cross-examination or presenting countervailing testimony.

Once a physician is found qualified to testify about allegedly harmful effects of a particular drug, he or she will be asked to state with reasonable medical certainty, or similar parlance, that the drug was wrongfully prescribed and that this wrongful prescription was a direct cause of the athlete's injury. Merely stating that a prescription was careless does not provide a basis for a judicial finding of liability. The statement must be coupled with an opinion that negligent prescription was a substantial factor in producing the athlete's injury or that, but for the negligence, no harm would have occurred. Thus, to support a claim that wrongful prescription of amphetamines caused major harm, an expert must state that the effect of amphetamines was to cause an athlete to sustain an otherwise improbable injury. If the harm was sudden death from cardiac failure in a young and previously healthy bicyclist, the expert's assertion of a causal relationship would be persuasive. But if the harm was a severe knee injury common among football players not taking amphetamines, the opinion about causation is more vulnerable to a contrary opinion that prescription of amphetamines had nothing to do with causing the injury.

Defending Against Charges of Improper Prescribing

Aside from attacking opinions of expert witnesses for injured athletes, team physicians may offer various other justifications for prescribing drugs to the athletes. They might assert that use of a particular drug was reasonable for a given athlete. Thus, prescription of anabolic steroids to a football lineman or weight lifter might be justified as an appropriate means of preparing them for competition in their chosen sports. The legal weight accorded this argument would depend on what evidence is developed about the actual utility of steroids in enhancing performance and their safety when prescribed in conventional doses (see Chapter 4).[37] Or the physicians might present evidence that athletes were duly informed about risks of the drugs and willingly assumed these risks.[38] They might also be able to establish that the athletes themselves were negligent because they unreasonably failed to follow instructions about dosage or failed to notify the physicians when side effects began to appear. Such contributory negligence might defeat their claims.[39]

The circumstances of contemporary athletic competition lend special importance to the legal doctrine of assumption of risk. Conventional statement of the doctrine is that one who knowingly and freely accepts a risk is barred from recovering against others if the risk indeed materializes. For this doctrine to constitute an effective defense, however, a defendant must prove that a claimant understood the nature and extent of the risk and nevertheless willingly accepted it.[38] This requirement that the claimant must have voluntarily accepted the risk is a major obstacle to applying the doctrine in the context of highly competitive sports. For example, to suggest that a professional football player who receives anabolic steroids from a team physician freely accepts the risks of their side effects ignores the possibility that the player feels he must take steroids to protect his livelihood. In this sense, an element of duress exists when a team physician suggests to a professional athlete that he take anabolic steroids or some other drug the physician bills as ergogenic. The implication of duress cannot be overcome simply by arguing that an athlete is free to choose some other occupation if he doesn't wish to take certain drugs that are lawfully prescribable by physicians. In other vocational contexts, courts have decided that employees who subject themselves to certain occupational risks out of fear of loss of employment do not voluntarily assume those risks.[40,41] Professional athletes are, if anything, under greater pressure than most employees to assume occupational risks of harm. Most recognize their maximal earning potential will only last a few years at best and that they must perform at a consistently high level in order to remain in professional sports. This leaves them susceptible to

suggestions they will perform better if they take particular drugs. Indeed they may avidly seek such drugs, not because they want to be bigger or more aggressive, but because they want to keep their jobs. This "choice" to accept drugs, even if informed by awareness of potential adverse reactions, may therefore be seen as less than voluntary.

If coercion is discounted as a factor in an athlete's taking a prescribed drug, it must still be shown that the athlete accepted a specific materialized risk before the assumption of risk doctrine applies.[42] For example, an athlete who takes prescribed amphetamines before a competition with the knowledge that it may make him play more aggressively and thereby increase his risk of injury does not, unless specifically informed, assume the risk he may develop life-threatening elevations of blood pressure or cardiac arrhythmias (see Chapter 6). The assumption of risk doctrine thus blends with the doctrine of informed consent in medical malpractice law by its focus on what risks were in fact disclosed. In both situations, the physician is protected from unfavorable legal consequences only if the specific materialized risk has been disclosed to the patient.

Team Physicians and Confidentiality

While providing care to athletes, team physicians may gather information the athletes want held in confidence (see Chapter 17). This may include admissions that the athletes are users of alcohol or other "recreational" drugs, or are taking ergogenic drugs provided by persons other than team physicians. In traditional doctor-patient relationships, a patient expects the physician will hold such information in confidence, and its unauthorized disclosure may be viewed as defamatory or otherwise wrongful.[7,8,43,44] Moreover, various state laws and administrative regulations make it unlawful for physicians to release information obtained from patients during the course of medical treatment unless patients consent.[7,8] Where physicians are employees or contractors of sports teams, however, athletes whom they treat may have less reason to expect the physicians to maintain confidentiality about usage of drugs, especially where the drugs might impair athletic performance or increase the risk of injury. Athletes can't help but know that a vital part of a team physician's role is to serve the team's interest in keeping athletes fit to compete. Knowing this, they should also realize that the physician may feel pressured to share information bearing on fitness with coaches or other team managers, and may not confine reporting to an unvarnished statement that an athlete is or is not ready to play.

Even if athletes have diminished expectations of confidentiality, team physicians are not necessarily free to disclose their knowledge about the athlete's drug usage. There does not appear to be specific legal authority for the proposition that employee physicians are justified in breaching confidentiality because they believe this promotes the interests of their employers. Unauthorized disclosures of confidential information are ordinarily justifiable only on a showing that disclosure is necessary to protect patients or others from danger or to serve an important public interest.[7,8] For example, the California Supreme Court ruled a psychologist had a duty to warn a young woman she was in danger where a patient had told him that he intended to kill her.[45] But the court was careful to state that this ruling represented a limited exception to legal doctrines that bar nonconsensual disclosure of confidential communications.

In a legal system that places a high value on protecting confidentiality in doctor-patient relationships, it would seem that a team physician's response to an athlete's admission of drug use should have a therapeutic orientation. Without notifying team management, a physician might refer an athlete to a drug treatment program or to a physician who specializes in treating drug users, and confine his or her role to determining if the athlete is fit to compete despite usage of drugs. A team physician who finds an athlete is not fit to play must of course advise the employer of this finding. A physician who believes the athlete's drug usage should also be disclosed to management should probably seek the athlete's consent before making this disclosure. If the athlete accepts the team physician's judgment of unfitness for play but does not consent to disclosure of drug use, nonconsensual disclosure cannot be justified as necessary to protect the athlete or others from injury. On the other hand, because the ability of the athlete to perform on

behalf of the team has been impaired by drug use, the legal interest of the athlete in preserving confidentiality about drug usage may not be regarded as compelling enough to support a claim for breach of confidentiality. A scenario such as this is increasingly unlikely in professional sports where player contracts are coming to deal explicitly with drug matters, including teams' rights to investigate drug usage among players. But it might occur in some intercollegiate and other amateur sports where systematic approaches to drug usage have not been developed.

Failure to Detect Drug Usage

Rather than disclose use of ergogenic or recreational drugs, athletes may seek to hide their drug usage from team physicians. Successful concealment will depend on what drugs they are using, how heavy the usage, and how alert team physicians are to signs of drug usage. The athlete who is often agitated or euphoric, who has a persistently rapid pulse, or who has lost weight may be abusing stimulant drugs such as amphetamines, cocaine, or "look-alikes" (see Chapters 6, 7, and 8). One who has chronic rhinorrhea and seems emotionally labile may be abusing cocaine, one who appears excessively bland or sedated may be abusing marijuana (see Chapter 13) or "downers" (e.g., barbiturates, benzodiazepines [see Chapter 10]), and one who frequently appears "hung over" may be abusing alcohol (see Chapter 11) or other depressant drugs. The physician who perceives these possibilities has an opportunity to explore further and determine if the athlete is indeed being affected by drugs. While a team physician may not feel an obligation to delve into this issue, especially where an athlete is performing at a level satisfactory to coaches or team managers, he may be seen as having a legal duty to do so.

The argument for imposing a legal duty to diagnose drug abuse runs something like this: drug abuse and dependency are a form of sickness that may be amenable to medical treatment; society has entrusted physicians with responsibility to diagnose sickness; patients who present to physicians with signs of sickness are entitled to have these signs heeded; and physicians who fail to attend to these signs are not behaving as physicians. Couched in more legalistic terms, the argument would be that part of a physician's duty to a patient is to diagnose illnesses that are detectable by exercise of reasonable standards of medical practice. Thus, once the physician suspects drug abuse or dependency, he is obligated to try to investigate further (e.g., additional history taking, urine testing [see Chapter 17]). However, if the athlete-patient denies drug usage and rejects testing that would establish this fact, thereby defeating the physician's diagnostic efforts, it is difficult to justify holding the physician responsible for the consequences of the patient's continuing abuse of drugs. Moreover, it is likely that most team physicians will lack the training or experience needed to evaluate drug abuse or dependency. Under conventional malpractice doctrines, physicians are held to standards appropriate for physicians in their particular area of specialization or activity, and are not judged by standards that apply to physicians in other areas.[30] One might argue that it would be unreasonable to expect a team physician whose specialty is orthopedics to meet the same standards that apply to a psychiatrist specializing in treatment of drug abuse and dependency. However, epidemiologic data suggest considerable drug use and abuse among athletes (see Part II). This information, coupled with the detailed discussions in this text on the psychophysiologic makeup of the athlete, the drugs used by athletes and the therapeutic, ergogenic, and adverse effects of these drugs, and the principles of recognition and management of drug-related problems, present a compelling argument that team/sports medicine physicians should accept responsibility for recognizing and ensuring proper treatment of athletic drug-related problems.

If it is somehow established that a team physician's failure to diagnose drug usage was inconsistent with reasonable standards of medical practice, liability would hinge on evidence that this diagnostic failure caused harm to the athlete or those foreseeably endangered by the athlete. For example, if a physician negligently failed to determine that an athlete was abusing amphetamines or cocaine and the athlete died of a cardiac arrhythmia during competition, the rationale of a claim against the physician might be that an appropriate diagnosis would have led to the athlete being barred from the competition that helped trigger the fatal disturbance of cardiac rhythm. Similarly, an opposing player seriously injured by a hyperaggressive drug-abusing athlete might assert that the physician's negligence was a substantial factor in causing his injury. One can only speculate about whether such claims would succeed in the face of the athlete's own intervening misconduct in using drugs. But the mere fact that they can be envisioned suggests that team physicians should be knowledgeable about and sensitive to recognizing and initiating the management of certain types of drug usage in athletes for whom they are responsible.

CONSTRAINING DRUG USE IN SPORTS

Deterrents

Several factors may operate to deter athletes from using drugs. If drugs are seen as having adverse short-term or long-term effects on health or performance, athletes may conduct their own risk-benefit analysis and conclude it is not in their best interests to use drugs. This sort of rational calculation may be reinforced by religion, familial attitudes, educational exposures, and influences of peers and mentors who regard nearly any form of drug usage as unacceptable (see Chapter 2). For those whose internal controls are less well-developed, threats of criminal prosecution with respect to use of regulated drugs or threats of banishment from competition for use of regulated or prescription-only drugs may suffice to prevent or limit drug usage. For professional athletes who see nothing inherently wrong about taking ergogenic or recreational drugs, specific contractual provisions permitting screening for certain drugs and league or team policies that allow firing, suspension, or banning for drug use may be effective dissuaders.

That these deterring factors have not eliminated drug usage among athletes should not be surprising. Contemporary American athletes have been nurtured in a society that tolerates the advertisement, sale, and widespread use of alcohol and tobacco, drugs that by any objective measure are at least as addictive and otherwise harmful as some regulated drugs.[46] That society also condones extensive prescribing by physicians of psychoactive drugs (e.g., benzodiazepines, barbiturates) whose potential for abuse is significant.[34] This atmosphere of permissiveness with respect to drug usage is reinforced by publicity about uneven enforcement of drug laws and about prominent athletes and other public figures who admit to abuse of regulated drugs but who are never brought to the bar of criminal justice. Indeed, before recent declarations of "war" against drugs, many young athletes might have been excused for believing that using certain drugs (excepting narcotics and "crack") is not morally culpable enough to deserve worried social attention, much less banning from competition or criminal punishment.

Athletes as Role Models

While athletes may be as vulnerable to inducements to use drugs as are nonathletes, and may be even more vulnerable because of pressures to maximize physical performance, the question arises if they have a special obligation to be more abstemious than nonathletes. Thus, one argument of the NCAA in the case of the Stanford athletes was that its drug-testing program was needed in order to assure the public that college athletes were competing fairly with one another. Even if one accepts the arguable proposition that use of drugs on the NCAA's long list might in fact provide a competitive edge for some athletes, one can also ask why athletic competition should be off-limits to pharmacology. If performers in other areas can take propranolol to avert "stage fright" (see Chapter 15), sedatives to assure adequate sleep before a major performance, tranquilizers to reduce anxiety or other symptoms that interfere with optimal functioning, and antihistamines or catecholamines to relieve airway congestion, what is so distinctive about athletic competition as to require participants to refrain from taking drugs whose use by nonathletes is accepted or tolerated? The answer is not self-evident.[47]

A cynical response is that the public often gambles on the outcome of athletic events, and gamblers can't tolerate the uncertainties that might be introduced if athletes are subject to pharmacologic manipulation. Thus, a federal court upheld a New Jersey law mandating that jockeys at state-regulated tracks submit to random urine testing for drugs.[14] The court justified its ruling in part on the basis of the public's interest in fair horse races. A more principled response is that the ideal of "pure" competition represents an important social value and that those who control sporting competitions should be given wide latitude in defending against pernicious influences, such as drug use. But even if one accepts that the ideal is worth defending, the hypocrisies should not be ignored. Incident to trying to win, boxers, football players, and hockey players harm their opponents, baseball pitchers employ "chin music" to keep batters from "digging in" and sometimes cause grievous head injuries when their pitches misfire, and a well-placed surreptitious elbow is a potent weapon for some basketball players. It seems hard to draw a fine moral line between the athlete who uses ergogenic drugs to try to gain an edge and one who depends on tricks or outright attempts to frighten or injure. Neither is much of a role model, but the latter may receive praise for being a "tough competitor" or some such categorization. In any event, it may be that the best rationale for a campaign to limit drug usage by athletes is not to perpetuate a myth that athletes behave more honorably than the rest of us, but to take advantage of the visibility of athletes to demonstrate in particular ways that certain drugs adversely effect human physiology or threaten permanent harm to those who take them.

Contractual Limitations on Drug Use

As more sports become professionalized, more athletes will find themselves negotiating with teams or sponsors about terms and conditions of employment. If athletes are members of a players' union or equivalent unit, they are usually represented by the organization's attorney and/or elected players' representative. If athletes are not members of such an organization, their personal attorneys or agents will represent them. Where negotiations involve testing for drugs or other drug-related issues, those representing the athletes and their employers will have an opportunity to reach an agreement that accommodates the athletes' interests in personal privacy and employers' interests in controlling drug usage. Discussion can be had about whether random testing is allowable, what testing procedures and technologies are mutually acceptable, what quantum of suspicion will justify an employer in requiring testing beyond agreed-upon scheduled testing, what rights of appeal or retesting athletes have if they test positive for prohibited drugs, and what sanctions or requirements an employer can impose on athletes who test positive.

The balance struck on these and other issues will depend on relative strengths of bargaining positions of the parties. If they are not members of a union, rookies and relatively less-accomplished competitors may have to accept whatever drug policies a team has devised if they wish to compete. Union members and highly rated athletes are in a better position to protect themselves against overly intrusive or arbitrary policies relating to drugs, and may even be able to negotiate contracts that restrict testing to only those situations where employers can show reasonable cause to believe they are taking prohibited drugs. On the other hand, powerful teams or their representatives may unilaterally attempt to impose testing on employee-athletes without regard to contractual limitations.[48] They may justify this on the basis of a compelling need to protect the integrity of their "product" (i.e., sporting competition). But if their conduct is inconsistent with provisions of agreements negotiated with players' unions, they may be vulnerable to charges of unfair labor practices under federal labor laws or to grievance claims under the agreements.[48]

The notion they have a social duty to control drug usage may appeal to some owners and managers of professional athletic teams. This may encourage attempts to conduct random testing, to hire private investigators, and to recruit informers, all in the name of combating the plague of drug abuse. But if teams choose to act like the prosecutorial arm of the criminal justice system, then it would seem appropriate that their activities be subject to safeguards analogous to those applicable to government prosecutors. In other words, teams should respect their players' privacy and develop procedures providing a measure of fairness or due process for those whom they investigate.[28]

Government Regulation of Testing by Sports Teams

If teams use superior bargaining power or other measures to impose intrusive or unfair requirements on athletes whose drug use they seek to control, it may be appropriate to consider legislation to limit such exploitation. This legislation could take several forms, ranging from an outright ban on drug testing to regulation of the technology of testing.[17] A complete ban would imply that a team has no legitimate interest in trying to determine if its employee-athletes are using certain drugs, and for this reason seems indefensible. Teams, especially professional ones, should not be absolutely barred from trying to identify drug use where they have reasonable cause to believe a player's fitness to compete or performance is being adversely affected by drugs. On the other hand, legislation designed to assure that testing is reliably performed and that those who test positive are entitled to confirmatory testing before action is taken to fire or suspend them would provide a minimum basic safeguard to the rights of those who can't otherwise protect themselves.

More contentious are legislative efforts to limit random testing. Unless there is some empirical or observational basis for believing that athletes are using drugs, random testing seems objectionable as a disproportionate response to a problem whose contours are amorphous. On the other hand, if teams have nontrivial evidence that a particular player is using drugs or that drug use among players generally is substantial, then random testing of the individual player or the suspect group may be defensible. Accordingly, it might be appropriate to enact legislation barring testing except that based on reasonable evidence of drug use by the targets of testing. Protective legislation might also require that athletes receive some sort of hearing before they are banned or suspended for drug use. This type of legislation would not deny teams an opportunity to rid themselves of drug users, but would aim to assure that the process leading to ban or suspension is fair. At present, there are few legislative restrictions on what private employers, including sports teams, can do in the realm of policies about drug users. This leaves many athletes in the position of relying on the uncertain application of labor laws or on constitutional and other legal doctrines whose applicability to drug use in sports remains open to question.

REFERENCES

1. *Hill and McKeever* v. *NCAA*, #619209, Cal Superior Ct, Santa Clara County, 11/19/87.
2. *Roe* v. *Wade*, 93 S Ct 705, 1973.
3. Beresford, HR: Legal aspects of decisions to reduce care. Ann Neurol 15:409, 1984.
4. McGovern, TL: Employee drug testing legislation: Redrawing the battlelines in the war on drugs. Stanford Law Rev 39:1453, 1987.
5. *Bowers* v. *Hardwick*, 106 S Ct 2841, 1986.
6. California State Constitution, Art I, section 1.
7. Areen, J, et al: Law, Science and Medicine. Foundation Press, Mineola, NY, 1984, p 417.
8. Waltz, JR and Inbau, FE: Medical Jurisprudence. Macmillan, New York, 1971, p 234.
9. *Jones* v. *McKenzie*, 833 F 2d 335 (DC Cir 1987).
10. *McDonnel* v. *Hunter*, 809 F 2d 1302 (8th Cir 1987).
11. *National Treasury Employees Union* v. *Von Rabb*, 816 F 2d 170 (5th Cir 1987).
12. Curran, WJ: Compulsory drug testing: The legal barriers. New Engl J Med 316:317, 1986.
13. *Div 241 Amalgamated Transit Union* v. *Suscy*, 538 F 2d 1264 (7th Cir 1976).
14. *Shoemaker* v. *Handel*, 508 F Supp 1151 (D NJ 1985), affd 795 F 2d 1136 (3d Cir 1986).
15. *Allen* v. *City of Marietta*, 601 F Supp 482 (ND Ga 1985).
16. *Ariosoroff* v. *NCAA*, 746 F 2d 1019 (4th Cir 1984).
17. Imwinkelreid, EJ: Some preliminary thoughts on the wisdom of governmental prohibition or regulation of private employee urinalysis testing. Clin Chem 33/11:19B, 1987.
18. *Howard University* v. *NCAA*, 510 F 2d 213 (DC Cir 1975).
19. *Parish* v. *NCAA*, 506 F 2d 1028 (5th Cir 1975).
20. *Behagen* v. *Intercollegiate Conference of Faculty Representatives*, 346 F Supp 602 (D Minn 1972).
21. *White* v. *Davis*, 13 Cal 3d 757, 1975.
22. *Patchogue-Medford Congress of Teachers* v. *Board of Education*, 517 NYS 2d 456, 1987.
23. *Colorado Seminary* v. *NCAA*, 417 F Supp 885 (D Colo 1976), affd per curiam 570 F 2d 320 (10th Cir 1978).
24. *Buckton* v. *NCAA*, 366 F Supp 1152 (D Mass 1973).
25. Friedmann, WG: Corporate power, government by private groups, and the law. Columbia Law Rev 57:155, 1957.
26. *O'Connor* v. *Ortega*, 107 S Ct 1492, 1987.
27. *King* v. *McMickens*, 501 NYS 2d 679, 1986.
28. Panner, MJ and Christakis, NA: The limits of science in on-the-job drug screening. Hastings Ctr Rep 16(12):7, 1986.
29. AMA Council on Scientific Affairs: Scientific issues in drug testing. JAMA 257:3110, 1987.
30. King, JH: The duty and standard of care for team physicians. Houston Law Rev 18:657, 1981.
31. *Johnson* v. *Borland*, 26 NW 2d 755 (Mich 1947).
32. *Betesh* v. *US*, 400 F Supp 238 (D DC 1974).
33. *Mendenhall* v. *Oakland Raiders*, #441-241, Cal Superior Ct, Alameda County, 9/28/73.
34. Shell, ER: First do no harm. Atlantic, May 1988, pp 83–84.
35. Federal Rules of Evidence, Rule 702.
36. Black, B: Evolving legal standards for the admissibility of scientific evidence. Science 239:1508, 1988.
37. AMA Council on Scientific Affairs: Drug abuse in athletes. Anabolic steroids and human growth hormone. JAMA 259:1703, 1988.
38. Restatement (Second) of Torts, sections 496A-496E.
39. Restatement (Second) of Torts, section 463.
40. *Hurd* v. *Hurd*, 423 A 2d 960 (Maine 1981).
41. *Kitchens* v. *Winter Co Builders*, 289 SE 2d 807 (Ga App 1982).
42. *Hackbart* v. *Cincinnati Bengals Inc*, 601 F 2d 516 (10th Cir 1979).
43. *Alberts* v. *Devine*, 479 NE 2d 113 (Mass 1985).
44. *Berthiaume's Estate* v. *Pratt*, 365 A 2d 792 (Maine 1976).
45. *Tarasoff* v. *Regents*, 551 P 2d 334 (Calif 1976).
46. Boffey, PM: Key drug problem: The user, not the seller. New York Times, April 12, 1988.
47. Fost, N: Banning drugs in sports: A skeptical view. Hastings Ctr Rep 16(8):5, 1986.
48. Lock, E: The legality under the National Labor Relations Act of attempts by National Football League owners to unilaterally implement drug testing programs. Univ Fla Law Rev 39:1, 1987.

Epilogue

Although abuse of drugs by athletes has often dominated headlines, two events served to focus national attention on this phenomenon. The first was the unexpected prevalence of anabolic steroid abuse at the 1983 Pan American Games. The second was the sudden death of collegiate basketball star Len Bias from cocaine, closely followed by the death of professional football player Don Rogers, also from cocaine. However, as can be seen from Table 1 in the Introduction, drug abuse in sports is widespread, is lethal, is not limited to professional sports, and is not limited to any particular sport or drug.

Preoccupation with illicit drug use by athletes has diverted attention from the abuse of licit drugs such as alcohol, nicotine, and caffeine. Preoccupation with recreational drugs has diverted attention from the abuse of therapeutic drugs such as benzodiazepines. Pigeonholing drugs into one category or another has tended to obscure the reasons for their abuse as well as the consequences of that abuse. Even categorizing drugs as recreational, therapeutic, and performance-enhancing suggests that the distinction between categories is well-defined, yet pharmacologic principles indicate otherwise. For example, does categorizing cocaine and nicotine as recreational drugs take into account their effect on performance? What justifies prohibiting medically recommended use of legally obtained therapeutic drugs, such as phenylpropanolamine or ephedrine, when nonsteroidal anti-inflammatory drugs, which allow an injured athlete to perform better, are permitted?

Such issues raise questions of definition. Most notable among these is the question: what is a performance-enhancing drug? In the purest sense, a performance-enhancing drug is one that permits the athlete to perform better in competition than if the drug were not taken. While seemingly a straightforward proposition, the data indicate it is quite the contrary. For example, how do laboratory criteria of performance, such as stance stability and angular visual tracking, correlate with on-field performance? Are correlations between these measures and performance close enough to justify banning a drug solely on the basis of such tests? Consider anabolic steroids and their effect on the athletic performance of a quarterback. In a laboratory setting, an athlete who uses anabolic steroids and is weight training on a high protein diet can perform better doing a single repetition of a weight-lifting maneuver. How does that translate to the competitive performance of a quarterback? Is he faster? Can he throw the ball farther? Can he backpedal as well? How about the lineman? Does his increased bulk impair agility and speed? Does his increased aggressiveness impair judgment? On the other hand, if perception is one's reality, does mere belief that a drug is ergogenic make it a performance-enhancing drug? Certainly it is an issue to be considered when discussing the ergogenicity of anabolic steroids.

The major difficulties in determining ergogenicity of drugs in the laboratory setting are the paucity of data and a lack of uniformity and standards in research design. On the other hand, determination of the ergogenicity of a drug in a competitive setting is even more difficult where there is a lack of information regarding pharmacologic parameters of dosage, frequency of administration, and potency of illicitly obtained and clandestinely used drugs. Although prospective studies similar in design to those of Smith and Beecher could theoretically answer many questions about ergogenicity in the competitive setting, approval of such studies for most drugs is unlikely, given the health risks involved.

Assuming ergogenicity of a drug in the competitive setting can be firmly established, then other issues come into focus. One is dose-response. For example, trace amounts of cocaine in the urine have different implications for performance than do moderate amounts. Can a residue of cocaine taken 4 days prior to athletic competition enhance performance? Undoubtedly no. Should the athletic community test for drugs such as cocaine in a quantitative fashion similar to caffeine? If performance enhancement is at issue, the answer is yes. But if the goal is to identify users of illicit drugs, quantification is less important.

As sensitivity of detection methods increases, the reasons for testing must be better defined. For example, if current technology allows detection of anabolic steroids in the urine at levels of 10 ng per ml, and thus for as long as 9 months after taking an oil-based anabolic steroid, what will be the detection window (the length of time after usage a drug can be detected) if improved technology permits detection of 1 ng per ml? Consider the athlete who may have experimented in a limited fashion with anabolic steroids 1 year prior to a sanctioned athletic event. For how long should he carry the burden of such indiscretion, especially if the detection window for parenteral steroids becomes greater than 1 year? Furthermore, is there sufficient evidence that steroids taken 1 year prior to an event can improve performance? The answer is by no means clear-cut.

Such issues serve to focus attention on the role of drug testing as a means of discouraging the use of ergogenic drugs. Given the shortage of unequivocal scientific data about ergogenicity of the many drugs covered by various athletic testing protocols, it is not surprising that drug testing for ergogenic drugs has evoked much dissent. Moral, ethical, and legal issues aside, the technology of drug testing has added another dimension to the debate. This technology has moved in two principal directions: increased specificity

and increased sensitivity. Increased specificity has added credibility to drug testing in competitive athletics. On the other hand, the scientific achievement of increased sensitivity may, in fact, be undermining acceptance of drug testing as a means of eliminating use of ergogenic drugs. Clearly, an argument could be advanced for raising rather than lowering detection limits if one objective of drug testing is to link drug use to athletic performance.

If a drug is taken to enhance performance, its use perverts the very intent of athletic competition—the pursuit of individual and/ or team excellence. Such perversions are banned in other aspects of sports. Thus, the banning of brass knuckles in boxing—or "spaghetti strings" in tennis—has philosophic roots similar to the banning of ergogenic drugs. On the other hand, should use of appropriately prescribed therapeutic drugs such as decongestants disqualify an athlete from a sporting event, especially when it has not been clearly shown that therapeutic doses of the drug are, in fact, ergogenic?

Preoccupation with the question of ergogenicity obscures the fact that it is not drug testing alone that deters use of ergogenic aids by the elite athlete. Rather, it is the intrinsic morality in most elite athletes that acts as a deterrent to the use of ergogenic drugs. For them, enhanced athletic performance is achieved by disciplined hard work, combined with application of principles and concepts derived from the physical and psychological sciences. Enhanced performance, as evidenced by continuously improved records since the turn of the century, correlates much more with improved training methods, better materials and equipment, improved nutrition, and improved psychological techniques than with the use of ergogenic drugs.

Performance enhancement aside, use of recreational drugs by athletes must be viewed within the context of the broader issue of drug abuse in society. Though cocaine has dominated the headlines in the 1980s, alcohol and tobacco are the most frequently used drugs in sports. Given the athlete's status as a highly visible role model, use of cocaine by the athlete is especially disturbing. Yet, it is ironic that organized athletics traditionally has been so overwhelmingly supported by the alcohol and tobacco industries. While the sudden death of an athlete from cocaine shocks the collective conscience of a nation, regular use of alcohol and tobacco accounts for more morbidity and mortality than use of all other drugs combined. Except for occasional criminal punishment for driving while intoxicated (DWI), the use of these drugs is too often treated with casual indifference.

As drug testing has increased throughout society, legal challenges notwithstanding, it has also increased in organized athletics. Issues of ergogenicity aside, there are those who claim that athletes should be scrutinized more closely than others in society and should be held to a higher standard. Some justify close scrutiny on the grounds that fame, fortune, and free time, as well as a sense of invincibility, make some athletes more vulnerable to drug abuse than others in society. Others point out that there is little question athletes serve as highly visible role models for our youth. However, any reasons given for close scrutiny must be complemented by a consistent and sound drug policy. Drug testing of athletes requires that the principles of science be rigorously adhered to and that the multitude of inconsistencies permeating the subject of drug abuse in sports be addressed. For example, if cocaine is to be tested for, then what about marijuana? If illicit drug use occurs distant in time and place from the field of play, is that the rightful concern of management? Since alcohol and tobacco are such major causes of morbidity and mortality, should they be banned in the sports setting? Should there be constraints on the sponsorship of sporting events by the alcohol and tobacco industries? Given the high attendance of youth at sporting events, should there be restrictions on the sale of tobacco and alcoholic beverages at such events?

A 1988 New York Times–CBS News survey indicated that 16 percent of the American public considered drug abuse to be the nation's most important problem. This was twice as great as the second and third problems of unemployment and the federal deficit, respectively. The untimely deaths of young athletic superstars from cocaine, or the forfeiture of Olympic gold for anabolic steroid use, together with revelations of widespread drug abuse in sports, have underscored the fact that the sports community shares in this worldwide problem. While nations grope for solutions, so does the sports community. These efforts have taken many forms—position papers, educational programs, drug testing protocols, employee assistance programs, suspensions, and banishments.

Some feel the athlete has been unduly scrutinized for what is, in fact, a worldwide problem. However, given the ubiquity of sports in society, its impact on youth, its prominence in educational institutions, its dominance in the media, in sum, its role as a national pastime, one may reasonably suggest that the athlete should be held to a higher standard as a symbol of the solution rather than as a symbol of the problem.

Though there are no easy solutions to the problem of drug abuse and the athlete, one point remains clear. Any approach to remediation requires that candor replace dogma, that science replace myth, and that testing programs be consistent and even-handed. Our hope for this text is that it will assist the implementation of policies and programs consistent with this approach.

Appendices

APPENDIX I

International Olympic Charter Against Doping in Sport

(Adapted with permission of the IOC Medical Commission)

This charter was drafted at the First Permanent World Conference on Antidoping in Sports, co-hosted by the International Olympic Committee and the Government of Canada, and held in Ottawa June 26–29, 1988. Attending were representatives of international sports organizations from 28 countries and senior government officials from the same nations, to ensure a coordinated sport and government solution to the problem of doping in sport.

A. PRINCIPLES IN THE ELIMINATION OF DOPING IN SPORT

Solutions for the problems posed by the abuse of drugs in sport will emerge only as the result of a thoughtful, systematic and coordinated activity on the part of all involved. This process might be accelerated if agreement can be reached on the underlying principles which should govern the development of any approach to this subject. For purposes of discussion, they might be considered to include:

1. Acknowledgment of the Problem:

A recognition that the use of drugs and other substances to enhance performance occurs in some sports and that the potential for such practices exists in virtually every sport. Furthermore that pharmacological developments may precipitate other problems in the future.

"The use of drugs and other substances and banned methods to enhance or accentuate athletic performance is a tragic reality that must be eliminated from modern sport."

2. Health and Safety Concerns:

A recognition that the health and well-being of athletes may be compromised by an involvement in doping practices.

"A concern for the health, safety and well-being of athletes underlies the desire to eliminate doping from sport."

252

3. The Integrity of Sport:

The development of an attitude that sport is "tainted" at any level ultimately destroys a respect for, and the perceived value of, sport at every level. Sport is too important and too valuable a component of our cultures to permit it to be diminished in this way.

"The inherent integrity of sport, a positive cultural force in modern society, must not be compromised by the activities of those who indulge in doping practices."

4. "Fair Play" Concerns:

Sport should take place on a "level playing field." As such, it should reflect competition between athletes, not biological preparations.

"Fair athletic competition is dependent upon the integrity of all members of the sporting community. The use of drugs in contravention of the rules of sport is cheating and thus contravenes the most basic principles of fair play and sportsmanship."

5. A Uniform Approach:

The programmes and processes designed to eliminate doping from sport should operate consistently and uniformly throughout the world of sport with variation only as the nature of a particular sport warrants it.

"A consistent, coordinated approach should be developed to combat the problem of doping in sport, this should be reflected in all the elements of any antidoping programme."

6. The Rights and Roles of the Athlete:

The vast majority of athletes train and compete in a manner consistent with the highest standards of sportsmanship. Athletes should be involved in all aspects of antidoping activity. Programmes and policies to eliminate doping from sport should be carried out in a manner which safeguards the rights of all athletes, including the right to be presumed innocent.

"Athletes should be encouraged to participate in the development and implementation of antidoping activity at all levels. Measures to eliminate doping from sport must safeguard the rights of all athletes and be applied in accordance with accepted standards of natural justice and principles of jurisprudence."

7. Sporting Values:

It should be recognized that success in eliminating doping from sport will be achieved when all involved in sport behave in a manner consistent with accepted standards of fair play—thus education, counselling and the encouragement of positive sporting values are as important as drug testing and the development of sanctions in securing dope-free sport.

"The development and nurturance of positive sporting values is as important as programmes of testing and sanctions in securing drug free sport."

8. Shared Responsibilities:

A recognition that all in the sporting family have responsibilities for the elimination of doping in sport. Administrators, coaches, physicians, sport-scientists, national and international federations, as well as athletes must address these responsibilities. Fundamental to the solution of doping in sport is the principle of cooperation between the Sport and Government sectors.

"All in sport have responsibilities to work for the elimination of doping from sport. Similarly, responsibility for the use of drugs in sport should be shared."

9. An Internationally Accepted Definition:

It is essential that a clearly articulated and internationally accepted definition of the term "Doping in Sport" be established. Such a definition must reflect an appreciation of the following:

Medical/Clinical concerns. In the preparation of any definition of doping or list of banned substances and methods, consideration must be given to the effect that the inclusion of any medication or substance may have on the provision of medical care or treatment to athletes.

Scientific/Analytical concerns. In the preparation of any definition of doping or designation of a banned list of substances and methods, consideration must be given to the ability of current laboratory techniques to provide qualitative and quantitative analyses, thus, for example, permitting the determination of threshold limits for certain substances.

Ethical considerations. Any definition of doping should provide for the banning of practices or processes which while not specifically delineated, contravene the standards of what would be considered ethical behaviour in sport.

Legal considerations. In the preparation of any definition of doping consideration should be given to the ability of such a definition to withstand legal scrutiny from a variety of perspectives.

"A clear unequivocal definition of doping should be developed which reflects an appreciation of medical/clinical, scientific/analytical and ethical considerations."

10. Concerns Re: Testing:

It is recognized that testing carried out only in association with competition has limitations. Thus programmes of testing should be expanded in scope. In addition, it is essential that the disposition of all positive test results be verifiable.

"Programmes of testing should be carried out in association with competition *and* on a year round without-prior-notice basis. The results of all positive analyses must be tracked to ensure that the appropriate sanctions are imposed."

11. Containing the Problem:

Sport is a powerful social force by virtue of its profile and popularity. Thus the potential for the spread of sporting problems is significant.

"Efforts to prevent the spread of doping to regions of the world where the problem is nonexistent or of a lesser magnitude are important components of any antidoping campaign."

B. FUNDAMENTAL ELEMENTS OF THE INTERNATIONAL ANTIDOPING CHARTER

1. Role of the Sport Community

Regulations. Antidoping regulations of sports organizations should be consistent with, and not less effective than, those of the IOC. They should include lists of prohibited classes of drugs and banned methods, procedures for testing and imposition of penalties, recognition of the rights of athletes, coordination between national and international organizations, clear eligibility criteria for athletes, and encouragement for athletes to participate in antidoping policies.

Doping controls. Testing should be carried out at major competitions, particularly whenever a regional or world record is claimed, as well as on a year-round basis. National sports organizations and governments should cooperate in testing athletes training or competing in another country.

Penalties and disciplinary procedures. Realistic and effective penalties should be imposed for offenses, applied consistently between different sports and federations, and between athletes and all others implicated, including coaches, officials, and medical personnel.

2. Role of Governments

Legislative and financial measures. Governments should ensure that effective antidoping programs are implemented at the national level, to include the application of existing or new legislation regarding possession of prohibited drugs or material, and financial inducements for regulations and doping controls.

Laboratories. Doping control laboratories of the highest standard, to be accredited by the IOC, should be set up, maintained, and used fully. Research into new control techniques should be encouraged.

Distribution of doping agents. Government and its agencies should cooperate to restrict the movement and distribution of prohibited classes of drugs. They should also cooperate internationally to reduce the exploitation of differing national regulations, such as those concerning over-the-counter sales.

3. Shared Responsibilities

Education. Governments and sports organizations should agree on preventive educational strategies for schools and clubs. They also should cooperate in research on ways to improve performance without unethical aids. To assist the athlete's need for certain necessary medications, national sports organizations should provide lists of permissible pharmaceutical preparations.

C. MODEL FOR A NATIONAL ANTIDOPING PROGRAM

National antidoping programs vary from nation to nation depending on the particular government and sport structure of the country. The following elements were adopted as an Annex to the Charter, to be considered fundamental to any national antidoping program:

1. A published national policy, to include medical and ethical principles and guidelines for penalties.
2. National coordination mechanisms to ensure that the practices of various agencies and sport organizations are standardized both nationally and internationally. The national coordinating agency should ensure that only sample analysis for doping control organized by national and international sport bod-

ies in keeping with the IOC code of ethics occurs within or outside the country.

3. An advisory group of antidoping experts representing various areas of expertise should be formed to provide guidance.

4. Individual national sport federations should be required to submit annual antidoping plans which fit within the national program.

5. An IOC-accredited laboratory should be established; if not practical to do so, contractual arrangements should be made with one in another country.

6. Testing should be conducted both at scheduled competitions and without prior notice. Guidelines for proper procedure must be followed during all stages of the sampling process, and analysis must be undertaken only in IOC-accredited laboratories.

7. Review and appeal mechanisms must be available to those involved in alleged infractions.

8. Education programs should be implemented, aimed at specific target groups and should include both technical information and ethical dimensions.

9. Research concerning doping agents and practices, detection, behavioral aspects, and health consequences should be carried out.

10. The national antidoping program should cooperate with civil authorities, especially in criminalization of trafficking in certain classes of banned substances, notably anabolic steroids.

11. Countries should establish agreements to ensure that their athletes training in other countries are tested regularly, to assist countries without an IOC-accredited laboratory, and to foster relations with countries that have signalled their commitment to the antidoping cause.

U.S. Olympic Committee Division of Sports Medicine and Science

Drug Education & Control Policy, 1988

(Reproduced by permission of the U.S. Olympic Committee, Substance Abuse Research and Education Committee, Colorado Springs, CO 80909)

The International Olympic Committee (IOC) defines "Doping" as "the administration of or use by a competing athlete of any substance foreign to the body or of any physiological substance taken in abnormal quantity or taken by an abnormal route of entry into the body with the sole intention of increasing in an artificial and unfair manner his/her performance in competition. When necessity demands medical treatment with any substance which because of its nature, dosage, or application is able to boost the athlete's performance in competition in an artificial and unfair manner, this too is regarded by the IOC as doping." To implement this concept, the IOC has derived a list of banned substances and a testing program at the Olympics and related competitions to deter the use of these substances.

An athlete's misuse of drugs on the IOC banned list threatens the health of the athlete, the dignity of amateur sport, and public support of the Olympic movement. Drug education and positions on the ethics of sport, especially with respect to anabolic steroids, have not been effective deterrents to this practice unless accompanied by the threat of public disclosure and punitive action via drug testing. The complexities of implementing a credible drug testing program require a merging of commitment and operations of USOC and NGB that is mutually feasible and agreeable.

The USOC agrees to keep operational a complete drug testing program for NGBs that is equivalent to the IOC program, to distribute the official banned list and provide a Toll Free Hotline (1-800-233-0393) for accurate clarification of any related question.

Essentially the USOC observes the IOC list of banned drugs for its drug control program. Before taking any medication prior to competition, have it verified by the head physician for the event or a knowledgeable USOC medical staff member, or call the USOC Hotline. In addition, always declare every drug or substance that you are taking to the officials at drug testing.

Be especially alert to the exact name of your medication because many sound alike. For example, Tylenol and Afrin are acceptable medications to take. On the other hand, Co-Tylenol and Afrinol are banned medications. Chlor-Trimeton, a common antihistamine is safe, but any combination of Chlor-Trimeton with a Decongestant is banned. New products of this type appear on the market almost monthly, so beware of this caution. This list is always subject to change and will be revised and updated annually.

LIST OF DOPING CLASSES AND METHODS

I. DOPING CLASSES
    A. STIMULANTS
    B. NARCOTICS
    C. ANABOLIC STEROIDS
    D. BETA-BLOCKERS
    E. DIURETICS
II. DOPING METHODS
    A. BLOOD DOPING
    B. PHARMACOLOGICAL, CHEMI-CAL AND PHYSICAL MANIPU-LATION OF THE URINE.
III. CLASSES OF DRUGS SUBJECT TO CERTAIN RESTRICTIONS
    A. ALCOHOL
    B. LOCAL ANESTHETICS
    C. CORTICOSTEROIDS
    * HUMAN CHORIONIC GONAD-OTROPHIN

Note: The doping definition of the IOC Medical Commission is based on the banning of pharmacological classes of agents. The definition has the advantage that also new drugs, some of which may be especially designed for doping purposes, are banned.

The following list represents examples of the different dope classes to illustrate the doping definition. Unless indicated, all substances belonging to the banned classes may not be used for medical treatment, EVEN IF THEY ARE NOT LISTED AS EXAMPLES. If substances of the banned classes are detected in the laboratory, the IOC Medical Commission and the USOC will act and penalty will be imposed.

It should be noted that the presence of the drug in the urine constitutes an offense, irrespective of the route of administration.

Note: Certain Federations have their own list of banned substances. When the USOC Program is requested by the National Governing Body, substances on the Federation list, even though not found on the IOC list, will be added to the substances to be tested.

---

*Due to the frequent misuse of this substance in order to increase the production of androgenic steroids, the use of human chorionic gonadotrophin or compounds with related activity is now banned.

I. DOPING CLASSES

A. Stimulants

Stimulants comprise various types of drugs which increase alertness, reduce fatigue and may increase competitiveness and hostility. Although these drugs produce both psychological and physical stimulus to athletic performance, they also cause physiological side effects that can be detrimental. They produce aggressiveness, anxiety and tremor which can lead to poor judgment, placing the individual at risk of injury. Heart rate and blood pressure can be increased. Dehydration and decreased circulation may also result. Complications from these side effects include the risk of cerebral hemorrhage (stroke), cardiac arrhythmias (heart-beat irregularities), that can result in cardiac arrest. Death has resulted even when normal doses have been used under conditions of maximum physical activity.

Amphetamines and related compounds have the most notorious reputation for producing problems in sport. There is no medical justification for the use of stimulants (i.e.: Amphetamines, Cocaine and related substances) in sport.

Caffeine

An amount greater than 12 mcg/ml in the urine is considered doping. As an example, to reach this limit one would have to consume approximately 6–8 cups of coffee in one sitting and be tested within 2–3 hours. However, there are other sources of caffeine. The following examples are listed to indicate how excessive levels might be inadvertently accumulated:

Product	Amt/Dose	Equiv. in Urine Within 2–3 Hrs.
Decaffeinated coffee	2–3 mg	.03–.04 mcg/ml
One cup coffee	100.0 mg	1.50 mcg/ml
1 Coca-Cola, Diet Coke	45.6 mg	.68 mcg/ml
1 Tab	46.8 mg	.70 mcg/ml
1 Dr. Pepper	39.6 mg	.59 mcg/ml
1 Diet Pepsi, Pepsi Light	36.0 mg	.54 mcg/ml
1 No Doz	100.0 mg	1.50 mcg/ml
1 Vivarin	200.0 mg	3.00 mcg/ml
1 APC, Empirin or Anacin	32.0 mg	.48 mcg/ml
1 Excedrin	65.0 mg	.97 mcg/ml
1 Midol	32.4 mg	.48 mcg/ml

Beta 2 Agonists

The choice of medication in the treatment of asthma and respiratory ailments has posed many problems. Some years ago, ephedrine and related substances were administered quite frequently. However, these substances are prohibited because they are classed in the category of "sympathomimetic amines" and therefore considered as stimulants.

The use of the following beta 2 agonists is permitted in the AEROSOL or INHALANT FORM ONLY:

Bitolterol	- Tornalate
Orciprenaline	- Metaproterenol
	Alupent
	Metaprel
Rimiterol	- (Not presently available in the United States)
	Pulmadil, Asmaten
Salbutamol	- Albuterol = Ventolin, Proventil
Terbutaline	- Brethaire

One group of stimulants is the sympathomimetic amines of which ephedrine is an example. Ephedrine and its derivatives (pseudoephedrine, phenylpropanolamine, norpseudoephedrine) are often present in cold and hay fever preparations as decongestants which can be purchased in pharmacies and sometimes from other retail outlets without the need of a medical prescription. Because of their availability and common use, athletes must be careful not to be caught inadvertently or innocently taking banned substances.

THUS NO PRODUCT FOR USE IN COLDS, FLU OR HAY FEVER PURCHASED BY A COMPETITOR OR GIVEN TO HIM SHOULD BE USED WITHOUT FIRST CHECKING WITH A DOCTOR OR PHARMACIST THAT THE PRODUCT DOES NOT CONTAIN A DRUG OF THE BANNED STIMULANTS CLASS.

OVER THE COUNTER DRUGS FOR COLDS & SINUS CONTAINING STIMULANTS

CAUTION!! THIS IS NOT A COMPLETE LIST. THERE ARE NEW PRODUCTS ON THE MARKET ALMOST MONTHLY AND ALL PRODUCTS CARRYING THE NAME "DECONGESTANT" GENERALLY CONTAIN BANNED SUBSTANCES. The following are only a few examples:

Pseudoephedrine

Actifed, Ambenyl, Anamine, Afrinol, Co-Tylenol, Deconamine, Dimacol, Emprazil, Fedahist, Fedrazil, Histalet, Isoclor, Lo-Tussin, Nasalspan, Novafed, Nucofed, Poly-Histine, Pseudo-Bid, Pseudo-Hist, Rhymosyn, Ryna, Sudafed, Triprolidine, Tussend, Chlorafed, Chlor-Trimeton-DC, Disophoral, Drixoral, Polaramine Expectorant, Rondec.

Phenylephrine

Coricidin, Dristan, NTZ, Neo-Synephrine, Sinex.

Phenylpropanolamine

ARM, Allerest, Alka-Seltzer Plus, Contac, Dexatrim, Dietac, 4-Way, Formula 44, Naldecon, Novahistine, Arnex, Sine-Aid, Sine-Off, Sinutab, Triaminic, Triaminicin, Sucrets Cold Decongestant, and related products.

Prophylhexedrine

Benzedrex Inhaler.

Ephedrine

Bronkaid, Collyrium with Ephedrine, Pazo Suppository, Wyanoid Suppository, Vitronol Nose Drops, Nyquil Nighttime Cold Medicine, Herbal Teas and Medicines containing Ma Huang (Chinese Ephedra).

Some products containing Ma Huang: Bishop's Tea, Brigham Tea, Chi Powder, Energy Rise, Ephedra, Excel, Joint Fir, Mexican Tea, Miner's Tea, Mormon Tea, Popotillo, Squaw Tea, Super Charge and Teamster's Tea.

I. Examples of the Doping Classes:

A. Stimulants

Generic Name	Example
Amfepramone	Apisate, Tenuate, Tepanil
Amfetaminil	AM-1 (Germany)

Amiphenazole	Dapti, Daptizole, Amphisol
Amphetamine	Delcobese, Obetrol, Benzedrine, Dexedrine
Bemigride	Megimide
Benzphetamine	Didrex
Caffeine	12 mcg/ml (see p. 258)
Cathine	(Norpseudoephedrine) Adiposetten N (Germany)
Chlorphentermine	Pre Sate, Lucofen
Clobenzorex	Dinintel (France)
Clorprenaline	Vortel, Asthone (Japan)
Cocaine	Surfacaine
Cropropamide	(component of "Micoren")
Crothetamide	(component of "Micoren")
Diethylpropion HCL	Tenuate, Tepanil
Dimetamfetamine	Amphetamine
Ephedrine	Tedral, Bronkotabs, Rynatuss, Primatene
Etafedrine	Mercodal, Decapryn, Nethaprin
Ethamivan	Emivan, Vandid
Etilamfetamine	Apetinil (Netherlands)
Fencamfamine	Envitrol, Altimine, Phencamine
Fenetylline	Captagon (Germany)
Fenproporex	Antiobes Retard (Spain), Appeitzugler (Ger)
Furfenorex	Frugal (Arg.), Frugalan (Spain)
Isoetharine HCL	Bronkosol, Bronkometer, Numotac, Dilabron
Isoproterenol	Isuprel, Norisodrine, Metihaler-ISO
Meclofenoxate	Lucidril, Brenal
Mefenorex	Doracil (Arg), Pondinil (Switz), Rondimen (Ger)
Metaproterenol	Alupent, Metaprel (Oral Form-Tablets)
Methamphetamine*	Desoxyn, Met-Ampi
Methoxyphenamine	Ritalin, Orthoxicol Cough Syrup
Methylamphetamine	Desoxyn, Met-Ampi
Methylephedrine	Tzbraine, Methep (Germany, G.B.)
Methylphenidate HCL	Ritalin
Morazone	Rosimon-Neu (Germany)
Nikethamide	Coramine
Pemoline	Cylert, Deltamin, Stimul
Pentetrazol	Leptazol
Phendimetrazine	Phenzine, Bontril, Plegine
Phenmetrazine	Preludin
Phentermine HCL	Adipex, Fastin, Ionamin
Phenylpropanolamine	Sinutab, Contac, Dexatrim
Picrotoxine	Cocculin
Pipradol	Meratran, Constituent of Alertonic
Prolintane	Villescon, Promotil, Katovit
Propylhexedrine	Benzedrex Inhaler
Pyrovalerone	Centroton, Thymergex
Strychnine	Movellan (Germany)

AND RELATED SUBSTANCES.

*VICKS INHALERS CONTAINING L-DE-SOXYEPHEDRINE (FOREIGN PRODUCED INHALERS DO NOT CONTAIN THIS IN-GREDIENT, BUT THOSE SOLD IN THE USA DO) USED IN EXCESSIVE, NON-REC-OMMENDED DOSES CAN PRODUCE THE METABOLITE METHAMPHETAMINE IN THE URINE. THEREFORE, CAUTION—VICKS INHALER SHOULD NOT BE USED 48 HOURS BEFORE COMPETITION. AFRIN NASAL SPRAY IS AN ACCEPTABLE SUBSTITUTE IF NEEDED.

B. Narcotic Analgesics or Pain Killers

Narcotic Analgesics or pain killers produce a sensation of euphoria or psychological stimulation, a false feeling of invincibility, and illusions of athletic prowess beyond the athlete's inherent ability. They also increase the pain threshold so that the athlete may fail to recognize injury thus leading to more serious injury. The athlete may also perceive dangerous situations as safe thus placing himself and others at risk for injury. These drugs also produce physical dependence, leading to the many problems associated with addiction and withdrawal.

The drugs belonging to this class are represented by morphine and its chemical and pharmacological analogs. Most of these drugs have major side effects, including dose-related respiratory depression, and carry a high risk of physical and psychological dependence. There exists evidence indicating that narcotic analgesics have been and are abused in sports, and therefore the IOC Medical Commission has issued and maintained a ban on their use during the Olympic Games. The ban is also justified by international restrictions affecting the movement of these compounds and is in line with the regulations and recommendations of the World Health Organizations regarding narcotics.

Furthermore, it is felt that the treatment of slight to moderate pain can be effective using drugs—other than the narcotics—which have analgesic, anti-inflammatory and anti-pyretic actions. Such alternatives, which have been successfully used for the treatment of sports injuries, include Anthranilic acid derivatives [such as Mefenamic acid (Ponstel), Floctafenine (Idalon), Glafenine (Gilfanan), etc.], Phenylakanoic acid derivatives [such as Diclofenac (Voltaren), Ibuprofen (Advil, Motrin), Ketoprofen (Orudis), Naproxen (Anaprox), etc.] and compounds such as Indomethacin (Indocin) and Sulindac (Clinoril). The Medical Commission also reminds athletes and team doctors that Aspirin and its newer derivatives [such as Diflunisal (Dolobid)] are not banned, but cautions against some pharmaceutical preparations where Aspirin is often associated to a banned drug such as Codeine. The same precautions hold for cough and cold preparations which often contain drugs of the banned classes.

Note: Dextromethorphan (LABELED DM—IN COUGH MEDICINES) IS NOT BANNED AND MAY BE USED AS AN ANTI-TUSSIVE (ANTI-COUGH). DIPHEN-OXYLATE, COMMONLY CALLED LOMO-TIL, AN ANTI-DIARRHEA MEDICINE, IS ALSO PERMITTED.

I. Examples of the Doping Classes:

B. Narcotic Analgesics

Generic Name	Example
Alphaprodine	Misentil
Anileridine	Leritine, Apodol
Buprenorphine	Buprenex
Codeine	Codicept (Ger), Codipertussin (Ger)
Dextromoramide	Palfium, Jetrium, D-Moramid, Dimorlin
Dextropropoxyphen	Palfium, Jetrium, D-Moramid, Dimorlin
Diamorphine	Heroin
Dihydrocodeine	Synalogos DC, Paracodin
Dipipanone	Pipadone, Diconal, Wellconal
Ethoheptazine	Panalgin (Italy)
Ethylmorphine	Diosan Comp (Sp), Trachyl (Fr)
Levorphanol	Levo-Dromoran
Methadone HCL	Dolophine, Amidon
Morphine	Cyclimorph 10, Duromorph, MST-Continus
Nalbuphine	Nubain
Pentazocine	Talwin
Pethidine (Eur.)	Demerol, Centralgin, Dolantin, Dolosol, Pethold
Phenazocine	Narphen, Primadol
Trimeperidine	Demerol, Mepergan

And related compounds, ie:

Hydrocodone	Hycodan, Tussionex
Oxocodone	Percodan, Vicodan
Oxomorphine	Narcan
Hydromorphone	Dilaudid
Tincture Opium	Paregoric

C. Anabolic Steroids

These drugs are derivatives of the male hormone testosterone, which is also included in this banned class. They increase protein synthesis which may, with training, create an increase in lean muscle mass. This is perceived by athletes to increase strength and endurance. These drugs, being hormones, greatly interfere with the normal hypotha-lamic-pituitary-gonadal thermostat of hormonal balance. This interference in normal hormone function produces detrimental side effects.

SIDE EFFECTS OF STEROID USE:

Adult Male

- Acne
- Increase in aggressiveness and sexual appetite—sometimes resulting in aberrant sexual and criminal behavior, but after repeated use leads to impotence.
  - Kidney dysfunction
  - Reduction of testicular size (testicular atrophy)
  - Reduction of sperm production (cessation of spermatogenesis)
  - Breast enlargement
  - Premature baldness
  - Enlargement of the prostate gland
  - Prostatitis (inflamed prostate gland)

Adolescent

- Severe facial and body acne
- Premature closure of the growth centers of long bones which may result in stunted growth.

Female

- Masculinization
- Abnormal menstrual cycles (suppression of ovarian function and menstruation)
- Excessive hair growth on the face and body*
  - Enlargement of the clitoris*
  - Deepening of the voice*

I. Examples of the Doping Classes:

C. Anabolic Steroids

Generic Name	Example
Bolasterone	
Boldenone	Vebonol
Clostebol	Sternanobol
Dehydrochlormethyl-Testosterone	Turnibol
Fluoxymesterone	Android F, Halotestin, Ora-Testryl
Ultandren	

---

*MAY CAUSE PERMANENT EFFECTS.

Generic Name	Example
Mesterolone	Androviron, Proviron
Metandienone	Danabol, Dianabol
Metenolone	Primobolan, Primonabol-Depot
Methandrostenolone	Dianabol
Methyltestosterone	Android, Estratest, Methandren, Oreton, Testred
Nandrolone	Durabolin, Deca-Durabolin, Kabolin
Nandrobolic	
Norethandrolone	Nilevar
Oxandrolone	Anavar
Oxymesterone	Oranabol, Theranabol
Oxymetholone	Anadrol, Nilevar, Anapolon 50, Adroyd
Stanozolol	Winstrol, Stroma
Testosterone*	Malogen, Malogex, Delatestryl, Oreton

AND RELATED COMPOUNDS, i.e.: Danazol - Danocrine

*Testosterone

The definition of a positive depends upon the following:

The administration of testosterone or the use of any other manipulation having the result of increasing the ratio in urine of testosterone/epitestosterone to above six (6).

Human Growth Hormone

The use of Human Growth Hormone, Synthetic Growth Hormone or Growth Hormone Releasing Hormone is considered doping by the U.S. Olympic Committee and is therefore prohibited.

The USOC adopts this position irrespective of the fact that we do not formally test for Growth Hormone at this time. Any evidence confirming, after appropriate investigation, that Growth Hormone was administered to an athlete will be cause for punitive action, comparable to that for using a banned substance. The same punitive action policies will apply to anyone implicated by that evidence (i.e.: Athlete, Coach, Sports Official, Medical Personnel, and any others).

D. Beta-Blockers

Beta-blockers are drugs commonly used for heart disease to lower blood pressure, decrease the heart rate and block stimulatory responses. They are used in sports such as shooting, to steady the trigger finger and nerves. This is considered doping and they are therefore banned.

The IOC Medical Commission has reviewed the therapeutic indications for the use of beta-blocking drugs and noted that there is now a wide range of effective alternative preparations available in order to control hypertension, cardiac arrythmias, angina pectoris and migraine. Due to the continued misuse of beta-blockers in some sports where physical activity is of no or little importance, the IOC Medical Commission reserves the right to test those sports which it deems appropriate. These are unlikely to include endurance events which necessitate prolonged periods of high cardiac output and large stores of metabolic substrates in which beta-blockers would severely decrease performance capacity.

At a meeting of the IOC Medical Commission in September of 1987 it was determined that only certain sports would be tested for beta-blockers at the Olympic Games, they are as follows:

Winter Games	Summer Games
Biathlon	Archery
Bobsled	Diving & Sync. Swimming
Figure Skating-compulsory event	Equestrian
Luge	Fencing
Ski Jumping	Gymnastics
	Mod. Pent.—shooting only
	Sailing
	Shooting

I. Examples of the Doping Classes:

D. Beta Blockers

Generic Name	Example
Acebutolol	Sectral
Alprenolol	Aptine (FR), Betacard (AUSTR), Sinalol (JAP)
Atenolol	Tenormin
Labetalol	Normodyne, Trandate
Metoprolol	Lopressor
Nadolol	Corgard
Oxprenolol	Apsolox, Oxanol (SP), Trasacor (JAP)
Pindolol	Visken
Propranolol	Inderal
Sotalol	Betacardone (ARG), Sotalex (GER)
Timolol	Blocadren

AND RELATED SUBSTANCES

E. Diuretics

Diuretics have important therapeutic indications for the elimination of fluids from the tissues in certain pathological conditions. However, strict medical control is required.

Diuretics are sometimes misused by competitors for two main reasons, namely: To reduce weight quickly in sports where weight categories are involved and to reduce the concentration of drugs in the urine by producing a more rapid excretion of urine to attempt to minimize detection of drug misuse. Rapid reduction of weight in sport cannot be justified medically. Health risks are involved in such misuse because of serious side-effects which might occur.

Furthermore, deliberate attempts to reduce weight artificially in order to compete in lower weight classes or to dilute urine constitute clear manipulations which are unacceptable on ethical grounds. Therefore, the IOC Medical Commission has decided to include diuretics on its list of banned classes of drugs.

Note: For sports involving weight classes, the IOC Medical Commission reserves the right to obtain urine samples from the competitor at the time of the weigh-in.

I. Examples of the Doping Classes:

E. Diuretics

Generic Name	Example
Acetazolamide	Diamox, AK-ZOL, Dazamide
Amiloride	Midamor
Bendroflumethiazide	Naturetin
Benzthiazide	Aquatag, Exna, Hydrex, Marazide, Proaqua
Bumetanide	Bumex
Canrenone	Aldactone (GER), Phanurane (FR), Soldactone (SWIT)
Chlormerodrin	Orimercur (SP)
Chlorthalidone	Hygroton, Hylidone, Thalitone
Diclofenamide	Daranide
Ethacrynic Acid	Edecrin
Furosemide	Lasix
Hydrochlorothiazide	Esidrix, Hydro Diuril, Oretic, Thiuretic
Mersalyl	Mersalyl Injection
Spironolactone	Alatone, Aldactone
Triamterene	Dyrenium, Dyazide

AND RELATED SUBSTANCES

II. DOPING METHODS

A. Blood Doping

Blood transfusion is the intravenous administration of red blood cells or related blood products that contain red blood cells. Such products can be obtained from blood drawn from the same (autologous) or from a different (non-autologous) individual. The most common indications for red blood transfusion in conventional medical practice are acute blood loss and severe anemia.

Blood doping is the administration of blood or related red blood products to an athlete other than for legitimate medical treatment. This procedure may be preceded by withdrawal of blood from the athlete who continues to train in this blood depleted state.

These procedures contravene the ethics of medicine and of sport. There are also risks involved in the transfusion of blood and related blood products. These include the development of allergic reactions (rash, fever, etc.) and acute haemolytic reaction with kidney damage if incorrectly typed blood is used, as well as delayed transfusion reaction resulting in fever and jaundice, transmission of infectious diseases (viral hepatitis and AIDS), overload of the circulation and metabolic shock.

Therefore, the practice of blood doping in sport is banned by the IOC Medical Commission.

B. Pharmacological, Chemical and Physical Manipulation of the Urine

The IOC Medical Commission bans the use of substances and of methods which alter the integrity and validity of urine samples used in doping controls. Examples of banned methods are catheterization, urine substitution and/or tampering, inhibition of renal excretion (e.g., by Probenecid and related compounds).

III. CLASSES OF DRUGS SUBJECT TO CERTAIN RESTRICTIONS

A. Alcohol

Alcohol is not prohibited. However, breath or blood alcohol levels may be determined at the request of an International Federation.

B. Local Anesthetics

Injectable local anesthetics are permitted under the following conditions:

1. that procaine, xylocaine, carbocaine

without epinephrine, etc. are used, but not cocaine.

2. only local or intra-articular injections may be administered; (intra-vascular injections are not permitted);

3. only when medically justified (i.e. the details including diagnosis, dose and route of administration must be submitted immediately in writing to the IOC Medical Commission).

C. Corticosteroids

The naturally occurring and synthetic corticosteroids are mainly used as anti-inflammatory drugs which also relieve pain. They influence circulating concentrations of natural corticosteroids in the body. They produce euphoria and side-effects such that their medical use, except when used topically, require medical control.

Since 1975, the IOC Medical Commission has attempted to restrict their use during the Olympic Games by requiring a declaration by the team doctors, because it was known that corticosteroids were being used non-therapeutically by the oral, intramuscular, and even the intravenous route in some sports. However, the problem was not solved by these restrictions and therefore stronger measures designed not to interfere with the appropriate medical use of these compounds became necessary.

The use of corticosteroids is banned except for topical use (aural ophthalmological and dermatological), inhalational therapy (asthma, allergic rhinitis) and local or intra-articular injections.

ORAL, INTRAMUSCULAR AND INTRAVENOUS USE OF CORTICOSTEROIDS IS BANNED. ANY TEAM DOCTOR WISHING TO ADMINISTER CORTICOSTEROIDS INTRA-ARTICULARLY OR LOCALLY TO A COMPETITOR MUST GIVE WRITTEN NOTIFICATION TO THE IOC MEDICAL COMMISSION.

LETTER OF NOTIFICATION FOR LOCAL OR INTRA-ARTICULAR CORTICOSTE-ROID INJECTION: Include—athlete name, sport, diagnosis, medication, dose, site of injection, date of administration. Send to:

Robert O. Voy, M.D., Director
Division of Sports Medicine & Science
U.S. Olympic Committee
1750 East Boulder Street
Colorado Springs, Colorado 80909

SUMMARY

In summary, if use of any of these banned drugs is detected by USOC drug testing, loss of eligibility will result for at least six months if the first offense, and at least four years if a repeated offense, or as the existing policies of the National Governing Body shall determine. Further, any person who helped a disqualified athlete take a banned substance will be subject to equivalent penalties to the extent the USOC has prerogative.

PENALTIES

USOC Sanctions:

1. First Offense—loss of eligibility for at least 6 months
2. Repeated Offense—loss of eligibility for at least 4 years
3. Positive Test at Olympic Trials—disqualification

IOC Sanctions for Games:

1. Anabolic steroids, amphetamine-related and other stimulants, caffeine, diuretics, beta-blockers, narcotic analgesics and designer drugs:
   a) 2 years for the first offense
   b) Life ban for the second offense
2. Ephedrine, phenylpropanolamine, codeine, etc., (when administered orally as a cough suppressant or painkiller in association with decongestants and/or antihistamines):
   a) A maximum 3 months for the first offense
   b) 2 years for the second offense
   c) Life ban for the third offense

International Amateur Athletic Federation (IAAF) Doping Control Regulations, 1986

(Reprinted with permission of IAAF)

The IAAF strongly condemns the use of "dope" by athletes on both fair-play and health grounds. Apart from the immediate health hazards, there is considerable risk that the use of dope may have serious long-term side-effects.

Doping is, therefore, expressly forbidden and any athlete offending the IAAF Doping Rule (Rule 144) renders himself ineligible to take part in competitions under IAAF Rules or the Rules of his Member Federation.

There is provision for an appeal to the Council for re-instatement. *It should be noted, however, that the Council has ruled that, under normal circumstances, any such re-instatement may not come into force within 18 months of the date of the declaration that the athlete has rendered himself ineligible.*

This document supersedes all previously published Regulations.

PART I—IAAF RULE 144—"DOPING":

1. Doping is the use by or distribution to an athlete of certain substances which could have the effect of improving artificially the athlete's physical and/or mental condition and so augmenting his athletic performance.

2. Doping is strictly forbidden.

3. Doping substances, for the purpose of this rule, comprise the following groups:

(a) Stimulants: e.g.

amiphenazole	cocaine	ethylamphetamine
amphetamine	cropopamide*	fencamfamin
amphetaminil	crotethamide*	fenethylline
benzphetamine	diethylpropion	fenproporex
cathine	dimethylamphetamine	furfenorex
chlorphentermine	ephedrine	meclofenoxate
clobenzorex	etafedrine	mefenorex
clorprenaline	ethamivan	methoxyphenamine

methylamphetamine	pentetrazol	prolintane
methylephedrine	phendimetrazine	propylhexedrine
methylphenidate	phenmetrazine	pyrovalerone
morazone	phentermine	strychnine
nikethamide	phenylpropanolamine	
pemoline	pipradol	

and chemically or pharmacologically related compounds.

(b) Narcotic Analgesics: e.g.

alphaprodine	diamorphine	morphine
anileridine	dihydrocodeine	nalbuphine
buprenorphine	dipipanone	pentazocine
codeine**	ethylmorphine	pethidine
dextromoramide	levorphanol	phenazocine
dextropropoxyphene	methadone	trimeperidine

and chemically or pharmacologically related compounds.

(c) Anabolic Steroids: e.g.

bolasterone	mesterolone	norethandrolone
boldenone	methandienone	oxandrolone
chlordehydromethyl-	methenolone	oxymesterone
testosterone	methyltestosterone	oxymetholone
clostebol	nandrolone	stanozolol
fluoxymesterone		testosterone***

and chemically and pharmacologically related compounds.

This list is not necessarily comprehensive. Cases of doubt shall be referred to the Medical Committee for decision.

Before Any Penalties Are Imposed Under This Rule, the Actual Doping Substance Will Be Identified

4. The practice of "Blood Doping" is forbidden.

5. Doping controls conducted under IAAF Doping Control Regulations shall take place at IAAF Meetings under Rule 12, paragraph 1(a), (b) and (e) and whenever possible 1(c). In addition, doping controls shall be held if ordered by the IAAF, or by the Area or National Governing Body responsible for organising or sanctioning a meeting. Doping Control shall also be conducted on any athlete who is deemed to have broken a world record.

Doping controls shall be carried out under the supervision of a Doping Committee for the meeting. At meetings held under Rule 12, paragraph 1(a), (b) and (c), this Committee must be composed internationally with representatives from at least two countries, and it must be composed in such a way that the interests of all Members remain protected. At meetings under Rule 12, paragraph 1(a) and (b), this Doping Committee shall include:

   (i) The Medical Delegate (Chairman) appointed by IAAF or Regional Association;

---

*Component of "Micoren"
**Permitted for the treatment of a disorder
***And any other substance which has the effect of increasing the testosterone/epitestosterone ratio.

    (ii) A member or representative of the IAAF Medical Committee, appointed by the IAAF;

    (iii) A qualified medical officer of the organising country.

The IAAF Representative will supervise doping control at meetings under Rule 12, paragraph 1(c), (d), (e), (f) and (g).

Before the event, the criteria for selecting the athletes to be controlled shall be determined by the Doping Committee. This should be either on a final position basis and/or a random basis, but not by selection of named individuals. The total number of athletes tested may depend on the capacity of the Laboratory.

Additional controls may be ordered at the discretion of the Doping Committee.

6. An athlete who takes part in a competition must, if so requested in writing by the responsible official, submit to a doping control (see Appendix 1). Failure to do so will result in disqualification from the competition and the athlete will be deemed to have rendered himself ineligible for competition as if a positive result had been obtained. He shall be reported to the IAAF and his National Governing Body by the Doping Committee Chairman.

7. To facilitate the analysis, any form of medication, administered by any route during the two days prior to the state of the competition or event, should be declared on the Doping Control Form. (See Appendix 2.)

8. A competitor found to have a doping substance and/or a metabolite of a doping substance present in his urine at an athletics meeting shall be disqualified from that moment and the case reported to the IAAF and his National Governing Body (See Rule 53 (iv)).

Likewise, any person assisting or inciting others to use doping substances shall be considered as having committed an offence against IAAF Rules, and thus renders himself liable to disciplinary action.

Any offences under this Rule arising from competition at a national level shall be reported by the National Governing Body to the IAAF.

9. The procedural guidelines for the conduct of tests, including the collection of urine samples, the method of analysis and the use of accredited laboratories, shall be determined by the Medical Committee of the IAAF. Copies of the current recommended procedures shall be supplied on request by the IAAF.

PART II—PROCEDURAL GUIDELINES FOR DOPING CONTROL

(To be followed as closely as possible)

1. General:

(a) Meeting organisers must ensure that adequate control station facilities are provided, e.g., a waiting room, WCs (men and women), a private room (secure from intruders).

(b) The control station must be clearly marked and signposted from the Stadium.

(c) Before a meeting, the members of the Doping Committee will ensure that all the necessary equipment is available in the doping control room. This will include IAAF standard bottles, where provided, numbering and sealing equipment.

(d) All officials concerned should acquaint themselves with the procedures. In particular, team officials should ensure that athletes in their delegation are warned in advance that they may be required to undergo doping control.

(e) Athletes selected for doping control must be handed a Notice (Appendix 1) as soon as possible after the event and, in any case, not later than 30 minutes after the event. The handing over of this Notice shall be carried out as discreetly as possible, and the athlete shall acknowledge receipt on the relevant section of the Notice.

2. Collection and Recording of Urine Samples:

(a) The athlete must report to the control station within one hour of the completion of his event and he may be accompanied by a team doctor or team official. A urine sample shall be collected. The competitor shall have fulfilled his duty to submit to the doping control only after having delivered the necessary volume of urine, irrespective of the time required for this.

(b) In addition to the competitor and any accompanying team official, only the following persons may be present in the control station:
- Members of the Doping Committee;
- the Official in charge of the Station;
- the officials in charge of taking samples;
- an interpreter.

(c) At no time should there be more than one competitor in the room or WC when urine is collected.

A minimum of 70 ml of urine must be collected from a competitor to be tested.

(d) The competitor shall be allowed the choice of two glass bottles from a number of clean unused bottles.

(e) The urine sample collected shall then be divided by an official in the presence of the competitor into the two chosen glass bottles, both of which must bear the distinctive code, eg—
No 1A (test sample)—40 ml minimum
No 1B (reserve sample)—30 ml minimum

(f) The two glass bottles shall be sealed in the presence of the competitor who should check that the code on each bottle is the same as the official's entry against the competitor's name on the Doping Control Form (see Appendix 2). This code shall be scratched on the bottles; any other method must receive prior approval from the Chairman of the Doping Committee.

(g) The signatures of the competitor and an official of the control station must appear on the Doping Control Form, confirming that the above procedures have been carried out.

The Control Form will generally be so devised that 3 duplicate forms are produced at the same time.

The Chairman of the Doping Committee shall retain the top copy, and transmit the first duplicate copy to the relevant authority (eg IAAF or Regional Association). The second duplicate copy shall be given to the controlled athlete and the third duplicate sent to the Laboratory which will conduct the tests.

The duplicate Control Form which is sent to the laboratory will not contain any information which could identify the athlete who provided the sample.

3. Storage and Disposal of Samples:

(a) Before the bottles containing the urine are packed, it will be confirmed that all samples taken are present and that the numbering is in accordance with the list of code numbers.

(b) The samples and reserve samples shall be placed in a suitable container for transportation to the laboratory.

(c) If at all possible, the sealed containers shall not be opened during transit to the laboratory. IAAF will provide identification labels if required for customs purposes.

(d) The samples for analysis shall be dispatched to the laboratory as soon as possible after the end of the competition and by the quickest method.

(e) The reserve samples may only be destroyed:
(i) when the results of the first analysis are negative
or (ii) in a case where the first test shows the presence of a substance of the banned classes, after the second test has been completed
or (iii) when advised by IAAF.

(f) It is important that all samples should be securely stored in a refrigerator or freezer before testing.

4. Analysis of Samples:

(a) Only laboratories accredited or approved by the IAAF may be used to carry out the analysis in connection with Doping Control.

Access to the laboratory during the analysis is restricted to members of the Doping Committee for the meeting, members of the IAAF Medical Committee and to authorised observers (see 5(d)).

5. Communication of Results and Protests:

(a) The results of the controls are strictly confidential and must be communicated by the laboratory to the IAAF and the Chairman of the Doping Committee or his nominee in a sealed envelope.

(b) The evidence which has led to a definitive identification of the presence of a doping substance must be made available.

(c) If the first analysis indicates the presence of a doping agent, the athlete's Federation shall be informed immediately. The athlete shall then be informed by a representative of his Federation. It is recommended that the Federation should allow the athlete the opportunity of a hearing, before the second test is conducted. The Federation shall then be informed of the date and time of the analysis of the reserve sample which will be conducted in the same laboratory as soon as possible after the first test.

(d) The athlete and one or two of the Federation's representatives may be present during the testing procedure which shall be conducted in the presence of a neutral observer designated by the IAAF.

(e) If the analysis of the reserve sample confirms the result of the analysis of the first sample, this fact shall be reported immediately to the IAAF by the Head of the laboratory or his representative.

(f) The IAAF shall then inform the athlete's Federation that the athlete has contravened IAAF Rule 144, has been disqualified from the competition and is ineligible for further competition under IAAF Rules.

Until such action is taken, all details concerning the investigation are to be treated as confidential by all persons connected with the control.

6. Subsequent Action:

(a) The athlete shall remain ineligible until such time as the IAAF Council reinstates him following an application from the athlete's Federation. Under normal circumstances, reinstatement may not come into force with 18 months of the date of the declaration that the athlete has rendered himself ineligible.

(b) It is desirable that the athlete's National Federation should carry out an investigation to ascertain:

(i) the source of the illegal substance(s);

(ii) any earlier use of illegal substance(s);

(iii) the identity of any persons inciting him to take drugs.

A report of such findings should be made to the IAAF

* * * * * *

NOTE: *Where appropriate in these Regulations, the masculine shall include the feminine and the singular shall include the plural.*

APPENDIX 1—SPECIMEN NOTICE TO ATHLETES

Notice to Athletes
IAAF Doping Control

Competitor's Name . . . .

Number . . . .

Date of competition . . . .

Please note that you are required to report to the Doping Control Station not later than . . . .
(one hour after the competition)

Failure to report may result in disqualification. You may be accompanied by an attendant (e.g. Team Official or Doctor).

At this test, a urine sample will be taken under supervision.

Acknowledgment Form for Signature by the Athlete

I acknowledge receipt of a Doping Control Notice and agree to attend not later than the time stated.

Signature . . . . .Date . . . . .Time . . . .

APPENDIX 2—INTERNATIONAL AMATEUR ATHLETIC FEDERATION DOPING CONTROL FORM

NAME OF MEETING . . . . VENUE . . . .

NAME OF ATHLETE . . . . COUNTRY . . . .

EVENT . . . . COMPETITOR'S NUMBER . . . .

TIME OF EVENT . . . . TIME OF URINE SAMPLING . . . .

NUMBER—BOTTLE (A) . . . . NUMBER—BOTTLE (B) . . . .

AMOUNT OF URINE (IN ML) . . . . MALE/FEMALE . . . .

DRUGS DECLARED TO HAVE BEEN USED . . . .

. . . .

. . . .

SIGNED—OFFICIAL OF DOPING CONTROL . . . .

I DECLARE THAT I AM/AM NOT* SATISFIED WITH SAMPLE COLLECTION PROCEDURE (*Delete as appropriate)

SIGNED—ATHLETE . . . . DATE . . . .

REMARKS . . . .

. . . .

The NCAA Drug-Testing Program, 1988–1989

(Reprinted with permission of the National Collegiate Athletic Association. This material is subject to annual review and change)

I. PREFACE

With their approval of Proposal No. 30 at the January 1986 Convention and Proposal No. 80 at the January 1988 Convention, NCAA member institutions reaffirmed their dedication to the ideal of fair and equitable competition at their championships and postseason certified events. At the same time, they took another step in the protection of the health and safety of the student-athletes therein competing. So that no one participant might have an artificially induced advantage, so that no one participant might be pressured to use chemical substances in order to remain competitive and to safeguard the health and safety of participants, this NCAA drug-testing program has been created.

The program involves urine collection on specific occasions and laboratory analyses for substances on a list of banned-drug classes developed by the NCAA Executive Committee.* This list is comprised of substances generally purported to be performance enhancing and/or potentially harmful to the health and safety of the student-athlete. The drug classes specifically include stimulants (such as amphetamines and cocaine) and anabolic steroids as well as other drugs.

II. DRUG-TESTING LEGISLATION

Constitution 3-6-(b)

Staff members of the athletics department of a member institution or others employed by the intercollegiate athletics program who have knowledge of the use contrary to Bylaw 5-2 by a student-athlete of a substance on the list of banned drugs set forth in Executive Regulation 1-7-(b), and who fail to follow institutional procedures dealing with drug abuse, shall be subject to disciplinary or corrective action as set forth in Section 7-(b)-(12) of the NCAA enforcement procedure. *(Adopted: 8/1/86)*

Constitution 3-9-(g)

The student-athlete annually, prior to participation in intercollegiate competition during the academic year in question, shall sign a statement in a form pre-

---

*This list was approved initially by the 1986 NCAA Convention.

scribed by the NCAA Council in which the student-athlete submits information related to eligibility, recruitment, financial aid, amateur status and involvement in organized gambling activities concerning intercollegiate athletics competition under the governing legislation of this Association, and consents to be tested for the use of drugs prohibited by NCAA legislation. Failure to complete and sign the statement annually shall result in the student-athlete's ineligibility for participation in all intercollegiate competition. *(Adopted: 8/1/75, Revised: 8/1/84, 8/1/86)*

Bylaw 2-2-(f)

The eligibility rules governing individual participation and drug usage shall be as demanding as those governing participation in NCAA-sponsored meets and tournaments. *(Revised: 1/12/82, 8/1/86)*

Bylaw 5-2

A student-athlete who is found to have utilized (in preparation for or participation in an NCAA championship or certified postseason football contest) a substance on the list of banned drugs set forth in Executive Regulation 1-7-(b) shall not be eligible for further participation in postseason competition. Subject to the ineligibility provisions of the following paragraph, the certifying institution may appeal to the Eligibility Committee for restoration of the student-athlete's eligibility if the institution concludes that circumstances warrant restoration. *(Adopted: 1/13/73, Revised: 1/12/77, 8/1/86)*

A student-athlete who tests positive in accordance with the testing methods authorized by the Executive Committee shall remain ineligible for postseason competition for a minimum of 90 days after the test date. If the student-athlete tests positive after being restored to eligibility, he or she shall be charged with the loss of one season of postseason eligibility in all sports and shall remain ineligible for postseason competition at least through the succeeding academic year.

The Executive Committee shall adopt a list of banned drugs; shall authorize methods for drug testing of student-athletes who compete in NCAA championships and certified postseason football contests, and, in conjunction with the Council, may provide guidelines for drug testing of student-athletes by member institutions during the regular season. The list of banned drugs and the authorized methods for drug testing at NCAA championships shall be set forth in Executive Regulation 1-7. *(Adopted: 1/13/73, Revised: 1/12/77, 8/1/86)*

In the sport of football, and on a voluntary basis with the institution, the NCAA may test a member institution's student-athletes for the use of anabolic steroids between January 1 and the end of the member institution's academic year. The association shall utilize the drug-testing methods established pursuant to Executive Regulation 1-7 on a random-selection basis in the administration of this legislation, and the NCAA shall pay the costs. Any use of anabolic steroids by student-athletes discovered pursuant to this program shall be reported to the member institution upon its request, but no individual or institutional eligibility sanctions shall be applied by the NCAA. *(Adopted: 1/13/88)*

Executive Regulation 1-7-(a)

The Executive Committee shall authorize methods for drug testing of student-athletes who compete in NCAA championships and certified postseason football contests. The authorized methods, and any subsequent modifications, shall be published in The NCAA News, and copies of the report shall be available to member institutions. The Executive Committee shall determine those championships and certified postseason football contests for which drug tests shall be made and the procedures to be followed in disclosing its determinations.

Executive Regulation 1-7-(b) and 1-7-(c)

[Note: Paragraphs (b) and (c) of Executive Regulation 1-7 consist of the list of banned-drug classes and substances and procedures given special consideration. This information is included as Part IV of this program.]

Executive Regulation 1-7-(d)

Exceptions for categories (4) and (5) of paragraph (b) of Executive Regulation 1-7 may be made by the Executive Committee for those student-athletes with a documented medical history demonstrating the need for regular use of such a drug.

Legislation regarding funding of the drug-testing program may be found in the Executive Regulations pertaining to distribution of net receipts for championships and approved special events.

III. STUDENT-ATHLETE CONSENT FORM

Each year, student-athletes will sign a consent form demonstrating their understanding of the NCAA drug-testing program and their willingness to participate. This consent statement is part of a total Student-Athlete Statement required of all student-athletes prior to participation in intercollegiate competition during the year in question. Failure to complete and sign the statement annually shall result in the student-athlete's ineligibility for participation in all intercollegiate competition.

The text of the Student-Athlete Statement follows:

NATIONAL COLLEGIATE ATHLETIC ASSOCIATION STUDENT-ATHLETE STATEMENT

1988–89 Academic Year

This form has three parts: a statement concerning eligibility, a Buckley Amendment consent and a drug-testing consent. You must sign all three parts to participate in intercollegiate competition.

Before you sign this form, you should read the Summary of NCAA Regulations provided by your director of athletics or read the sections of the NCAA Manual that deal with your eligibility. If you have any questions, you should discuss them with your director of athletics.

The conditions that you must meet to be eligible and the requirement that you sign this form are spelled out in the following sections of the NCAA Manual:

- Sections 3-1, 3-3, 3-4, 3-6 and 3-9 of the NCAA Constitution
- Sections 1-1, 1-2, 1-4, 1-5, 1-6, 1-7, 1-9, 1-10, 4-1, 5-1, 5-2 and 5-6 of the NCAA Bylaws
- Section 7 of NCAA Executive Regulation 1

Statement Concerning Eligibility

By signing this part of the form, you affirm that, to the best of your knowledge, you are eligible to compete in intercollegiate competition.

You affirm that you have read the Summary of NCAA Regulations or the relevant sections of the NCAA Manual and that your director of athletics gave you the opportunity to ask questions about them.

You affirm that you meet the NCAA regulations for student-athletes regarding eligibility, recruitment, financial aid, amateur status and involvement in organized gambling.

You affirm that you have reported to the director of athletics of your institution any violations of NCAA regulations involving you and your institution.

You affirm that you understand that if you sign this statement falsely or erroneously, you violate NCAA legislation on ethical conduct and you will further jeopardize your eligibility.

_____ _____
Date   Signature of student-athlete

                         _____
                         Home address

                         _____

Buckley Amendment Consent

By signing this part of the form, you certify that you agree to disclose your education records.

You understand that this entire form and the results of any NCAA drug test you may take are part of your education records. These records are protected by the Family Educational Rights and Privacy Act of 1974, and they may not be disclosed without your consent.

You give your consent to disclose only to authorized representatives of this institution, its athletics conference (if any) and the NCAA, the following documents:

- this form
- results of NCAA drug tests
- any transcript from your high school, this institution, or any junior college or any other four-year institutions you have attended
- records concerning your financial aid
- any other papers or information obtained by this institution pertaining to your NCAA eligibility

You agree to disclose these records only to determine your eligibility for intercollegiate athletics, your recruitment by this institution and your eligibility for athletically related financial aid.

_____ _____
Date   Signature of student-athlete

Drug-Testing Consent

By signing this part of the form, you certify that you agree to be tested for drugs.

You agree to allow the NCAA, during this academic year, before, during or after you participate in any NCAA championship or in any postseason football game certified by the NCAA, to test you for the banned drugs listed in Executive Regulation 1-7-(b).

You reviewed the procedures for NCAA drug testing that are described in the NCAA Drug-Testing Program brochure.

You understand that if you test positive (consistent with NCAA drug-testing protocol), you will be ineligible to participate in postseason competition for at least 90 days.

If you test positive and lose eligibility, and then test positive again after your eligibility is restored, you will lose postseason eligibility in all sports for the current and the next academic year.

You understand that this consent and the results of your drug tests, if any, will only be disclosed in accordance with the Buckley Amendment consent.

Date	Signature of student-athlete

Date	Signature of parent if the student-athlete is a minor

IV. NCAA BANNED DRUG CLASSES 1988–89

Executive Regulation 1-7-(b)

The following is the list of banned drugs:

(1) Psychomotor and Central Nervous System Stimulants:

amiphenazole
amphetamine
bemigride
benzphetamine
caffeine[1]
chlorphentermine
cocaine
cropropamide
crothetamide
diethylpropion
dimethylamphetamine
doxapram
ethamivan
ethylamphetamine
fencamfamine

meclofenoxate
methamphetamine
methylphenidate
nikethamide
norpseudoephedrine
pemoline
pentetrazol
phendimetrazine
phenmetrazine
phentermine
picrotoxine
pipradol
prolintane
strychnine
AND RELATED COMPOUNDS

(2) Sympathomimetic Amines [2]:

clorprenaline
ephedrine
etafedrine
isoetharine
isoprenaline

methoxyphenamine
methylephedrine
phenylpropanolamine
pseudoephedrine
AND RELATED COMPOUNDS

(3) Anabolic Steroids:

boldenone
clostebol
dehydrochlormethyl-testosterone
fluoxymesterone
mesterolone
methenolone
methandienone

nandrolone
norethandrolone
oxandrolone
oxymesterone
oxymetholone
stanozolol
testosterone[3]
AND RELATED COMPOUNDS

(4) Substances Banned for Specific Sports:

Rifle:

alcohol

atenolol

metoprolol

nadolol

pindolol

propranolol

timolol

AND RELATED COMPOUNDS

(5) Diuretics:

acetazolamide

bendroflumethiazide

benzthiazide

bumetanide

chlorothiazide

chlorthalidone

ethacrynic acid

flumethiazide

furosemide

hydrochlorothiazide

hydroflumethiazide

methyclothiazide

metolazone

polythiazide

quinethazone

spironolactone

triamterene

trichlormethiazide

AND RELATED COMPOUNDS

(6) Street Drugs:

heroin

marijuana[4]

THC (tetrahydrocannabinol)[4]

Definition of positive depends on the following:

[1]for caffeine—if the concentration in urine exceeds 15 micrograms/ml.

[2]refer to Section No. 3.5 of the drug-testing protocol or Executive Regulation 1-7-(c)-(5).

[3]for testosterone—if the ratio of the total concentration of testosterone to that of epitestosterone in the urine exceeds 6.

[4]for marijuana and THC—if the concentration in the urine of THC metabolite exceeds 25 nanograms/ml.

Executive Regulation 1-7-(c)

The use of the following drugs and/or procedures will be given special consideration and may or may not be permissible, depending on limitations expressed in these guidelines and/or quantities of these substances used:

1. **Blood doping and growth hormone.** The practice of blood doping (the intravenous injection of whole blood, packed red blood cells or blood substitutes), as well as the use of growth hormone (human, animal or synthetic), is prohibited and any evidence confirming use may be cause for punitive action.

2. **Local anesthetics.** The NCAA Executive Committee will not be opposed to the limited use of local anesthetics under the following conditions:

(i) That procaine, xylocaine, carbocaine without epinephrine or any other vasoconstrictor may be used, but not cocaine;

(ii) That only local or topical injections can be used (i.e., intravenous injections are not permitted);

(iii) That use is medically justified only when permitting the athlete to continue the competition without potential risk to his or her health.

(iv) The NCAA crew chief in charge of testing must be advised in writing by the team physician if an anesthetic has been administered within 24 hours of the competition. He also must be advised of time, route and dose of administration.

3. **Asthma or exercise-induced bronchospasm.** The use of five beta-agonists—bitolterol, metaproterenol, orciprenaline, salbutamol (albuterol) and terbutaline—for the treatment of asthma is approved under the following condition: The team doctor must notify the crew chief beforehand of which student-athletes on the team are asthmatics and are using, or may require the use of, either one or all of these drugs. Requests must be in writing, identifying the drugs, dose and frequency of administration. All other sympathomimetic amines are banned subject to the provisions of Executive Regulation 1-7-(c)-5. Drugs such as cromolyn sodium, aminophylline and theophylline, beclomethasone and atropine sulfate may be used.

4. **Corticosteroids.** The NCAA has become increasingly concerned by the misuse of corticosteroids in some sports. The Executive Committee has determined that the use of these drugs at NCAA championships or certified football bowl games must be declared. A doctor using them must state in writing to the crew chief the name of the competitor being treated; the name, dose and route of administration of the drug; the reason for this use; the date of administration; the time of administration, and the name and signature of the doctor.

5. **Sympathomimetic amines.** The use of a banned substance from the sympathomimetic amine category (some of which are over-the-counter cold and diet medications) must be declared by the student-athlete on the Student-Athlete Signature Form at the time of collection. A decision on eligibility will be made based on declaration consistent with concentration levels determined by laboratory analysis and other data.

6. **Nicotine.** The NCAA is concerned about the use of tobacco products (including smokeless tobacco) by student-athletes at NCAA championships and certified football bowl games; therefore, drug screening for nicotine may be conducted for nonpunitive research purposes.

V. PROTOCOL

1.0. Medical Code.

1.1. Any use of a substance belonging to a class of drugs currently banned by the NCAA may be cause for loss of eligibility.

1.2. Evidence of use of a banned substance will be from analysis of the student-athlete's urine and confirmation by gas chromatography/mass spectrometry by an NCAA-certified laboratory.

1.3. The current NCAA list of banned-drug classes is in Part IV of this brochure. In addition, other substances may be included in the screening process for nonpunitive research purposes in order to gather data for making decisions as to whether other drugs should be added to the list. The NCAA Executive Committee will be responsible for reviewing and revising the list of banned-drug classes.

2.0. Organization.

2.1. The NCAA Executive Committee has final authority over the procedures and implementation of the NCAA drug-testing program.

2.2. An NCAA committee responsible for drug testing will recommend policies and procedures to the Executive Committee.

2.3. The NCAA staff will support, coordinate and be responsible for the general administration of the drug-testing program under the supervision of the assistant executive director for administration.

2.3.1. The NCAA staff will be responsible for administration of the program. This will include training the crew chiefs who will take responsibility for respective drug-testing occasions and who will be responsible for appointing their crew members under the direction of a committee responsible for drug testing and the approval of the Executive Committee.

2.3.2. Crew chief assignments will be part of the administrative responsibility of the NCAA staff.

2.3.3. No member of a drug-testing crew may concurrently be serving at an NCAA championship in any other capacity or should serve as crew chief if representing an institution being tested.

2.4. The sports committee for an NCAA championship or postseason certified football bowl game will recommend an individual to serve as site coordinator with the NCAA and the crew chief assigned to that testing site.

2.5. The NCAA executive director will approve the contractual arrangements necessary for an effective specimen forwarder service and laboratory analysis.

2.5.1. The drug-testing laboratory(ies) will be required to demonstrate, to the satisfaction of the NCAA committee responsible for drug testing, proficiency in detection and confirmation of the banned substance categories on the NCAA list of banned-drug classes. A periodic quality control check of the laboratory(ies) will be maintained.

2.5.2. Members of the NCAA committee responsible for drug testing and/or its consultants may be called upon to interpret test results.

2.5.3. The specimen forwarder system will have the capability of expeditious and efficient service with complete signature confirmation from testing site to laboratory.

3.0. Causes for Loss of Eligibility.

3.1. According to Constitution 3-9-(g), "The student-athlete annually, prior to participation in intercollegiate competition during the academic year in question, shall sign a statement in a form prescribed by the NCAA Council in which the student-athlete submits information related to eligibility, recruitment, financial aid, amateur status and involvement in organized gambling activities concerning intercollegiate athletics competition under the governing legislation of this Association, and consents to be tested for the use of drugs prohibited by NCAA legislation. Failure to complete and sign the statement annually shall result in the student-athlete's ineligibility for participation in all intercollegiate competition." *(Adopted: 8/1/75, Revised: 8/1/84, 8/1/86.)*

3.2. All student-athletes found to be positive for a substance belonging to a banned-drug class are subject to loss of eligibility consistent with existing policies, as designated in NCAA Bylaw 5-2-(a).

3.3. Student-athletes who fail to sign the notification form, fail to arrive at the collection station within one hour without justification, fail to provide an adequate urine sample, or alter the integrity or validity of the urine specimen will be treated as if there were a positive for a banned substance.

3.4. Staff members of the athletics department of a member institution or others employed by the intercollegiate athletics program who have knowledge, contrary to Bylaw 5-2, of the use by a student-athlete of a substance on the list of banned-drug classes set forth in Executive Regulation 1-7-(b), and who fail to follow institutional procedures dealing with drug abuse, will be subject to action as set forth in Section 7-(b)-(12) of the NCAA enforcement procedure.

3.5. The use of a banned substance from the sympathomimetic amine category (some of which are over-the-counter cold and diet medications) must be declared by the student-athlete on the Student-Athlete Signature Form at the time of collection. A decision on eligibility will be made based on declaration consistent with concentration levels determined by laboratory analysis and other data.

3.6. Causes of ineligibility may also be found in Section No. 5.3.1. of the protocol.

4.0. Student-Athlete Selection.

4.1. The method for selecting student-athletes will be recommended by the NCAA committee responsible for drug testing, approved by the Executive Committee in advance of the testing occasion, and implemented by the NCAA staff and assigned crew chiefs. All student-athletes entered in the event are subject to testing.

4.2. At NCAA individual/team championships events, choice of student-athletes may be based on NCAA-approved random selection, position of finish, or suspicion. Crew chiefs will be notified which method or combination of methods have been approved by the Executive Committee or the executive director acting for the Executive Committee.

4.3. In team championships and certified football bowl games, student-athletes may be selected on the basis of playing time, positions, suspicion and/or NCAA-approved random selection.

4.4. If the use of a banned substance is suspected, the NCAA will have the authority to select specific additional student-athletes to be tested.

4.5. Persons who test positive at one championship automatically will be tested at the next championship at which they appear and at which drug testing is being conducted.

4.5.1. It is the responsibility of an institutional representative at an NCAA championship or postseason football bowl testing site to notify the drug-testing crew chief that a student-athlete is present who must be tested to satisfy the re-testing requirement as outlined in Section No. 4.5.

4.6. Student-athletes may be tested more than once during a championship (but no more than once on a given day). Student-athletes will be tested following their final competition on any given day.

4.7. Student-athletes may be tested prior to, during or after NCAA championships and certified postseason football bowl games.

5.0. Specimen-Collection Procedures.

5.1. At NCAA championship events, immediately following participation of the student-athlete selected for drug testing, the student-athlete will be handed a Student-Athlete Notification Form by an official courier. The notification form will instruct the student-athlete to accompany the courier to the collection station within one hour, unless otherwise directed by the crew chief or designate.

5.1.1. The time of notification will be recorded by the courier and the notification form will be signed by the student-athlete.

5.1.2. Upon return to the collection station, the courier will give the crew chief (or designate) the form. The student-athlete will be given a copy at the completion of the collection process.

5.1.3. During an NCAA competition, if the student-athlete competes in another event that day, the student-athlete must report to the collection station within one hour following completion of his or her last event of the day unless this time is modified by the crew chief.

5.1.4. A witness may accompany the student-athlete to the collection station to certify identification and observe processing of the forms and the specimen.

5.1.5. Only those persons authorized by the crew chief will be allowed in the collection station.

5.2. Upon entering the collection station, the student-athlete will provide adequate identification to the crew chief or a designate. The time of arrival is recorded on the Student-Athlete Signature Form and a crew member will be assigned to the student-athlete for observation within the station.

5.2.1. The student-athlete will select a beaker that is sealed in a plastic bag from a supply of such.

5.2.2. The student-athlete will select a personal code number. The number is recorded on the Student-Athlete Notification Form, the Student-Athlete Signature Form and the beaker.

5.2.3. A crew member will monitor the furnishing of the specimen by observation in order to assure the integrity of the specimen until a specimen of at least 100 ml, preferably 200 ml, is provided. This crew member will sign the Student-Athlete Signature Form.

5.2.4. Fluids given student-athletes who have difficulty voiding must be from sealed containers (certified by the crew chief) that are opened and consumed in the station. These fluids must be caffeine- and alcohol-free.

5.2.5. If the specimen is incomplete or inadequate, the student-athlete must remain in the collection station under observation of a crew member until the sample is completed. During this period, the student-athlete is responsible for keeping the collection beaker covered and controlled.

5.2.6. Once a specimen (at least 100 ml) is provided, the student-athlete will select a pair of new specimen bottles that are sealed in a plastic bag from a supply of such and will pour at least 75 ml of the specimen into the bottle marked "A" and the remaining amount into bottle "B," leaving a small volume in the beaker.

5.2.6.1. The student-athlete will place the seal and the cap on each bottle; the crew member will then seal each bottle in the required manner under the observation of the student-athlete and witness (if present).

5.2.6.2. The crew member will apply the student-athlete code number in a secure manner to each bottle under the observation of the student-athlete and witness (if present). Each bottle will be sealed in an envopak and the seal number recorded on the Student-Athlete Signature Form.

5.2.7. A crew member will check the specific gravity and the pH of the urine remaining in the beaker.

5.2.7.1. This finding is recorded on the Manifest and Student-Athlete Signature Form. If the urine has a specific gravity below 1.010 or is alkaline, the student-athlete must remain in the station until an adequate specimen is provided. The student-athlete will select a new code number, new beaker, and new bottles and a new Student-Athlete Signature Form will be utilized.

5.2.8. All specimens provided by the student-athlete will be appropriately identified and sent to the laboratory.

5.3. The student-athlete and witness (if present) will sign the Student-Athlete Signature Form, certifying that the procedures were followed as described in the protocol. Any deviation from the procedures must be described and recorded on the Student-Athlete Signature Form at that time. If deviations are noted, the student-athlete will be required to provide another specimen.

5.3.1. Failure to sign the Student-Athlete Notification Form, to appear within the one-hour period without justification or to provide an adequate urine specimen is cause for the same action(s) as evidence of use of a banned substance. The crew chief will inform the student-athlete of these implications (in the presence of witnesses) and record such on the Student-Athlete Signature Form if the student-athlete still will not sign. If the student-athlete is not available, the crew chief will notify the NCAA official responsible for administration of the event. The student-athlete will be considered to have withdrawn consent and will be ineligible on that basis.

5.3.2. The crew chief will sign the Student-Athlete Signature Form, give the student-athlete a copy and secure all remaining copies. The compiled Student-Athlete Signature Forms constitute the "Master Code" for that drug testing.

5.4. All sealed envopaks will be secured in an NCAA shipping case. When the case is full or complete, the crew chief will sign the laboratory manifest, put the original and one copy in the case, and prepare the case for forwarding.

5.5. After the collection has been completed, the cases will be forwarded to the laboratory in the required manner, the remaining supplies returned or discarded, and all copies of all forms mailed to the designated persons.

6.0. Chain of Custody.

6.1. An NCAA forwarder's agent will sign for the shipping cases at the collection station and deliver them to the air carrier.

6.2. A laboratory employee will sign that the shipping cases have been received.

6.3. The laboratory will register on the laboratory manifest whether the seals on each bottle arrived intact.

7.0. Notification of Results.

7.1. The laboratory will use a portion of specimen A for its initial analysis.

7.1.1. Positives for a banned substance will be confirmed by another laboratory staff member with another portion of specimen A before it is determined to contain a banned substance.

7.1.2. The laboratory director will review all results showing a banned substance in specimen A and provide the NCAA with information regarding the presence of a banned substance. The laboratory report shall be submitted to the NCAA assistant executive director for administration or a designate. Laboratory interpretations regarding level of substance and consistency with the student-athlete declaration may be reviewed by the committee responsible for drug testing.

7.1.2.1. If the results are to be reviewed by the committee responsible for drug testing, appropriate arrangements for review of information pertaining to the collection and declaration shall be made.

7.1.3. By telephone and telecopier, the laboratory will inform the NCAA of the results by each respective code number. Subsequently, the laboratory will mail to the NCAA assistant executive director for administration the original manifest or a copy with the respective finding recorded for each code number.

7.2. Upon receipt of the telephone call, the NCAA assistant executive director for administration or a designate will break the number code to identify any individuals with positive findings or any information that may be utilized by the institution to provide further drug education information to student-athletes.

7.2.1. If a member institution has not heard from the NCAA within 30 days after the specimen was provided, the test results will be assumed to be negative.

7.2.2. For student-athletes who have a positive finding, the NCAA assistant executive director for administration or a designate will contact the director of athletics or a designate by telephone as soon as possible. The telephone contact will be followed by "overnight/signature-required" letters (marked "confidential") to the chief executive officer and the director of athletics. The institution shall notify the student-athlete of the finding.

7.2.2.1. The NCAA assistant executive director for administration or a designate will, during the telephone conversation, advise the director of athletics that specimen B must be tested within 24 hours after the telephone notification, that any appeal must be held on the same day that specimen B results become known and that the student-athlete may be present at the testing of specimen B.

7.2.2.2. A positive finding may be appealed to the committee responsible for drug testing or a subcommittee thereof. Such an appeal may be conducted by telephone conference on the date that the laboratory's test results of specimen B are known, with the student-athlete being given the opportunity to participate therein. A technical expert may serve as a consultant to the committee in connection with such appeals. Notification by the institution of intent to appeal must be given to the NCAA within 12 hours of the initial notification.

7.2.2.3. The institution will be given the option to have the student-athlete represented at the laboratory for the testing of specimen B. Notification by the institution of intent to have the student-athlete represented for the testing of specimen B must be given to the NCAA within 12 hours of the initial notification.

7.2.2.4. If the institution cannot arrange for representation for the testing of specimen B in 24 hours, the NCAA will arrange for a surrogate to represent the student-athlete at the analysis of specimen B and will proceed with such testing.

7.2.2.5. The institution's representative or the surrogate will attest by signature as to the code number on the bottle of specimen B, that the bottle's seal has not been broken, and that there is no evidence of tampering.

7.2.2.6. Specimen B will be analyzed by a laboratory staff member other than the individual who analyzed that student-athlete's specimen A.

7.2.2.7. Specimen B findings will be final subject to the results of any appeal heard the same day. By telephone, laboratory personnel will inform the NCAA of the findings with respect to specimen B.

7.3. The NCAA will notify the institution's chief executive officer and director of athletics of the findings and the result of any appeal. This notification will be initiated by telephone to the director of athletics. This will be followed by another "overnight/signature-required" letter (marked "confidential") to the chief executive officer and the director of athletics. It is the institution's responsibility to inform the student-athlete. At this point, normal NCAA eligibility procedures will apply.

7.3.1. The NCAA may release the results of a student-athlete's final positive test to the involved institution's conference office upon the approval of the institution.

7.4. The NCAA assistant executive director for administration will send a confidential report of aggregate findings and the result of any appeal to the NCAA executive director for reporting to the Executive Committee. No report of aggregate data will be otherwise released without the approval of the NCAA Executive Committee.

7.5. The following is a recommended statement concerning a positive testing that results in a student-athlete's postseason ineligibility. If inquiries are received, this statement could be released:

"The student-athlete in question was found in violation of the NCAA eligibility rules and has been declared ineligible for postseason competition."

VI. OFF-SEASON STEROID TESTING

(Guidelines for administration of 1988–89 NCAA off-season steroid testing in the sport of football)

Proposal No. 80, as passed by the 1988 NCAA Convention, establishes a voluntary off-season testing program for anabolic steroids in the sport of football, using the NCAA drug-testing methods established pursuant to Executive Regulation 1-7.

The following are the guidelines under which the program will be administered.

1. Member institutions that wish to participate in the off-season testing program should contact, in writing, the NCAA director of sports sciences.
2. Written notification of intent to participate should be received no later than December 16, 1988, and should include the number of student-athletes to be tested and the method by which the institution will determine those student-athletes to be tested. In addition, the institution should recommend three possible dates for testing. [Note: Institutions should avoid recommending testing dates during winter and spring championship months (March and May).]

3. The institution may wish to consider selecting student-athletes for testing based on playing position (i.e., testing more at certain strength positions).

4. The NCAA will test no more than 24 student-athletes from any one institution.

5. Institutions may participate in NCAA off-season testing not more than once each year.

6. The institution must provide documentation that demonstrates that all student-athletes selected for NCAA off-season testing have signed a written consent form for such. The NCAA Drug-Testing Consent as part of the Student-Athlete Statement may be used as a model for the development of such a form.

7. The NCAA will provide drug-testing supplies and appropriate personnel for collection of specimens.

8. An NCAA testing crew will be assigned to administer the collection of specimens. Selection and assignment of testing crews will be the responsibility of the NCAA.

9. NCAA drug-testing protocol regarding chain of custody and specimen collection will be followed.

10. Institutions will be requested to provide adequate on-campus facilities for the drug-testing and beverages for consumption by student-athletes, to comply with Section No. 5.2.4. of the 1988–89 NCAA drug-testing protocol.

11. Specimens will be analyzed at one of three NCAA-certified laboratories.

12. Results will be reported to the institution upon request.

13. Expenses for testing crews, supplies, transportation and laboratory analyses will be charged to the NCAA.

VII. INSTITUTIONAL DRUG TESTING

(Suggested guidelines for consideration by NCAA member institutions contemplating a drug-testing program)

1. A member institution considering drug testing of student-athletes should involve the institution's legal counsel at an early stage, particularly in regard to right-to-privacy statutes, which may vary from one state and locale to another. With the use of proper safeguards such as those listed below, drug testing is considered legally acceptable; however, the legal aspects involved at each individual institution should be clarified.

2. Before initiating drug-testing activity, a specific written policy on drug testing should be developed, distributed and publicized. The policy should include such information as: (a) a clear explanation of the purposes of the drug-testing program; (b) who will be tested and by what methods; (c) the drugs to be tested, how often and under what conditions (i.e., announced, unannounced or both); and (d) the actions, if any, to be taken against those who test positive. (It is advisable that a copy of such a policy statement be given to all student-athletes entering the institution's intercollegiate athletics program and that they confirm in writing that they have received and read the policy. This written confirmation should be kept on file by the athletics department.)

3. At many institutions, student-athletes sign waiver forms regarding athletics department access to academic and medical records. It is recommended that specific language be added to such waiver forms wherein the student-athlete agrees to submit to drug testing at the request of the institution in accordance with the published guidelines. The NCAA student-athlete statement covers NCAA post-season drug testing.

4. An institution considering drug testing should develop a list of drugs for which the student-athlete will be tested. The NCAA list of banned-drug classes may be used if the institution wishes.

5. Any institution considering drug testing of student-athletes confronts several logistical, technical and economic questions. Among them are:
   a. When and how samples will be collected, secured and transported.
   b. Laboratory(ies) to be used.
   c. How samples will be stored and for how long before analysis.
   d. Analytical procedures to be utilized in the laboratory.
   e. Cost.
   f. Accuracy of tests and the false-positive and false-negative rates. (These will vary from one type of test to another and from one laboratory to another.)
   g. How will false-positives be identified and handled.
   h. Who will get the results and how the results will be used.

The NCAA recommends that each institution considering drug testing of student-athletes appoint a committee of representatives from various relevant academic departments and disciplines (e.g., pharmacy, pharmacology, chemistry, medicine) to deal with the issues.

The question of where the samples will be analyzed is critical. No matter where the analyses are done, data on false-positive and false-negative rates for the specific tests to be used should be provided. If the laboratory cannot provide such information, another laboratory should be considered.

There is one important consideration that must be dealt with by institutions that are planning to utilize the results of drug testing as a basis for action involving the student-athlete who tests positive. No matter what screening methods may be used, including thin layer chromatography and radioimmunoassay, there is a finite probability of a false-positive result (i.e., the test is positive even though the student-athlete is actually "clean"). The NCAA urges that before any action is taken on the basis of a positive result from such tests, the results should be confirmed by gas chromatography/mass spectrometry, with the latter test providing the definitive result.

The NCAA will continue to monitor guidelines and protocol in an effort to share new developments with the membership through The NCAA News.

American College of Sports Medicine Position Stands

(Adapted from the Position Stands of the ACSM; reproduced with permission of the ACSM)

A. BLOOD DOPING AS AN ERGOGENIC AID (1987)

A position statement on the use of blood doping must distinguish between scientific and sport applications of the procedure. Autologous RBC infusion is considered a scientifically valid and acceptable laboratory procedure to induce erythrocythemia for legitimate scientific inquiry under clinically controlled conditions. However, because RBC infusion (i.e., autologous and homologous) has attendant medical risks and violates doping control regulations, it is the position of the American College of Sports Medicine that *the use of blood doping as an ergogenic aid during athletic competition is unethical and unjustifiable.*

B. THE USE OF ANABOLIC-ANDROGENIC STEROIDS IN SPORTS (1984)

Based on a comprehensive literature survey and a careful analysis of the claims concerning the ergogenic effects and the adverse effects of anabolic-androgenic steroids, it is the position of the American College of Sports Medicine that:

1. Anabolic-androgenic steroids in the presence of an adequate diet can contribute to increases in body weight, often in the lean mass compartment.
2. The gains in muscular strength achieved through high-intensity exercise and proper diet can be increased by the use of anabolic-androgenic steroids in some individuals.
3. Anabolic-androgenic steroids do not increase aerobic power or capacity for muscular exercise.
4. Anabolic-androgenic steroids have been associated with adverse effects on the liver, cardiovascular system, reproductive system, and psychological status in therapeutic trials and in limited research on athletes. Until further research is completed, the potential hazards of the use of the anabolic-androgenic steroids in athletes must include those found in therapeutic trials.
5. Equitable competition and fair play are the foundation of athletic competition. If competition is to remain on this foundation, rules are necessary. The use of anabolic-androgenic steroids by athletes is contrary to the rules and ethical principles of athletic competition as set forth by many of the sports governing bodies. The American College of Sports Medicine supports these ethical principles and deplores the use of anabolic-androgenic steroids by athletes.

C. THE USE OF ALCOHOL IN SPORTS (1982)

Based upon a comprehensive analysis of the available research relative to the effects of alcohol upon human physical performance, it is the position of the American College of Sports Medicine that:

1) The acute ingestion of alcohol can exert a deleterious effect upon a wide variety of psychomotor skills such as reaction time, hand-eye coordination, accuracy, balance, and complex coordination.

2) Acute ingestion of alcohol will not substantially influence metabolic or physiological functions essential to physical performance such as energy metabolism, maximal oxygen consumption ($\dot{V}O_2$max), heart rate, stroke volume, cardiac output, muscle blood flow, arteriovenous oxygen difference, or respiratory dynamics. Alcohol consumption may impair body temperature regulation during prolonged exercise in a cold environment.

3) Acute alcohol ingestion will not improve and may decrease strength, power, local muscular endurance, speed, and cardiovascular endurance.

4) Alcohol is the most abused drug in the United States and is a major contributing factor to accidents and their consequences. Also, it has been documented widely that prolonged excessive alcohol consumption can elicit pathological changes in the liver, heart, brain, and muscle, which can lead to disability and death.

5) Serious and continuing efforts should be made to educate athletes, coaches, health and physical educators, physicians, trainers, the sports media, and the general public regarding the effects of acute alcohol ingestion upon human physical performance and on the potential acute and chronic problems of excessive alcohol consumption.

APPENDIX VI

Drug Policies of Major Sports Organizations

(All drug testing policies listed are subject to revision by the individual sports organizations.)

A. DRUG POLICY OF MAJOR LEAGUE BASEBALL, 1988
B. DRUG POLICY OF THE NATIONAL BASKETBALL ASSOCIATION, 1988
C. DRUG POLICY OF THE NATIONAL FOOTBALL LEAGUE, 1988
D. DRUG POLICY OF THE NATIONAL HOCKEY LEAGUE (LETTER, MARCH 14, 1988)
E. UNITED STATES POWERLIFTING FEDERATION DRUG CONTROL PROGRAM, 1988
F. DRUG POLICY OF THE NATIONAL ASSOCIATION FOR STOCK CAR AUTO RACING, 1988
G. DRUG POLICY OF THE INTERNATIONAL TENNIS FEDERATION, 1988
H. DRUG POLICY OF THE MEN'S TENNIS COUNCIL, 1988

A. Drug Policy of Major League Baseball, 1988

(Reprinted with permission of Major League Baseball)

TO: ALL MAJOR LEAGUE CLUBS

Baseball's Drug Abuse Program

March 1, 1988

The purpose of this memorandum is to reiterate the principal components of Baseball's ongoing drug abuse program. This memo restates in many respects the Commissioner's notice to all clubs of November 26, 1986. Baseball's fundamental drug policy has not changed since then but a reaffirmation of it is appropriate as we enter the 1988 season.

No Drugs in Baseball

The basic drug policy for the game is simply stated: There is no place for illegal drug use in Baseball. The use of illegal drugs by players, umpires, owners, front office personnel, trainers or anyone else involved in the game cannot be condoned or tolerated. It is the responsibility of all of us to see that the use of illegal drugs does not occur, or if it does to put a stop to it by the most effective means possible.

The health and welfare of those who work in Baseball will continue to be our paramount concern. No less compelling, however, is the need to maintain the integrity of the game. Drug involvement or the suspicion of drug involvement is inconsistent with maintaining these objectives.

These two guiding principles—the well-being of the individual and maintaining the integrity of the game—were set forth early in Peter Ueberroth's first season as Commissioner, and they will continue to serve as the basis for our actions.

Program Components

The following elements of our ongoing drug abuse prevention effort are to be maintained:

1. *Employee Assistance Programs.* Each club has already established an employee assistance program (EAP) for its major and minor league personnel. These programs are the backbone of our effort. They provide the means through which long-term, meaningful education and assistance can be provided.

You are all reminded that the fundamental objectives of the EAPs are twofold. First, they must provide basic educational information to players and other employees about the dangers of drug abuse. Second, they are to be a means of providing confidential, independent and expert counseling and, if needed, rehabilitative assistance.

2. *Testing.* Most clubs currently maintain a testing program for minor league players as part of their prevention effort. These testing programs are to be continued and encouraged as the most effective means available to deter and detect drug use. Any minor league player found by a club through testing to be involved in drugs must be given the opportunity for counseling and rehabilitation. No discipline can be imposed as a result of an initial positive test result.

As you all know, testing of Major League players can occur only under very precise circumstances. Before undertaking any testing for a Major League player, the details of the program must be reviewed and approved by the Player Relations Committee.

3. *Centralized efforts.* For a number of years, the Commissioner's Office and the PRC have undertaken efforts to provide all clubs with speakers and programs related to drug abuse. We have also allowed a team of agents from the FBI and Drug Enforcement Administration (DEA) to speak to our major and minor league players.

We will continue to provide and expand these programs. We will also continue to support the FBI/DEA presentations and have already been in contact with clubs concerning the 1988 program schedule.

For the past three years, we have also conducted an industry-wide testing program covering all major and minor league personnel except Major League players. Thousands of individuals have participated at every level of baseball. This has been done professionally and confidentially. Test results are known only to the doctors involved in the program. The program has run well and we will continue it in 1988. The policy and procedures governing this program are set forth in the attached Exhibit "A". We have also provided consulting and technical support to the Winter Leagues in testing programs they have operated for the past three seasons. We will continue to provide that support.

Finally, the PRC will again in 1988 distribute to all clubs a set of operative drug rules for the industry in its relations with its Major League players (a copy of which is attached for your information). All clubs must post these rules in their clubhouses.

Player Involvement with Drugs

We fully understand that despite these efforts, some of our players or other employees will find themselves involved with a drug use problem. In such a circumstance, help will be provided in an immediate and comprehensive fashion. This can be done either locally by the club or through resources which we can identify. It will be done with the welfare of both the individual and the game foremost in mind. The concern of an individual club about a player's services to that club will *not* be a meaningful consideration in the course to be followed. Indeed, the Commissioner has stated the unequivocal position that if any club covers up or otherwise fails to disclose to this office any information concerning drug use by a player, that club will be fined $250,000, the highest allowable amount under the Major League Agreement.

Discipline is a secondary consideration to the health of an individual involved in drug use. Nevertheless, this office is prepared to take significant disciplinary action as the circumstances warrant. We will always seek to find a positive and constructive method for dealing with drug cases, but we will not hesitate to impose such discipline as may be appropriate. Repeated offenses or refusals to participate in a recommended and appropriate course of treatment will be significant factors in disciplinary cases. Finally, for admitted or detected drug users, testing will be an after-care component for the balance of that individual's professional baseball career.

If any club has a question about any aspect of our efforts, please contact me.

Very truly yours,

Edwin M. Durso

POSSESSION OF ILLEGAL DRUGS BY EMPLOYEES IS STRICTLY PROHIBITED

1. Any Major League player involved in the illegal possession or use of drugs or illegal trafficking with drugs of any sort will be subject to discipline. In serious cases, the discipline may include suspension or dismissal and termination of contract guarantees.
2. The prohibition applies to all illegal drugs, including illegally obtained prescription drugs. This club will dispense prescription drugs only under the direction of the team physician and appropriate records of use will be maintained. All drugs on club premises will be kept under lock and key. During spring training or the championship season (including any League Championship or World Series), any player who is taking any prescription drug under the direction of any physician other than the team physician must notify the team physician of this fact and of the drug(s) prescribed.
3. Anyone with a drug use or addiction problem, who voluntarily comes forth and cooperates with the club in a program for treatment and rehabilitation, will not be subject to discipline. In such a case appropriate disciplinary action may, however, be considered in the event of continued or renewed involvement with illegal drugs after undertaking rehabilitation treatment.

March 1988

_____
Club General Manager or President

Exhibit "A"

MAJOR LEAGUE BASEBALL DRUG TESTING POLICY AND PROCEDURES, MARCH 1988

The principal objective of Baseball's drug prevention efforts had been and will remain the health, welfare and safety of those who work in the game. Our other obvious concern is the maintenance of the integrity of Baseball. Drug involvement or the suspicion of drug involvement is inconsistent with maintaining these essential goals and cannot be permitted.

Our commitment to an effective drug testing program is the strongest, most positive step we can take toward eliminating illegal drug use from Baseball. When properly administered, testing allows an effective deterrent to drug use.

The following are the operative guidelines for the testing program:

1. The program will be administered under the direction of Anthony F. Daly, Jr., M.D. and Kim Jasper, Pharm.D., both of Los Angeles, California. Both of

these individuals have been involved in this program since its inception in 1985 and have broad experience with respect to the drug testing of world-class athletes.

2. Individuals covered by the testing program include all club owners, all full-time administrative and management personnel employed in professional Baseball, all Major League and National Association managers, coaches, trainers and umpires and all National Association players.

3. Samples will be taken no more than four times per year for any individual covered in the program between March and October. Collection will take place at major and minor league ballparks or at the administrative offices of covered management personnel. All test results will be kept confidential.

4. Samples will be tested for the following controlled substances: cocaine, marijuana, heroin, morphine and PCP. Other drugs may be added to this list if they prove to be abused.

5. Fully competent laboratories will be used to analyze the samples. Each laboratory will utilize state-of-the-art equipment and methodologies. Thorough quality control procedures will be observed at all times.

6. Each specimen will be collected under the direct supervision of a trained medical technician. Each specimen will then be divided into two containers, sealed against tampering, coded to protect the anonymity of the individual involved and secured for transport to the testing laboratory. Once at the laboratory, one sample will be analyzed and the other stored for confirmatory tests, if necessary. Only two people will be able to match the code and the name of the person giving the sample: the individual who gave it and Dr. Daly.

7. All samples will be initially screened utilizing a procedure designed to determine the class of any drugs which may be present. If such a test gives a presumptive positive, the drug's presence is confirmed by a second definitive test using the gas chromatography/mass spectrometry (GC/MS) technique. This technique provides unequivocal proof of a drug's presence and its identity.

8. Positive test results will be communicated by the testing laboratory to Dr. Daly who will directly contact the individual involved. The course of action thereafter will include evaluation and rehabilitative treatment (if necessary) and possible follow-up testing. There will be no discipline or penalties imposed on any individual for a first confirmed positive test result. The test results will not be provided to anyone in league or club management. The Commissioner's Office may be advised of test results and take action only in the case of positive test results coupled with refusals to cooperate in evaluation or treatment if in the opinion of the medical experts this notice is necessary and appropriate to provide effective assistance.

March 1988

B. Drug Policy of the National Basketball Association, 1988

(Reprinted with permission of the National Basketball Association)

NATIONAL BASKETBALL ASSOCIATION EXHIBIT C TO COLLECTIVE BARGAINING AGREEMENT

AGREEMENT made this _____ day of October, 1983, by and between the National Basketball Association ("NBA") and the National Basketball Players Association ("Players Association").

WHEREAS, the NBA and the Players Association recognize that the illegal use and abuse of drugs has become a serious problem in our society and in professional sports, in particular; and

WHEREAS, the illegal use of drugs can adversely affect the performance of NBA players and threatens the image of and public confidence in NBA basketball; and

WHEREAS, the NBA and the Players Association have agreed that the illegal use of drugs is inconsistent with competing in the NBA and that anyone found to have engaged in the use of the substances set forth in Exhibit 1, annexed hereto, ought properly to forfeit any opportunity to play in the NBA;

NOW, THEREFORE, the NBA and the Players Association have agreed upon the following program, the purpose of which is to eliminate the illegal use of drugs in the NBA:

1. *Dismissal and Permanent Disqualification.* Any player who has been convicted of or has pled guilty to a crime involving the use, possession, or distribution of any of the substances set forth in Exhibit 1, annexed hereto (the "prohibited substances") or has been found through the procedures set forth in Paragraphs 6 or 7 below to have used, possessed, or distributed any of the prohibited substances, shall, without exception, immediately be dismissed and permanently disqualified from any further association with the NBA or any of its teams. Such dismissal and permanent disqualification shall be mandatory and may not be rescinded or reduced by the player's club or the NBA.

2. *Amnesty.* (a) From the date hereof through December 31, 1983 (the "Amnesty Period"), no player will be subject to the penalty set forth in Paragraph 1 hereof. During the Amnesty Period, the NBA and the Players Association will use their best efforts to inform all players, in writing and in person at team and/or individual meetings, of the details of this Agreement, including the procedures to be utilized and the penalties provided. In addition, the parties may notify certain player(s) that one or both of the parties has reason to believe that such player(s) may have used, possessed, or distributed a prohibited substance.

(b) During the term of this Agreement, any player, except a player referred to in Paragraph 10 below, who comes forward voluntarily to seek treatment of a problem involving the use of drugs, will be provided with appropriate counselling and medical assistance, at the expense of the club. No penalty of any kind will be imposed on such a player and, provided he complies with the terms of his prescribed treatment, he will continue to receive his salary during the term of his treatment, for a period of up to 3 months of in-patient care in a facility approved by the Life Extension Institute and such out-patient care as is required in a program approved by the Life Extension Institute.

3. *Appointment of Independent Expert.* The NBA and the Players Association shall jointly appoint an Independent Expert (the "Expert") who shall be a person experienced in the field of drug abuse detection and enforcement. The Expert shall serve for the duration of the Collective Bargaining Agreement, dated October 10, 1980, between the NBA and the Players Association, as amended by the Memorandum of Understanding, dated April 18, 1983 (The "Collective Bargaining Agreement"); provided, however, that as of each September 1, either the NBA or the Players Association may discharge the Expert by serving 30 days' prior written notice upon him and upon the other party. In the event the parties do not reach an agreement, within 45 days, as to who shall serve as the Expert, each party shall appoint a person who shall have no relationship to or be affiliated with that party. Such persons shall then have fifteen days to agree on the appointment of an Expert. The Expert's fees shall be paid in equal shares by the NBA and the Players Association.

4. *Authorization for Testing.* In the event that either the NBA or the Players Association has information which gives it reasonable cause to believe that a player may have been engaged in the use, possession, or distribution of a prohibited substance at a time after the conclusion of the Amnesty Period, such party shall request a conference with the other party and the Expert, which shall be held within 24 hours or as soon thereafter as the Expert is available. Upon hearing the information presented, the Expert shall immediately decide whether there is reasonable cause to believe that the player in question may have been engaged in the use, possession, or distribution of a prohibited substance. If the Expert decides that such reasonable cause to believe exists, the Expert shall thereupon issue an Authorization for Testing with respect to such player in the form annexed hereto as Exhibit 2.

5. *Sources of Information.* In evaluating the information presented to him, the Expert shall be entitled to use his independent judgment based upon his experience in drug abuse detection and enforcement. The parties acknowledge that the type of information to be presented to the Expert is likely to consist of reports of conversations with third parties of the type generally considered by law enforcement authorities to be reliable sources, and that such sources might not otherwise come forward if their identities were to become known. Accordingly, neither the NBA nor the Players Association shall be required to divulge to each other or to the Expert the names of their sources of information regarding the use, possession, or distribution of a prohibited substance, and the absence of such identification of sources shall not be considered by the Expert in determining whether to issue an Authorization for Testing with respect to a player. In conferences with the Expert, the player involved shall not be identified by name until such time as the Expert has determined to issue an Authorization for Testing with respect to such player.

6. *Testing.* Immediately upon the Expert's issuance of an Authorization for Testing with respect to a particular player, the NBA shall arrange for such player to undergo the testing procedures, as set forth in Exhibit 3, annexed hereto, no more than four times during the six-week period commencing with the issuance of the Authorization for Testing. Such testing procedures may be administered at any time, in the discretion of the NBA, without prior notice to the player. In the event that any of the testing procedures produces a positive result, the player shall be deemed to have used a prohibited substance and shall suffer the penalty set forth in Paragraph 1, above, and shall be so notified by the Commissioner. Any player refusing to submit to a testing procedure, pursuant to an Authorization for Testing, at the time set by the NBA, shall be deemed to have produced a positive result

for such testing procedure and shall suffer the penalty set forth in Paragraph 1, above.

7. *Dismissal Without Testing.* In the event that either the NBA or the Players Association determines that there is sufficient evidence to demonstrate that a player has engaged in the use, possession, or distribution of a prohibited substance at a time after the conclusion of the Amnesty Period, it may, in lieu of requesting the testing procedure set forth in Paragraphs 4 through 6, request a hearing on the matter before the Impartial Arbitrator under the Collective Bargaining Agreement. If the Impartial Arbitrator concludes that the player has used, possessed, or distributed a prohibited substance at a time after the conclusion of the Amnesty Period, the player shall suffer the penalty set forth in Paragraph 1, above, notwithstanding the fact that the player has not undergone the testing procedure set forth in Paragraph 6.

8. *Confidentiality.* The NBA and the Players Association agree that neither of them will divulge to any other party, including their respective members and the player and team involved (other than as required by the Testing Procedure set forth in Paragraph 6 above):

i) That it has received information regarding the use, possession, or distribution of a prohibited substance by a player;

ii) that it is considering requesting, has requested, or has had a conference with the Expert;

iii) any information disclosed to the Expert; and

iv) the results of any conference with the Expert.

9. *Amendment to Uniform Player Contract.* All forms of the Uniform Player Contract attached to the Collective Bargaining Agreement as exhibits and, in cases where a player and a Member are parties to a currently effective Uniform Player Contract each such contract, shall, upon execution of this Agreement, be deemed amended to include a new Paragraph 6(d), which shall provide as follows:

"The Player acknowledges that, in the event he is found in accordance with the terms of the Agreement between the Association and the National Basketball Players Association, dated October _____, 1983 to have engaged in the use, possession, or distribution of a "prohibited substance" as defined therein, it will result in the termination of this contract and the Player's immediate dismissal and permanent disqualification from any employment by the Association and any of its teams. Notwithstanding any terms or provisions of this contract (including any amendments hereto) in the event of such termination, all obligations of the Club, including obligations to pay compensation, shall cease, except the obligation of the Club to pay the Player's earned compensation (either current or deferred) to the date of termination. The Player hereby releases and waives every claim he may have against the Club, the Association, the National Basketball Players Association, and each of their respective members, directors, governors, officers, stockholders, trustees, partners, and employees, arising out of or in connection with the testing procedures or the imposition of any penalties set forth in the Agreement between the Association and the National Basketball Players Association dated as of October _____, 1983."

10. *Second Treatment.* Any player who, after previously requesting and receiving treatment for a drug problem, again comes forward voluntarily to seek such treatment, shall be suspended without pay during the period of such treatment, but shall not suffer the penalty set forth in Paragraph 1, above. Any subsequent use, possession, or distribution of a prohibited substance, even if voluntarily disclosed, shall result in the imposition of the penalty set forth in Paragraph 1, above.

11. *Application for Reinstatement.* Notwithstanding the provisions of Paragraph 1 above, after a period of at least two years from the time of a player's dismissal and permanent disqualification, such player may apply for reinstatement as a player in the NBA. However, such player shall have no right to reinstatement

under any circumstance and the reinstatement shall be granted only with the prior approval of both the Commissioner and Players Association. The approval of the Commissioner and the Players Association shall rest in their absolute and sole discretion, and their decision shall be final, binding and unappealable. Among the factors which may be considered by the Commissioner and the Players Association in determining whether to grant reinstatement are (without limitation): the circumstances surrounding the player's dismissal and permanent disqualification, whether the player has satisfactorily completed a treatment and rehabilitation program, the player's conduct since his dismissal, including the extent to which the player has since comported himself as a suitable role model for youth, and whether the player is judged to possess the requisite qualities of good character and morality. The granting of an application for reinstatement may be conditioned upon periodic testing of the player or such other terms as may be agreed upon by the NBA and the Players Association. A player who has been reinstated pursuant to this paragraph shall, immediately upon such reinstatement, notify the Club for which he last played. Such Club shall have 30 days to notify the player that it is prepared to accept his playing services under the terms and conditions of that portion of the term of the player's last player contract, for which services were not rendered because of such player's dismissal and permanent disqualification. If the Club notifies the player that it is prepared to accept his employment under such terms and conditions, the Club and the player shall immediately enter into a new Uniform Player Contract in accordance with those terms and conditions. If the Club does not so notify the player, the player shall be deemed to have completed the services called for under his last player contract and shall immediately be free to negotiate and sign an Offer Sheet with any NBA team, subject to the Right of First Refusal set forth in Article XXII, Section 1(d) of the Collective Bargaining Agreement.

12. *Incorporation in Collective Bargaining Agreement.* This Agreement shall be incorporated in and extend through the term of the Collective Bargaining Agreement.

13. *Limitation on Other Testing.* Except as expressly provided in Paragraph 6, above, there shall be no other screening or testing for the prohibited substances conducted by the NBA or NBA clubs, and no player shall be required to undergo such screening or testing. Notwithstanding the foregoing, any player who has acknowledged the use of a prohibited substance by entering a treatment program, shall be subject to such screening or testing as may be determined by the Life Extension Institute. The frequency and duration of any screening or testing, as determined by the Life Extension Institute hereunder, shall not exceed 3 times a week or a period of more than one year following in-patient treatment. Any player refusing to submit to a screen or test pursuant to this paragraph or for whom such screen or test produces a positive result, shall be subject to the provisions of Paragraph 10, above, as a player who "again comes forward voluntarily."

IN WITNESS WHEREOF, the parties have entered into this agreement as of the day and year first written above.

NATIONAL BASKETBALL ASSOCIATION

By _____
                    Commissioner

NATIONAL BASKETBALL PLAYERS ASSOCIATION

By _____
                    President

EXHIBIT 1

LIST OF PROHIBITED DRUGS

Cocaine
Heroin

March 1, 1988

EXHIBIT 2

AUTHORIZATION FOR TESTING

TO: _____
(Player)

Please be advised that on _____, you were the subject of a conference held pursuant to the Agreement between the NBA and Players Association, dated _____ ("Agreement"). Following the conference, I authorized the NBA to conduct the testing procedures set forth in the Agreement, and you are hereby directed to submit to these testing procedures, on demand, no more than 4 times during the next six weeks.

Please be advised that your failure to submit to these procedures will result in your dismissal and permanent disqualification from the NBA.

_____
Independent Expert

Dated:

EXHIBIT 3

TESTING PROCEDURES

Urinalysis. To be screened and tested through scientifically accepted analytical techniques, such as chromatography (gas and/or thin-layer), spectrophoto fluorometry, EMIT, and/or TLC.

C. Drug Policy of the National Football League, 1988

(Reprinted with permission of the National Football League)

FROM THE COMMISSIONER

The following pages detail the National Football League's current policy on drugs. All players and other League personnel should read this information carefully.

For many years the Commissioner's office has promulgated measures to deal with problems involving drugs, beginning in 1971 with efforts to counteract abuse of amphetamines and similar substances. This was followed by periodic strengthening and updating of the policies to meet new problems, such as cocaine and anabolic steroids, as they arose.

Of primary importance in the League's approach to this issue are the involvement of an expert drug advisor to foster consistency by centralized administration of all parts of the policy, and the use of urine testing to detect drugs and deal with them effectively and expeditiously.

The plain fact is that drug use can remain undetected until it is too late. This can lead to personal tragedy, diminished job performance, injury to drug-using players or others who come in contact with them, potentially disastrous financial ramifications for players and clubs, adverse fan reaction, and generally a blot on a profession whose participants, due to their public visibility and the nature of their work, should maintain high standards of conduct and a sound respect for physical health.

Drugs in our society are a scourge. While no one can be so blindly optimistic as to expect any particular group or business to be totally free of such ills, we should nevertheless aim for that goal. Drug abuse is fundamentally a *health* problem—threatening the health of players, of the League, and, indirectly, of American society. I am asking every person involved with the NFL to join in supporting our drug policy and to help make professional football a game in which all participants can take the fullest possible pride.

PETE ROZELLE
Commissioner

LEAGUE PERSONNEL COVERED BY POLICY

Although the League's drug policy is written to apply principally to player-employees, its rules and procedures also may affect other persons working for member clubs, the League office, and affiliate organizations. The Commissioner will take appropriate action if he determines that any non-playing employee is involved in improper use or distribution of drugs.

Special duties and responsibilities of member clubs are noted throughout this policy, e.g., adherence to the prescription drug monitoring system, reporting of drug incidents to the Drug Advisor, and cooperation in the urine testing program.

DRUG ADVISOR

The Drug Advisor for the National Football League is Forest S. Tennant, Jr., M.D., Dr. P.H. He is executive director of Community Health Projects, Inc., a group of drug-treatment clinics headquartered in West Covina, California, and an associate professor at the UCLA School of Public Health. An expert in the field of drug treatment and research, Dr. Tennant also serves as a consultant to the California State Department of Justice, the California Highway Patrol, the National Association for Stock Car Auto Racing (NASCAR), and the Los Angeles Dodgers baseball organization.

Dr. Tennant, working with physicians at each of the 28 member clubs, administers and coordinates drug testing, treatment, and education under the NFL's policy.

PROHIBITED SUBSTANCES

Players are prohibited from using, possessing, purchasing, selling and/or participating in the distribution of:

Illegal drugs, regardless of amount. Illegal drugs include, but are not limited to: marijuana, cocaine, opioids (heroin, methadone), and phencyclidine (PCP).

Anabolic steroids and similar growth- and performance-enhancing substances. (See separate section below for further information on anabolic steroids.)

Amphetamines and substances that may create similar affects, e.g., phenylpropanolamine (the active ingredient in many over-the-counter decongestants), unless the player can supply medication information to his club physician and the NFL's Drug Advisor which verifies the player's legitimate need for appropriate dosages of such substances to treat an existing medical condition. Where amphetamines or similar substances are found to be abused, the Drug Advisor will first provide the involved player with appropriate educational materials and counseling. If abuse continues, the player will then be subject to all procedures applicable to other prohibited substances under this policy.

Illegal acquisition, distribution, and/or misuse of any legal prescription or over-the-counter drug are strictly prohibited.

While the moderate use of alcohol, a legal substance, is not prohibited, any serious misuse of alcohol, including violations of the law while intoxicated, may result in disciplinary action by the Commissioner. (See separate section below.)

The League may, from time to time, modify its list of prohibited substances.

ANABOLIC STEROIDS

The substances known as anabolic steroids, and the related growth drugs (produced synthetically or extracted from glandular tissue), deserve special mention. Because in many areas they are obtainable by prescription for limited therapeutic applications, their misuse by NFL players has been impermissible ever since the League promulgated its policy on prescription drugs in the early 1970s.

Now, due to widespread misuse of anabolic steroids in recent years throughout much of the sports world, including football, they are listed among those drugs prohibited by the League under any circumstances. *To repeat, the League no longer merely condemns the misuse of these substances; they are prohibited in any quantity for any purpose.* The NFL Physicians Society is on record declaring that there are *no* legitimate medical purposes to prescribe anabolic steroids for NFL players.

Players should be aware that in addition to the ethical issue raised by the use of performance-enhancing drugs to gain competitive advantage, there is mounting evidence that anabolic steroids, particularly in the often large dosages taken by athletes, can cause high blood pressure, heart disease, high cholesterol, hepatitis, liver tumors, addiction, acne, baldness, and adverse personality changes. In addition, some users now complain of impotence and have testicles the size of a young boy. These users have low sperm counts and could be sterile, changes that may not be reversible. Other changes that have occurred include breast enlargement and higher voice pitch.

There also is growing concern that players using anabolic steroids can cause serious on-field injuries not only to others but to themselves. One major insurance underwriter, reportedly responsible for writing half of the sports policies in this country and concerned about the use of these substances, has stopped writing coverage against football injuries.

NFL players should also be aware that the federal government is concerned about these drugs and that criminal prosecution has resulted in cases of improper distribution of anabolic steroids. Thus the user, like the user of cocaine or marijuana, is often the final link in a chain of illegal activity.

The technology is now available for the League to test for anabolic steroids when large numbers of players undergo physical examinations, e.g., at preseason training camps. This means that off-season use of these drugs, many of which stay in the system for long periods of time, can be detected. Once a player has anabolic steroids identified in his body—for example, at a timing-and-testing session of draft-eligible players operated by NFL scouting organizations or at a preseason physical examination conducted by an NFL club—he is subject to reasonable-cause urine testing for prohibited substances at any time in the future.

The following procedures will be in effect for the 1988 season.

Any player who has a confirmed positive test for anabolic steroids at a 1988 preseason training camp or as a result of reasonable-cause testing will be informed of the test results. The player will then be scheduled for a re-test within two to four weeks. If the second test is positive, the player will undergo a medical evaluation under the direction of the club physician and the NFL Drug Advisor. This evaluation will include a complete evaluation of the toxic complications, a quantitative steroid urine test, and, if necessary, a medical detoxification treatment.

Each instance in which a second positive test for anabolic steroids is confirmed will be handled on a case-by-case basis. Involved players will be subject to appropriate discipline by the Commissioner.

Any player who has tested positive for anabolic steroids in an NFL preseason training camp, at a pre-draft physical examination conducted by NFL scouting organizations, or as a result of reasonable-cause testing will be subject to reasonable-cause testing at any time in the future.

Any player who tests positive for anabolic steroids and shows medical complications, including but not limited to high blood pressure, rapid heart beat, enlarged heart, hepatitis, tumors, and/or chemical abnormalities in the blood may be considered to be unfit to participate in football and may be placed in the category of Non-Football Illness (NFI) until all evidence of the complications has been resolved.

ADDENDUM TO NFL POLICY*

In 1989, the Commissioner of the NFL issued the following directive.

"All NFL players will be tested for anabolic steroids and related substances, *and* for masking agents used to try to suppress their detection, in 1989 pre-season training camps or at any later time they may report. If you are or have been taking any of the masking agents, you *must*, at the time of your pre-season training camp test, declare that fact *and* supply an appropriate written explanation from your physician; *if you do not do so, a positive result for any masking agent will be treated as positive for a banned steroid* and carry the same consequences.

A positive pre-season test this year will result in your being removed from your club's training facility, placed on Reserve/Non-Football Illness, and prohibited from any further participation with the club for a *minimum of 30 days* from the time you are advised of the test result, or until your system is shown to be clear of steroids and/or masking agents, whichever is *later*.

A positive test will also mean that you will be subject to frequent reasonable-cause testing in the future, as players who have previously tested positive already are. If you *again* test positive this year for steroids or related drugs, or for a masking agent, *you will be suspended for the rest of the season (inclusing any post-season play)*."

ALCOHOL

The League takes the position that although alcohol use is legal in society and is not, in moderate quantities, a prohibited substance under this policy, it is without question the most abused drug in our sport. If urine testing reveals an unusually high concentration of alcohol (above 40 mg/dl at the time of testing), or a player becomes involved in a case of serious misuse of alcohol, including violations of the law while intoxicated, he will be subject to reasonable-cause urine testing and the treatment procedures of this policy, in addition to whatever disciplinary action the Commissioner may deem appropriate.

Any player who tests positive for alcohol at a level below 40 mg/dl will be given specific education about the hazards of alcohol, since any amount of alcohol in the urine usually represents usage above normal social levels.

Alcohol beverages, including beer and champagne for postgame celebrations, are prohibited in NFL locker rooms. (See also the section entitled "Alcohol and Tobacco Advertising" at the end of this policy.)

TREATMENT

The central goals of the NFL's drug policy are to prevent improper drug use in our sport and, where detected, to eliminate it, preferably through medical treatment rather than discipline. Accordingly, each club in the League should continue to be affiliated with a treatment facility within that club's franchise areas.

In all cases where an NFL player must undergo drug treatment, the League's Drug Advisor will be involved on a consultative basis with the club physician. This applies whether the treatment has been directed by the Commissioner, the club, or the player has come forward on his own.

Any player who feels that he may need drug treatment or counseling about drug use is urged to contact a member of his club's medical staff, a coach, or any other person in management. Similarly, all clubs are asked to provide players with the telephone number of the NFL Drug Advisor.

---

*Reproduced with permission of Joe Browne, Director of Communications, National Football League, October 1989

EDUCATION

The NFL considers education to be an important part of its drug policy. The Drug Advisor is responsible for obtaining or developing educational materials for use by each member club, e.g., video tapes and literature on pertinent subjects. He will give consideration to recommendations by representatives of the NFL Players Association and the NFL Management Council concerning the development and utilization of particular educational materials, and he will provide copies of all educational materials to the representatives of both groups when they are completed. All club personnel, particularly head coaches, should cooperate in making sufficient time available during team meetings for any League-sponsored visual presentations and lectures. The Drug Advisor is available to speak to playing squads, coaching staffs, and any other groups within the club organization.

LABORATORY AND TESTING METHODOLOGY

The League has retained as its principal drug-testing facility SmithKline Bio-Science Laboratories, a nationwide network of clinical laboratories headquartered in Norristown, Pennsylvania. SKBL conducts the preason testing for drugs of abuse that involves entire teams at training camp. (See also the section below entitled "Reasonable-Cause and Follow-Up Testing.") SKBL technicians gather the urine samples for testing, which are then analyzed at the main lab in Norristown. In some circumstances, urine samples are obtained by personnel other than those from SKBL but under the direction of the NFL Drug Advisor and then sent to SKBL and/or another laboratory for analysis. Any subcontracting to another laboratory for analysis of certain substances, e.g., anabolic steroids, is done under the strict supervision of the Drug Advisor.

Club trainers and club physicians are not involved in the specimen-gathering process when entire teams are tested except to direct individual players to SmithKline technicians. All specimens are coded and sealed in the players' presence and receive careful chain-of-custody handling in shipping to the laboratory. Results of the tests are reported by SmithKline to the Drug Advisor, who in turn reports them to the applicable club physicians.

Specimens are analyzed by state-of-the-art technology. The following procedures are carried out to minimize any possibility of false test results:

All specimens which show the presence of a prohibited substance are tested by a second, unrelated technological method.

Any urine specimen which does not show the presence of the drug by two different technological methods will be considered a negative specimen.

Marijuana, cocaine, and alcohol urine tests are quantified to help assist in determination of whether the player may be a binge user or may be tolerant and dependent. Since marijuana is now sold in very potent forms (some varieties as much as 10 times stronger than that which was available only a few years ago), its use is considered a serious problem because it may influence playing ability, increase risks of injury, retard the healing of injuries, and may produce dependence and addiction. All players who have a positive test for marijuana but either claim passive inhalation or are shown not to be dependent are subject to reasonable-cause testing.

Cocaine in urine at any level is considered serious.

Alcohol urine levels will be quantified and considered indicative of abuse at levels of approximately 40 mg/dl.

Once drugs or alcohol are identified in urine, the Drug Advisor, in consultation with the player's club physician and, if appropriate, a drug physician locally affiliated with the club, seeks to determine whether casual use or dependence exists. Part of this evaluation includes a second urine test and a physical examination.

TESTING TIMES

Following are the times when the League conducts urine testing for the presence of drugs. *Clubs are on notice that the scheduling of and the results of all drug urine testing of players, including reasonable-cause testing, will be under the control of the NFL's Drug Advisor. There are no exceptions.*

Preseason Camp. All players participate in urine testing at or near the beginning of preseason training camp (normally in July or early August). Such testing includes all payroll players on each team, i.e., those who are on paid categories of the Reserve List as well as those on the Active List. If a player reports to his team after the entire squad has been tested, he must undergo testing at the time of reporting.

Reasonable Cause. The Drug Advisor will consult with the applicable club physician regarding the determination as to whether there is need to require a player to undergo reasonable-cause testing. It may be necessary that reasonable-cause testing take place immediately upon the determination that such testing is required, at regular intervals over a period of time that is deemed appropriate, or on an unscheduled basis (i.e., without prior notice to players) for an indefinite period. Circumstances which constitute reasonable cause include, but are not limited to, the following: current or past involvement with the criminal justice system for drug- or alcohol-related activities (including arrests for "Driving Under the Influence"), prior treatment for drug or alcohol problems, admission of a current drug or alcohol problem, prior positive test for any of the abusable drugs, physiological signs of possible impairment from drugs, or a pattern of aberrant behavior. The Drug Advisor is available to all club personnel to explain further the signs that may point to the need for reasonable-cause testing.

Scouting Combine Sessions. All draft-eligible players attending the sessions conducted by NFL scouting organizations (normally in late January or early February at a central location, followed by a smaller session exclusively for physical examinations on a date closer to the NFL college draft) participate in urine testing to check for prohibited substances. Before such tests, the players execute consent forms specifying that the results may be submitted to the NFL Drug Advisor and to each club in the League before the college draft of that year. A positive test at the scouting organizations' session is reasonable cause for the Drug Advisor to direct that any such involved player, once signed to an NFL Player Contract, participate in urine testing at any time in the future.

REASONABLE-CAUSE AND FOLLOW-UP TESTING

Beginning in 1988, all urine testing done as a follow-up to a positive preseason test or for any other reasonable purpose as defined above (see the paragraph on reasonable cause under "Testing Times"), will be conducted by the NFL Drug Advisor. He will engage a team of qualified independent collectors who will come to each NFL franchise location for gathering of specimens. The Drug Advisor will establish a testing schedule for each player subject to follow-up and reasonable-cause testing. Results of each test, which will be analyzed at the Drug Advisor's laboratory or other laboratory approved by him, will be reported to the applicable club physician.

FAILURE TO TEST

Cases of failure or refusal to participate in urine testing will be reviewed by the Drug Advisor immediately, in consultation with the involved player's club physician. Players who willfully refuse will be considered to have tested positive for a prohibited substance and are subject to appropriate disciplinary action by the Commissioner. Any club and/or individual employed by a club found to be involved in urging a player or players not to participate in urine testing and/or refusing to cooperate with the timely and orderly testing process is subject to discipline by the Commissioner.

PROCEDURES FOLLOWING POSITIVE TESTS

The Drug Advisor has been designated by all club physicians as a facility for analysis and treatment purposes and has been authorized by the club physicians to receive test results. As soon as the Drug Advisor receives notification that a particular urine specimen has tested positive for a prohibited substance, he matches the coded number from that specimen to a master list in his possession and notifies the player's club physician of the identity of the player. The master list showing the name and code number of each player must be provided to the Drug Advisor by the club. To determine the extent of his drug involvement, the player is then evaluated by the club's drug physician and possibly by an outside consultant. (Similarly, such an evaluation is made if a player tests positive under the reasonable-cause testing procedures of this policy. In that event, the same procedures detailed below apply.)

The Drug Advisor, in consultation with the club physician and others who may have evaluated the player, then decides whether the player is unfit to participate in football and should be admitted for inpatient treatment (hospitalized) or subjected to a structured program of treatment and monitoring on an outpatient basis (without hospitalization).

A player directed to inpatient treatment anytime between the opening of summer training camp and the end of his team's playing season will be removed from his team's active roster immediately and placed on Reserve/Non-Football Illness (NFI). A player directed to inpatient treatment anytime between the end of his team's playing season and the opening of the next succeeding summer training camp will not go on NFI, but his personal file maintained by the NFL Drug Advisor will appropriately record the dates and details of such inpatient treatment. Similarly, any player who has not yet been evaluated but whose system carries a concentration of a prohibited substance which, in the Drug Advisor's judgment, renders him unfit to participate in football and/or potentially dangerous to himself or others on the playing field must be placed on NFI immediately if the judgment is made anytime between the opening of summer training camp and the end of his team's playing season.

A player who is hospitalized anytime between the opening of summer training camp and the end of his team's playing season must remain on NFI for a minimum of 30 days, even if the hospitalization period is shorter than that time; although he will not be permitted to participate in games during the 30-day period, a player may return to practice sessions with his club before the 30 days have elapsed if such return is deemed advisable by the Commissioner, the NFL Drug Advisor, and the club physician. The Drug Advisor monitors the patient's progress frequently with the treatment center and the club physician. After inpatient treatment is completed and if the player has not been given special permission to return to practice before the 30 days have elapsed (see above), the Drug Advisor and the club physician then decide when the player is fit to return to NFL participation, provided such date of return is later than 30 days from the date of original hospitalization. (NOTE: Players in the category of NFI under the procedures of the NFL's drug policy—either as outpatients or inpatients—are not permitted to participate in games or practice sessions for their clubs nor otherwise use club facilities until removed from such category, i.e., added to the Active List or Inactive List. A player given special permission to return to practice only, as detailed earlier in this paragraph, must be removed from NFI and occupy a space on the Active or Inactive List. Compensation for players on NFI will be in accordance with the operative NFL Collective Bargaining Agreement.)

In addition, the Drug Advisor, in conjunction with the club physician, monitors a structured aftercare program for players who have been hospitalized, including urine testing for as long as the player remains with the club or until the Drug Advisor deems that such aftercare is no longer needed.

Players who complete the first period (Step 1) of hospitalization (a minimum of 30 days during the period from the opening of training camp to the end of the season) but subsequently test positive for a prohibited substance must at that point begin another period of a minimum of 30 days (Step 2), regardless of whether they require inpatient or outpatient treatment at that point. Step 2 will, if it occurs during the period from the opening of training camp until the end of the season, require that a player go into NFI. In either case, in-season or off-season, the dates and details of Step 2 will be appropriately recorded in the player's personal file maintained by the NFL Drug Advisor. If, after the Drug Advisor and club physician have certified that the player who has been in Step 2 may return to active participation (provided a minimum of 30 days has elapsed), the player again tests positive, he is permanently banned from future participation in the NFL.

Players who, upon their original positive test, are evaluated as not requiring hospitalization, receive counseling and education as outpatients for a period of 30 days and are subject to urine testing on a continuing and confidential basis at the discretion of the Drug Advisor and club physician. This period of 30 days as an outpatient in Step 1 under these procedures (see chart below) and the dates and details of such period will be recorded in the player's personal file maintained by the NFL Drug Advisor. Such players remain in the same roster category they were formerly in unless the club elects to make a normal player-personnel move under League rules. If, at any time after a player has completed the 30-day Step 1 as an outpatient, he tests positive, he goes into Step 2 for a minimum of another 30 days, regardless of whether he needs hospitalization at that point. If such entry into Step 2 occurs during the period from the opening of training camp to the end of the season, the player will be placed on NFI (see note in fourth paragraph of this section concerning special procedures applicable to NFI). Any further positive test after the expiration of Step 2 results in the player being permanently banned from NFL participation.

Despite the above procedures concerning Step 1 for players in outpatient treatment, if at any time during such outpatient treatment the player is deemed by his club physician and the NFL Drug Advisor to require inpatient treatment, he will immediately be subject to the procedures for inpatient cases described above.

NFL players may also enter or advance a step under the three-step progression of these procedures for reasons other than a positive test, e.g., involvement in drug- or alcohol-related criminal activity, or any hospitalization for chemical dependence.

To recap in chart form:

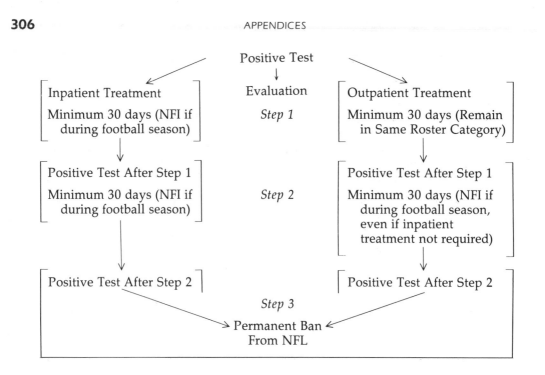

DISCIPLINE

As the above suggests, disciplinary action under this drug policy is viewed by the League as a last but sometimes necessary resort.

Any person in the League who violates this policy is subject to appropriate sanctions by the Commissioner, including fines, suspension from the League, and/or probation. Mandatory evaluation and rehabilitative treatment may also be required.

Any player disciplined under this policy has the right to appeal and a hearing before the Commissioner. If a ban is upheld, the player may apply to the Commissioner for reinstatement after one year.

Players are reminded that many of the drugs and most of the behavior concentrated on in this policy are illegal. Association with drug-related activity in a manner detrimental to the integrity of, or public confidence in, the National Football League is strictly forbidden. Moreover, involvement in the criminal justice system for a drug-related offense will be taken into account in disciplinary action imposed by the Commissioner. *Such involvement may also serve as an independent basis for Commissioner discipline, wholly outside the three-step program outlined above.* There can be no assurance that a period of judicially-imposed incarceration will obviate a subsequent period of suspension from the League.

ROSTER CHANGES BY CLUBS

Nothing in this policy prevents a club from making normal player-personnel decisions, e.g. requesting waivers on or trading a player, at any point after such player tests positive for a prohibited substance or abusable legal substance. Clubs are reminded that drug use is part of a player's health history and that such information must be included in the medical records sent to assignee clubs by assignor clubs. If a potential assignee club in a trade or waiver transaction wishes to obtain details of a player's health history from a potential assignor club, it is the responsibilty of management of the potential assignee club to direct its club physician to confer in a timely fashion with the club physician of the other involved club. A potential assignee club in these circumstances may also communicate with the Drug Advisor, through its club physician, to determine whether the involved player has any drug-use history, e.g. prior drug treatment and/or positive tests for a prohibited substance or an abusable legal substance. Any case in which an assignee club claims to have unknowingly acquired a drug-abusing player due to the assignor club concealing or misrepresenting medical records will be investigated by the Commissioner and appropriate discipline imposed if warranted.

If a player is assigned to another club in the League via trade or the waiver system, and such player has pending obligations under the procedures of this policy, he must meet those obligations with the assignee club. For example, if a player tests positive for a prohibited substance at the time of the preseason training camp, is immediately placed on waivers, and is assigned to another club before evaluation can take place, he must continue with that evaluation and all other required procedures when he reports to the assignee club.

CONFIDENTIALITY

Every effort must be made to protect the confidentiality of players under this policy, including those who test positive, undergo reasonable-cause testing, or enter treatment programs.

Neither the NFL Drug Advisor nor anyone in his employ is permitted to disclose publicly or allude publicly to any information acquired in his (or their) capacity as NFL Drug Advisor, whether or not it refers to identified players or clubs. Neither the NFL Drug Advisor nor anyone in his employ is permitted to comment publicly on the NFL Drug Advisor's (or their) activities as NFL Drug Advisor or communicate in any fashion with the news media concerning those activities.

The NFL Drug Advisor must periodically compile statistical reports on a League-wide basis regarding NFL players who have tested positive for each of the prohibited substances and abusable legal substances involved. Such statistical data must be maintained in confidence by the NFL Drug Advisor. Copies thereof must be provided by the NFL Drug Advisor in confidence only to the NFL Commissioner, the executive director of the NFL Management Council, and the executive director of the NFL Players Association.

One copy of the statistical data stamped "Confidential" must be delivered by the Drug Advisor to the Commissioner of the NFL and to the executive directors of the NFLMC and the NFLPA. No additional copies of the data are permitted to be made by any of the above-cited recipients or their agents or employees. Neither the data itself nor any information derived from the data is permitted to be publicly disclosed by any recipient or his agents or employees in any form, whether in whole or in part. Each copy of the statistical data must be maintained in a secure area. Access to the data must be restricted to those persons, employed by the recipients, who execute a pledge of non-disclosure, limited disclosure only to other signatories of the pledge under penalty of damages. Rosters of signatories must be maintained by the Drug Advisor, the NFL, the NFLMC, and the NFLPA and must be presented on request to the other parties.

Any club or club employee that publicly divulges, directly or indirectly, information concerning positive drug tests at the scouting organizations' sessions (including numerical summaries as well as specific names of persons) or otherwise breaches the confidentiality provisions of this policy is subject to a fine of up to $500,000 by the Commissioner.

REPORTING OF DRUG INCIDENTS

It is each club's responsibility to report immediately to the NFL Drug Advisor whenever the club becomes aware that a player is or is alleged to be involved in a drug- or alcohol-related incident. Incidents include, but are not limited to, involvement with the criminal justice system in drug- or alcohol-related activity, entry into drug treatment, reasonable-cause testing, and acts of violence away from the playing field. If not properly reported, such an incident could result in a player not getting necessary medical treatment. *Clubs are responsible for reporting each incident* regardless of whether it is made public or involves the criminal justice system. *Failure to do so will subject the club to disciplinary action by the Commissioner.*

MONITORING OF PRESCRIPTION DRUGS

All clubs are required to cooperate in the League's monitoring system for prescription drugs, which was established in the early 1970s. The system's intent is to guard against misuse or abuse of controlled substances (as defined by the Federal Controlled Substances Act) or performance-enhancing medications dispensed through member clubs. The data is compiled under the direction of the NFL Drug Advisor.

It is mandatory that a detailed inventory of each club's controlled substances be taken before and after the playing season and that all ordering, prescribing, and dispensing be accounted for. On-site audits of controlled substances are performed by security representatives of the League. It is also mandatory that all prescriptions of controlled substances written by club physicians be submitted to the NFL Drug Advisor on a quarterly basis. Through these procedures the League is able to verify the unit amount purchased and unit dose dispensed of all controlled substances handled. Clubs are also required to maintain all prescription drugs on site in a locked container, subject to approval by League security representatives.

Drugs which are not controlled substances but which are deemed by the NFL Drug Advisor to be abusable and/or to enhance athletic performance may also require the same inventory record-keeping and on-site audits as controlled substances. At a minimum, and unless otherwise stipulated by the NFL Drug Advisor, all non-controlled medications are to be ordered, prescribed/dispensed, and accounted for in records according to the state pharmacy laws where each individual NFL club is located.

The NFL Drug Advisor will notify the club physician if any discrepancies in controlled-substance audits or record-keeping are identified. He will advise on procedures to correct any deficiencies. Failure by clubs to properly account for controlled substances will result in appropriate disciplinary action by the Commissioner.

ALCOHOL AND TOBACCO ADVERTISING

NFL players, coaches, and other employees should not endorse or appear in advertisements for alcoholic beverages (including beer) or tobacco products.

While fully recognizing that the use of alcohol and tobacco is legal, the NFL nevertheless has long been of the view that participation in ads for such substances by its employees—particularly players, who are prohibited by federal law from appearing in such ads—may have a detrimental effect on the great number of young fans who follow our game. Endorsements or other close identification of NFL players with alcohol or tobacco could convey the erroneous impression that the use of such products is conducive to the development of athletic prowess, has contributed to their success, or at least has not hindered them in their performance.

For the above reasons, players and other club and League employees (including game officials) should not use alcohol or tobacco products while in the playing field area or while being interviewed on television.

D. Drug Policy of The National Hockey League (Letter, March 14, 1988)

(Reprinted with permission of John A. Ziegler, Jr., President, National Hockey League)

Our policy with respect to illegal drugs is quite simple. The use is forbidden. If you choose to use illegal drugs, you will be suspended. There are no exceptions. There are no excuses. To put it most bluntly, we have told our athletes they have a choice, they can pursue their careers in the NHL or they can use drugs. They may not do both.

John A. Ziegler, Jr.
President

E. United States Powerlifting Federation Drug Control Program, 1988

(Reprinted with permission of the United States Powerlifting Federation)

WHAT IS DRUG CONTROL?

- The education of athletes, coaches, administrative and medical personnel about appropriate uses of medications and the problems associated with misuse and abuse; plus
- Periodic drug-testing of athletes for banned substances to deter athletes from resorting to these substances; plus
- Support of research designed to produce effective educational and testing activities and reducing the health hazards of training and competition.

WHY DOESN'T THE USPF JUST EDUCATE INSTEAD OF DRUG TEST?

First, the USPF needs to give a clear message to athletes that its philosophy is not "to win at any price." Second, using drugs to increase performance is intrinsically unfair. Third, support of amateur sports in the U.S. by corporations and the public hinges on respectability and pride. Drug misuse clouds our message, promotes unfairness and erodes public support.

WHEN WILL I BE DRUG TESTED?

At any event so designated, presently the Senior Nationals, Women's Nationals, Natural Nationals and Regional and State Qualifying Meets, and Collegiate Nationals of the USPF, you may be subject to drug testing. All IPF World Championships, and some IPF-sanctioned regional meets, such as the Pan American Championships, are also drug tested.

If testing is planned for a competition, you will be notified when you register that testing will be conducted. You will be required to sign and return a release from liability and covenant not to sue, which should be sent to you with the meet entry form. USPF International team members, coaches, and officials will be required to sign and return a release from liability and covenant not to sue as a pre-condition to selection for the team.

FOR WHAT DRUGS WOULD I BE TESTED?

Testing is done to identify use of drugs in these major categories:

1) Anabolic steroids
2) Psychomotor stimulants

A list of banned anabolic steroids is attached as Schedule "A". A list of banned psychomotor stimulants is attached as Schedule "B". Schedule "C" provides a partial list of pharmaceutical brand names for some of these banned substances.

WHAT HARMFUL EFFECTS ARE ASSOCIATED WITH THE USE OF PSYCHOMOTOR STIMULANTS?

They give a false sense of ability, increase tolerance to pain (and thus can lead to high risk of serious injury), stimulate heart rate and raise blood pressure. This may produce an irregular heart rate and lead to heat illness, and could go as far as causing convulsions, stroke, heart attack, cardiovascular collapse, brain hemorrhage, and death.

WHY SHOULDN'T I USE STIMULANTS TO HELP ME TRAIN SO LONG AS THEY CLEAR THE SYSTEM BEFORE COMPETITION?

The stimulant effects are the same whether you are training or competing. Injuries and deaths from stimulant use occur just as frequently whenever used. Use of stimulants in competition is considered unethical and also considered "cheating."

CAN I BECOME DEPENDENT ON AMPHETAMINES AND OTHER PSYCHOMOTOR STIMULANTS?

Yes, and with regular use you may need larger doses to get the same effect.

WHAT ARE THE LONG-TERM EFFECTS OF USING STIMULANTS?

Malnutrition, skin disorders, ulcers, vitamin deficiencies, lack of sleep, weight loss, depression, brain damage, speech and thought disturbances, kidney damage, heart attacks and strokes.

DOES THE USPF OR IPF TEST FOR MARIJUANA?

No, marijuana is not generally considered a performance enhancing substance and therefore is not banned by the IOC, USPF, or IPF.

WHAT ABOUT ANABOLIC STEROIDS?

Anabolic steroids are drugs that act like testosterone, the male hormone. Natural testosterone regulates, promotes, and maintains physical and sexual development in normal males. The abuse of anabolic steroids may result in increased body hair, deepening of the voice, decreased sperm production and abnormal liver function. Many of the masculinizing changes also occur in the female and are apt to be irreversible. Their use has been implicated in the production of severe acne, increased atherosclerosis (hardening of the arteries) and heart disease, gynecomastia (bitch tits), high blood pressure, and kidney disease.

AREN'T ANABOLIC STEROIDS USED FOR SICK PEOPLE AND, IF SO, WON'T THEY BENEFIT HEALTHY PEOPLE?

Anabolic steroids promote protein synthesis. They have been used in cancer and other debilitated patients when a deficiency is present, but their use has generally been discontinued because of the potentially severe (liver and heart) side effects, associated with high dosages and prolonged usage. The only generally accepted therapeutic uses of anabolic steroids is to bring a testosterone-deficient male back to normal, to treat certain advanced cases of breast cancer, to treat a rare medical condition known as hereditary angioedema, and to stimulate the bone marrow in patients with unusual and rare anemias.

IF ANABOLIC STEROIDS BUILD MUSCLE, ISN'T THAT BENEFICIAL TO STRENGTH AND ENDURANCE?

Even though use of anabolic steroids causes weight gain and enlargement of muscle, this also leads to increased injuries like tendonitis and ruptured tendons and ligaments and, possibly, muscles as well.

THEN WHY DO SOME ATHLETES TAKE THEM?

Some athletes are convinced that anabolic steroids do increase performance and that without use of these drugs, they won't be competitive. It is irrelevant to argue that point. The key point is that even if they do work, all the other effects of these drugs must be accepted as well.

IS HUMAN AND THE NEW SYNTHETIC GROWTH HORMONE SAFE TO USE?

No. Use of the Human Growth Hormone (hGH) is also considered doping by the U.S. Olympic Committee and the International Olympic Committee. They are not presently being tested for, but probably will be in the near future.

WHAT ARE THE EFFECTS OF USING hGH?

Side effects are many and well documented. Not only does hGH cause muscle growth, but it also causes growth of other body tissues; i.e., increase in skin thickness, internal organs, bones and facial features. It also produces large, but weaker muscles than normal, and reduces the protective fat surrounding the abdominal organs. It causes the condition acromegaly, which consists of changes in the head and skull, enlargement of fingers, ears, nose, and toes; diabetes, heart disease, thyroid disease, menstrual disorders, decreased sexual desire, impotence, and shortened life span.

HOW WOULD I BE SELECTED FOR A DRUG TEST?

Every occasion for drug-testing by urinalysis at USPF-sanctioned meets has a pre-planned method for selecting athletes. *ALL* athletes who total at urinalysis-tested–national meets may be required to provide a urine sample. At most national meets, the samples of all 1st and 2nd place winners will be tested, but more may be tested, particularly if the 1st and 2nd place winners fail the drug test. At the Senior Nationals and Women's Nationals, every athlete who is apt to make the National Team, even as an alternate, is likely to be tested. Prospective Junior World Team members may also be tested.

Athletes participating in the USPF's Natural Program may be selected for polygraph testing at random, by lot, at the Natural Nationals and the Regional and State Qualifying meets. The outstanding lifters, as determined by formula, or 1st place winners may also be selected for polygraph testing.

The common feature to all urinalysis-tested and polygraph-tested meets held under USPF sanction is that a drug testing notice will explain the planned drug testing procedure. With respect to the IPF-sanctioned meets, the USPF will provide a drug testing notice setting forth as much information as the IPF releases in advance of the meet.

WHAT IS RANDOM TESTING?

"Random Testing" means that only a fraction of the athletes registered at an occasion in which drug testing is conducted will be selected and that the selection process is determined by lot. For example, at a World Championship, perhaps, one-fifth of the athletes may be selected, with the selections made in an impersonal manner which gives every registrant equal opportunity to be chosen.

WHEN SHOULD I BE NOTIFIED THAT I WILL BE TESTED?

If selected, you would customarily be notified after your event is completed, asked to report to the testing station, and then continuously observed until you report. At Natural meets, polygraph testing may be done before or after you compete.

WHAT HAPPENS AT THE TESTING STATION?

If selected for urinalysis, you will be asked to do the following:

1) Select a container for your urine sample.
2) Select a number to be used to identify your sample.
3) Tell the physician of every medication you have taken in the past few days.
4) Give a urine sample.
5) Pour your sample into two bottles, specimen "A" and specimen "B", place a seal on the mouth of each specimen bottle, observe its being crimped, place sealed and crimped bottles in a plastic bag, observe the bag being heat sealed, place the sealed bag in a locked anvil chest for shipment to the laboratory.
6) Sign a statement that the test was done properly.
7) Then you can leave.

DOES "UNDER CONSTANT SUPERVISION" MEAN THAT SOMEONE WILL BE WATCHING ME EVEN WHEN GIVING MY URINE SAMPLE?

Yes, you will be observed at *all* times. A member of your same gender will observe you while you are urinating. This protects you by assuring that the urine sample you give is indeed your own, and by assuring that the urine sample that each of your competitors gives is indeed his or her own.

HOW LONG DO I HAVE TO GIVE THE URINE SAMPLE?

As long as it takes. Beverages will be on hand to help. Alcoholic containing beverages are not allowed at the Collegiate Nationals.

WHAT HAPPENS IF MY SPECIMEN "A" TEST IS POSITIVE?

The second bottle, Specimen B, will be analyzed later, possibly with you or your representative present to check the code number, and the seal of the bottle. The finding of Specimen B is final.

The precise terms and conditions for testing Specimen "B," at USPF-sanctioned meets will be explained in a drug-testing notice that will be sent to you, along with the release from liability and covenant not to sue. This will include the cost to be borne by the athlete for testing the "B" sample—to be refunded to the lifter if the "B" sample proves to be negative. The terms and conditions for testing Specimen "B" at IPF-sanctioned meets, to the extent that the USPF is notified, will be included in the drug-testing notice that will be sent to all team members.

WHAT ABOUT MY RIGHT TO APPEAL?

Analysis of Specimen B is an automatic appeal on your behalf to be sure that the original finding was accurate. A lab technician, other than the one who analyzed specimen A, analyzes Specimen B. You have no other right of appeal at urinalysis-tested meets. At polygraph tested meets, if you dispute the test results, the meet director may, in his discretion, allow a re-test, but you will be required to sign a release that waives any legal or equitable rights to appeal the final results of the polygraph test.

HOW LONG DOES IT TAKE FOR ME TO GET BANNED SUBSTANCES OUT OF MY BODY?

The elimination time for drugs that appear on the banned list is a major factor in the testing program. There are significant biological and physiological variances between individuals. Only a broad generalization can be made in answering this question. Individual metabolism, amount of substance used, frequency of use, length of time used, and nominal biodegradation process in any given individual varies. In addition, many drugs are stored by the body and have longer elimination times. In general, the following can be used as a guideline:

Drug	Approximate Range of Elimination Times
Stimulants, i.e. amphetamines & derivatives	1 to 7 days
Anabolic steroids	
fat-soluble injectable types	6 to 18 weeks
Oral or water soluble types	3 to 6 weeks
Deca-Durabolin	6 to 14 months

WHAT IF I REFUSE TO TAKE THE TEST?

You will be disqualified. Refusal to be tested will be acted upon as if the test were positive and subject to the same penalties as a positive test.

COULDN'T I OR MY COMPETITORS USE SOMEBODY ELSE'S URINE?

No! Each athlete will be observed at all times, including while giving the sample.

AREN'T DRUGS PRESCRIBED BY MY DOCTOR OKAY TO TAKE?

Not necessarily! A banned substance is still banned even if prescribed by your doctor. All medications should be reviewed by the U.S.P.F. Medical Staff to be sure they do not contain banned substances. Your personal physician is not likely to be aware of the complicated drug restrictions in amateur sports. YOU SHOULD NOT TAKE ANY DRUG UNLESS IT HAS BEEN APPROVED BY THE U.S.P.F. TEAM PHYSICIAN!

HOW CAN I BE SAFE?

1) Don't take any medication or questionable substance prior to or at the meet that has not been approved by the U.S.P.F. Medical Staff. The sooner you can seek their advice, the better.

2) Discuss with the U.S.P.F. Medical Staff all medicines that you have taken within the past year.

3) If there is any doubt, do not take the medicine or drug.

4) Remember that medications on the banned list are not all oral medications.

WHY CAN'T I HAVE A LIST OF DRUGS THAT WON'T CAUSE A POSITIVE TEST?

No list can be complete. New names come on the market constantly. Foreign medicines may not appear on the U.S. drug reference books. The list of banned substances is subject to change. For any of these reasons, you cannot rely on a "safe list"—drugs not listed may also not be safe. However, there are medications that can be used. The following are only examples:

Mild pain (analgesics)
    Aspirin
    Tylenol
Anti-inflammatory
(arthritis, tendonitis, bursitis)
    Ibuprofen
      Advil
      Motrin
    Feldene
    Naprosyn
    Butazolidin
    Indocin
Muscle Relaxants
    Flexeril
    Soma
    Norflex
    Parafon
Antihistamines
(Sinus Medicines)
    Benadryl
    Chlor-Trimeton
    Seldane
Decongestants
    Oxymetazoline (Afrin, Sinex Long Acting Nasal Spray)
Asthma
    Aminophylline (Theophylline)
    Cromolyn
    Albuterol (aerosol form only)
    Terbutaline (aerosol form only)
Antibiotics—all
    Eye and Ear Medicines
      Topical use acceptable
Cough Medicines—Non-Narcotic
    and Dextromethorphan

Diarrhea
  Imodium
  Kaopectate
  Lomotil
  Pepto-Bismol
Laxatives—all laxatives

These are just a few examples. Experience tells us that there are no medical conditions for which a non-banned substance cannot be used in place of a banned substance.

ARE SUBSTANCES SUCH AS GAURANA, OCTACOSANOL, GINSENG, PROTEOLYTIC ENZYMES, DMSO AND ALOE VERA BANNED?

No, and generally there is no scientific evidence available to support their claims of performance enhancement or efficacy.

SO WHAT'S THE BOTTOM LINE ON DRUG TESTING? IT MAY BE YOUR DISQUALIFICATION, OR THE DISQUALIFICATION OF YOUR ENTIRE TEAM?

The decision to risk any use of drugs is to risk your health, your future, the reputation of you and your teammates, and public support of the entire powerlifting movement. Rely on your own talent, training, confidence, and determination to produce the performance level for which you are capable. Do not take or use any medications or drugs, prescriptions or otherwise, or any other health items that have not been approved by the USPF Medical Staff.

WHAT ARE THE PHYSICAL SIGNS OF DRUG USE?

It varies with the drug, i.e.:

Stimulants: dilated pupils, increased sweat, nervousness, anxiety, paranoid behavior, hand tremor, weight loss, insomnia, rapid heart rate, increased blood pressure.

Anabolic steroids: Changing moods, generally paranoid and hostile, increased sexual appetite, darkening skin, acne—face and back, patchy hair growth, enlargement of breasts and reddened nipples, lowered voice, abdominal pain, particularly right side; pain and blood on urination, atrophy of testicles, amenorrhea (loss of menstrual periods), swollen face (cushingoid or half-moon appearance), increased blood pressure.

ATHLETES RIGHT TO PRIVACY

Following USPF-sanctioned meets, all positive laboratory results will be made known, utilizing code numbers only, *not* the athlete's name, directly to the Chairman of the USPF Sports Medicine Committee, and *only* to him. The Chairman will then decode the results and provide this information to the President of the USPF, who will then be responsible for contacting the individual athlete.

The results from U.S. athletes following IPF-sanctioned meets, are made known using the athlete's names, directly to the President of the USPF, who then is responsible for contacting the individual athlete.

SCHEDULE A

BANNED ANABOLIC STEROIDS

bolasterone
boldenone
chloroxomesterone
   (dehydrochlormethyltestosterone)
clostebol
fluoxymesterone
mesterolone
methandienone
   (methandrostenolone)
methenolone

methyltestosterone
nandrolone
norethandrolone
oxandrolone
oxymesterone
oxymetholone
stanozolol
testosterone*
and related compounds

SCHEDULE B

BANNED PSYCHOMOTOR STIMULANTS

amphetamine
benzphetamine
cathine
chlorphentermine
clortermine
cocaine
diethylpropion
dextroamphetamine
dimethylamphetamine
ethylamphetamine
femcamfamine

meclofenoxate
methamphetamine
methylphenidate
norpseudoephedrine
pemoline
phendimetrazine
phenmetrazine
phentermine
pipradol
prolintane
and related compounds

SCHEDULE C (ADAPTED)

AMPHETAMINE SULFATE

Amphetamine Sulfate (Lannett)

DEXTROAMPHETAMINE SULFATE

Dextroamphetamine Sulfate
(Various)
Dexampex (Lemmon)
Dexedrine (SKF)

Ferndex (Ferndale)
Dexedrine Spansules (SKF)
Spancap No. 1 (Vortech)

METHAMPHETAMINE HCl (DESOXYEPHEDRINE HCl)

Desoxyn (Abbott)
Desoxyn Gradumets (Abbott)
Methampex (Lemmon)

---

*A testosterone/epitestosterone ratio of greater than six to one will be considered a positive test result.

AMPHETAMINE COMPLEX (RESIN COMPLEX OF AMPHETAMINE AND DEXTROAMPHETAMINE)

Biphetamine 12½ (Pennwalt)
Biphetamine 20 (Pennwalt)

AMPHETAMINE MIXTURES

Obetrol-10 (Obetrol)

PHENTERMINE HCl

Phentermine HCl (Various)
Phentrol (Vortech)
Tora (Reid-Provident)
Phentermine HCl (H.L. Moore)
Phentermine HCl (Camall)
Fastin (Beecham Labs)
Obe-Nix (Holloway)
Obephen (Mallard)
Obermine (Forest Pharm)
Obestin-30 (Ferndale)
Phentamine (Major)

Phentrol 2 (Vortech)
Unifast Unicelles (Reid-Provident)
Wilpowr (Foy Labs)
Adipex-P (Lemmon)
Dapex-37.5 (Ferndale)
Ionamin (Pennwalt)
Parmine (Parmed)
Phentrol 4 (Vortech)
Phentrol 5 (Vortech)

BENZPHETAMINE HCl

Didrex (Upjohn)

PHENMETRAZINE HCl

Preludin (Boehringer-Ingelheim)

PHENDIMETRAZINE TARTRATE

Phendimetrazine Tartrate (Various)
Adphen (Ferndale)
Bacarate (Reid-Provident)
Bontril PDM (Carnrick)
Di-Ap-Trol (Foy)
Melfiat (Reid-Provident)
Metra (Forest Pharm)
Obalan (Lannett)
Obeval (Vale)
Phenzine (Mallard)
Plegine (Ayerst)

Sprx-1 (Reid-Provident)
Statobex (Lemmon)
Statobex-G (Lemmon)
Trimstat (Laser)
Trimtabs (Mayrand)
Weightrol (Vortech)
Anorex (Dunhall)
Sprx-3 (Reid Provident)
Weh-less (Hauck)

NIKETHAMIDE

Coramine (Ciba)

DOXAPRAM HCl

Dopram (Robins)

METHYLTESTOSTERONE

Methyltestosterone
  (Various)
Android-10 (Brown)
Metandren (Ciba)
Metandren Linguets (Ciba)

Oreton Methyl (Schering)
Testred (ICN)
Virilon (Star)
Android-25 (Brown)
Android-5 (Brown)

FLUOXYMESTERONE

Fluoxymesterone (Bolar)
Halotestin (Upjohn)
Ora-Testryl (Squibb)
Fluoxymesterone (Various)
Android-F (Brown)

STANOZOLOL

Winstrol (Winthrop-Breon)

NANDROLONE PHENPROPIONATE

Nandrolone Phenpropionate
  (Various)
Androlone (Keene)
Durabolin (Organon)
Hybolin Improved (Hyrex)

Nandrobolic (Forest Pharm)
Nandrolin (Reid-Provident)
Anabolin I.M. (Alto)
Androlone 50 (Keene)

OXYMETHOLONE

Anadrol 50 (Syntex)

OXANDROLONE

Anavar (Searle)

ETHYLESTRENOL

Maxibolin (Organon)

METHANDROSTENOLONE

Methandrostenolone (Various)
Methandroid (Goldline)

NANDROLONE DECANOATE

Nandrolone Decanoate (Various)
Analone-50 (Reid-Provident)
Androlone D-50 (Keene)
Deca-Durabolin (Organon)
Hybolin Decanoate (Hyrex)
Neo-Durabolic (Hauck)

Anabolin LA 100 (Alto)
Analone-100 (Reid-Provident)
Androlone-D 100 (Keene)
Hybolin Decanoate (Hyrex)
Nandrobolic L.A. (Forest Pharm)

TESTOSTERONE (IN AQUEOUS SUSPENSION)

Testosterone Aqueous (Various)
Bay Testone-50 (Bay Pharm)
Histerone 50 (Hauck)
Testaqua (Kay)
Testoject-50 (Mayrand)

Andro 100 (O'Neal)
Android-T (Brown)
Bay Testone-100 (Bay Pharm)
Histerone 100 (Hauck)

TESTOSTERONE ENANTHATE (IN OIL)

Testosterone Enanthate (Various)
Android-T (Brown)
Everone (Hyrex)
Testate (Savage)
Testone LA 100 (Ortega)
Andro L.A. 200 (O'Neill)
Andryl 200 (Keene)

Anthatest (Kay)
Delatestryl (Squibb)
Testone LA 200 (Ortega)
Testostroval-P.A. (Reid-P)
Testrin PA (Pasadena)
Testoject-E.P. (Mayrand)

TESTOSTERONE CYPIONATE (IN OIL)

Depo-Testosterone (Upjohn)
Testosterone Cypionate (Various)
Andro-Cyp 100 (Keene)
Andronate 100 (Pasadena)
depAndro 100 (O'Neal)
Duratest-100 (Hauck)
Testoject-LA (Mayrand)

Andro-Cyp 200 (Keene)
Andronate 200 (Pasadena)
depAndro 200 (O'Neal)
Duratest-200 (Hauck)
Testa-C (Vortech)
T-lonate P.A. (Reid-P)

TESTOSTERONE PROPRIONATE (IN OIL)

Testosterone Propionate (Various)
Testex (Pasadena)
Testosterone Cypionate and Estra-
diol Cypionate (Various)
Andro/Fem (Pasadena)
De-Comberol (Schein)
depAndrogyn (Forest Pharm)
Depo-Testadiol (Upjohn)
Depotestogen (Hyrex)
Duo-Cyp (Keene)
Duratestrin (Hauck)
Monoject-LA (Mayrand)
T.E. Ionate P.A. (Reid-Provident)
Testadiate-Depo (Kay Pharm)
Test-Estra-C (Vortech)
Test-Estro Cypionates (Rugby)
Testosterone Enanthate and Estra-
diol Valerate (Various)
Andrest 90-4 (Seatrace)

Andro-Estro 90-4 (Rugby)
Androgyn L.A. (Forest Pharm)
Deladumone (Squibb)
Ditate (Savage)
Duo-Gen L.A. (Vortech)
Duoval PA (Reid-Provident)
Estra-Testrin (Pasadena)
Teev (Keene)
Testradiol 90/4 (Schein)
Valertest No. 1 (Hyrex)
Deladumone OB (Squibb)
Ditate-DS (Savage)
Valertest No. 2 (Hyrex)
Halodrin (Upjohn)
Premarin with Methyltestosterone
(Ayerst)
Estratest (Reid-Provident)
Estratest H.S. (Reid-Provident)
Tylosterone (Lilly)

F. Drug Policy of the National Association for Stock Car Auto Racing, 1988

(Reprinted with permission of the NASCAR)

PREAMBLE

Since its inception, NASCAR has endeavored to make stock car auto racing in the United States safe for competitors as well as spectators. In the interest of maintaining the safety of stock car racing, NASCAR takes seriously the prevalence of drugs in America's society and, more particularly, their threat to the safety of motorsports. The use of illegal drugs at any time, or the abuse of alcohol during a NASCAR Event, can endanger competitors, officials and fans, and such conduct cannot be permitted by NASCAR. High speed racing and drugs are not compatible. Although NASCAR's drug policy is intended to apply principally to drivers, mechanics and crew members (hereinafter "designated competitors"), as well as NASCAR officials (hereinafter "officials"), it may also be applied to other participants in a NASCAR event.

The success of NASCAR racing has been based upon the cooperation between NASCAR officials and competitors. The success of NASCAR's Substance Abuse Policy will be equally dependent upon such cooperation, and NASCAR encourages all NASCAR members to support this policy and to cooperate with NASCAR in its implementation and application.

1. DRUG ADVISOR

The Drug Advisor for NASCAR is Dr. Forest S. Tennant, Jr., M.D. He is executive director of Community Health Projects, Inc., a group of drug-treatment clinics headquartered in West Covina, California, and an associate professor at the UCLA School of Public Health. An expert in the field of drug treatment and research, Dr. Tennant also serves as a consultant to the National Football League, the California State Department of Justice, the California Highway Patrol, and the Los Angeles Dodgers baseball organization.

2. PROHIBITED ACTS AND SUBSTANCES

Designated competitors and officials are prohibited from using, possessing, purchasing, selling and/or participating in the distribution of prohibited substances, regardless of amount, at any time. Prohibited substances include, but are not limited to: marijuana, cocaine, opioids (heroin), and phencyclidine (PCP). NASCAR may, from time to time, modify its list of prohibited substances.

Illegal acquisition, distribution, and/or misuse of any legal prescription or over-the-counter drug, at anytime, are strictly prohibited.

On the day of a NASCAR Event (or at any other time when a designated competitor or official is involved in track activities), a designated competitor or official is prohibited from being under the influence of alcohol at any time prior to or during a qualifying race, a practice run, a time trial or a designated race of a NASCAR Event (or at any other time when the designated competitor or official is involved in track activities). A designated competitor or official is deemed to be under the influence of alcohol, for purposes of a NASCAR Event or other track activity, if a test reveals a breath, urine, or blood alcohol level above 40 mg per 100 ml (.04%) at the time of testing. Nothing in this paragraph shall preclude a NASCAR official from determining that a designated competitor or an official with a breath, urine, or blood alcohol test level below 40 mg per 100 ml (.04%) is physically unfit for race driving, participating, or officiating in a NASCAR event and taking such action as the official may deem appropriate under the NASCAR Rulebook.

3. URINE, BLOOD, BREATH, AND EYE TESTING FOR REASONABLE SUSPICION OF DRUG/ALCOHOL USE

NASCAR may require designated competitors or officials to submit to a urine, blood, breath and/or eye test if a NASCAR official has reasonable suspicion that the designated competitor or official (a) has used a prohibited substance at any time or (b) is under the influence of alcohol at any time on the day of a qualifying race, a practice run, a time trial or the designated race of a NASCAR Event (or at any other time when the designated competitor or official is involved in track activities). Some of the conditions, observations, and/or reports that may cause a NASCAR official to have such a reasonable suspicion are as follows:

A. When a designated competitor or official is found or observed in possession of drugs or drug paraphernalia at any time.
B. Observation of two or more of the following signs, symptoms and behaviors known to accompany repeated drug and alcohol use:
    1. Physical signs of red or droopy eyes, dilated or constricted pupils;
    2. Slurred speech, stumbling, or hyperactivity;
    3. Needle marks;
    4. Sudden, repeated disappearances from an Event;
    5. Nose constantly runs, appears red, or persistent sniffling;
    6. Time distortion, including repeated tardiness and missed appointments;
    7. Chronic forgetfulness or broken promises;
    8. Frequent accidents during Events;
    9. Inability to concentrate, remember, or maintain attention;
    10. Mental confusion or paranoia or presence of bizarre thoughts or ideas;
    11. Violent tendencies, loss of temper, or irritability;
    12. Extreme personality change or mood swings;
    13. Deteriorating personal hygiene or appearance as observed over a period of time.
C. Receipt of a specific report from any reliable source that a designated competitor or official is using, possessing or selling drugs, or is under the influence of alcohol.
D. An examination or test, as provided by the NASCAR Rulebook, which shows evidence of drug use or alcohol abuse.
E. Aroma of alcohol on breath or body.

In addition, NASCAR may require a designated competitor or official to submit to a urine, blood, breath and/or eye test following a serious accident during an Event or following an incident in which safety precautions were violated or careless acts were performed during an Event.

4. AUTHORIZATION FOR TESTING AND RELEASE

If a designated competitor or official refuses to execute the authorization for testing and release form attached to this policy, that competitor or official will not be issued a NASCAR competitor's or official's license and, if already issued, the license will be suspended until the competitor or official executes the above authorization and release. If a NASCAR official directs a designated competitor or official to submit to a urine, blood, breath and/or eye test, the competitor or official must consent to and participate in the test. If the competitor or official refuses to consent to and participate in such a test or tests, the NASCAR official may eject the competitor or official from the racing premises or take such other emergency action as may be appropriate, and the competitor or official will be subject to disciplinary action pursuant to the NASCAR Rulebook.

5. COLLECTION AND TRANSPORT OF SPECIMENS

NASCAR will designate specific NASCAR officials to be in charge of body fluid collection or eye testing and they will carry out the following procedures:

1. Insure that body fluid specimen is from the competitor or official in question.
2. Label, secure, and transport the specimen in such a manner as to insure that the sample is not misplaced or relabeled.

6. LABORATORY FOR TESTING

All testing will be done at a laboratory or laboratories selected by NASCAR, and according to testing methodology selected by NASCAR.

7. TECHNOLOGICAL ASPECTS OF TESTING

The testing laboratory will determine whether and in what amount a particular specimen tests positive with respect to a prohibited substance and/or alcohol. All positive test results will be confirmed at the laboratory by a second test before the test results are to be considered a "true positive result."

8. REVIEW AND REPORTING OF TEST RESULTS

The results of the above tests will be reviewed for accuracy by NASCAR's Drug Advisor to determine whether they are a "true positive result" or not. After this review, NASCAR's Drug Advisor will advise NASCAR of the test results.

9. PROCEDURES IF A URINE, BLOOD OR OTHER TEST SHOWS THE PRESENCE OF DRUG OR ALCOHOL

A. With respect to prohibited substances other than alcohol:
1. Upon being notified by the Drug Advisor that a designated competitor or official has tested "true positive" for a prohibited substance, NASCAR's Vice President for Competition or his designee will suspend the competitor's or official's NASCAR license for an indefinite period.
2. If the competitor or official wishes to return to racing or officiating during or after the suspension period, the competitor or official must submit to a re-test by urine and/or blood. This will be done at a time and place and under conditions specified by NASCAR at the competitor's or official's expense, which expense will include lab fees and all other direct and indirect costs incurred by NASCAR in connection with each test. If and when a competitor's or official's body fluid analysis shows no evidence of a prohib-

ited substance, the competitor or official may return to racing or officiating, assuming he is not otherwise ineligible *and* if the competitor or official is agreeable to future random urine and/or blood tests for any 'substance at such times and places as may be determined by NASCAR, at the expense of the competitor or official as described above. Such future tests need not be based upon "reasonable suspicion."

B. With respect to alcohol:

1. Upon being notified by the Drug Advisor that a competitor or official has been determined to have an alcohol content in this breath, blood or urine in excess of the alcohol level permitted under this policy, the NASCAR Vice President for Competition or his designee may suspend the competitor's or official's NASCAR license for an indefinite period and/or take such other action as he deems appropriate under the circumstances.

2. If a competitor or official wishes to return to racing or officiating during or after the suspension period, the competitor or official must agree to future random urine, blood and/or breath tests for any substances at such times and places as may be determined by NASCAR, at the expense of the competitor or official. Such future tests need not be based upon "reasonable suspicion."

10. FALSIFICATION OR WITHHOLDING INFORMATION

Any designated competitor or official who attempts to or does falsify, alter, or otherwise tamper with a urine or blood specimen, will be subject to disciplinary action by NASCAR.

11. DISCIPLINARY ACTION IN THE EVENT OF PROHIBITED ACTS WHERE THERE IS NO EVIDENCE OF OR TESTING FOR DRUG OR ALCOHOL USE

With respect to any "prohibited act" described herein, other than drug use or alcohol abuse, if a NASCAR Official determines that a designated competitor or official has engaged in any such prohibited act, the Official may eject the competitor or official from the racing premises or take such other emergency action as is appropriate, and the competitor or official will be subject to disciplinary action pursuant to the NASCAR Rulebook.

12. TREATMENT FOR DRUGS AND ALCOHOL

NASCAR does not recommend or provide specific drug or alcohol rehabilitation programs, rather NASCAR strongly encourages self-help and treatment for those afflicted with a drug problem or alcohol abuse. Many programs, both public and private, are available for quality care and treatment for drugs and alcohol, and NASCAR's Drug Advisor will provide anyone who needs help with a list of such programs. NASCAR will continue in its efforts to support a drug-free America and a society in which alcohol is not abused.

13. APPLICABILITY OF THE NASCAR RULEBOOK

This substance abuse policy is a supplement to the provisions of the NASCAR Rulebook, as it may be amended from time to time, and will be interpreted and applied by NASCAR Officials. This substance abuse policy is binding upon all NASCAR members in the same manner and to the same extent as are the provisions of the NASCAR Rulebook.

AUTHORIZATION FOR TESTING AND RELEASE

I, _____,
hereby give my consent to the National Association for Stock Car Auto Racing,
Inc. ("NASCAR") and its designated agents to collect blood and/or urine samples
from me; and to test those samples for the presence of alcohol and/or the prohibited substances set forth in NASCAR's Substance Abuse Policy; and to conduct
such other tests as NASCAR deems necessary from time to time to determine
whether or not my ability to race in, participate in, or officiate at a NASCAR Event
may be influenced by the use of drugs or alcohol; all as set forth in the NASCAR
Substance Abuse Policy as it may be amended from time to time. I have received,
read, and understand the current NASCAR Substance Abuse Policy dated January
1988.

I ALSO HEREBY RELEASE AND AGREE TO HOLD HARMLESS NASCAR,
its designated agents and any other persons or entities against whom I might have
a claim through NASCAR, for any claims, damages, loss, or expenses of any kind
arising out of NASCAR's Substance Abuse Policy, its implementation or application by NASCAR, or any other actions taken by NASCAR in connection with
the implementation or application of that policy as it may be amended from time
to time.

I have received a copy of this document.

_____   _____
(Date)   (Print Name of Designated Competitor or Official)

                                     _____
                                     (Signature)

G. Drug Policy of the International Tennis Federation, 1988

(Reprinted with Permission of the International Tennis Federation)

INTERNATIONAL TENNIS FEDERATION

The International Tennis Federation created a Medical Commission in 1985 as an IOC requirement resulting from tennis' re-appearance in the Olympic movement. Comprised of three eminent physicians, this Commission studied amongst other topics, the complexities of performance enhancing drugs related to the game of tennis.

This year, the ITF Committee of Management agreed to the Medical Commission's recommendation to invite medical representatives from both the Men's Tennis Council and the Women's International Professional Tennis Council to send their own medical experts to participate in their deliberations. The joint collaboration of all parties resulted in a special "Drug and Health Seminar" being held during the French Championships in Paris at which a variety of topics were addressed, particularly the need for tennis to discipline itself with regard to performance enhancing drugs.

Although not yet applicable to the professional tennis circuits, 141 National Tennis Associations unanimously adopted the following rules at the ITF Annual General Meeting in July 1988 to provide the much-needed direction for all other aspects of the game worldwide.

RULES OF THE INTERNATIONAL TENNIS FEDERATION DRUG (DOPE) TESTING, 1988

A. Medical Code

Players are prohibited from using any drug (dope) or doping method which is either:

  i) Illegal according to the laws of the place at which it is used; or,
  ii) Of a nature intended to enhance or stimulate training and/or performance.

The basic principle is to prevent drug misuse with the minimum of interference to the correct therapeutic use of drugs in treating medical conditions.

Any player or official who refuses to submit to a medical control or examination or who is found guilty of using any such drug or doping method is liable to exclusion from the competition concerned and may be excluded from future competitions, including the Olympic Games.

B. Doping Classes and Methods

Prohibited classes of doping shall include:

- stimulants
- narcotics
- anabolic steroids
- diuretics

Banned procedures shall include blood doping and pharmacological, chemical and physical manipulation.

Alcohol, local anaesthetics and corticosteroids are also subject to certain restrictions.

The definition of such doping classes and methods shall be as codified by the Committee of Management based on the recommendation of the ITF Medical Commission in accordance with the current medical code of the International Olympic Committee (IOC).

C. Testing

The Committee of Management may order testing on a general or random basis to be conducted in strictest confidence at any ITF approved event except those events sanctioned, recognized or governed by either the Men's Tennis Council or the Women's International Professional Tennis Council. National Associations may only order testing within their own territories providing such testing complies with the procedures referred to as herein.

The ITF Medical Commission in collaboration with the organizing committee of the event concerned shall be responsible for arrangements to conduct any drug test and shall ensure that analysis of samples takes place at a laboratory accredited for this purpose by the IOC.

Any player or official selected for a drug test shall be notified by a representative of the organizing committee who must observe him or her at all times and accompany him or her to the waiting room of the dope control station designated on the testing notification.

Testing shall then be conducted in accordance with the procedures as published by the International Olympic Committee in its booklet entitled "IOC Medical Controls".

D. Reports

The results of a test shall only be received by the Chairman of the ITF Medical Commission on a strictly confidential basis who shall report any findings on drug or doping misuse to the Committee of Management.

E. Review

The Committee of Management shall review all reports of drug or doping misuse by a player or official received from the Chairman of the ITF Medical Commission as duly verified by an IOC accredited laboratory's test, and shall conduct a thorough investigation into each case taking into account the Chairman's recommendations in assessing the nature of any offence that may have been committed against the Regulations.

Any necessary disciplinary action, including the possible suspension of the player or official concerned from competition, shall be taken by the Committee in accordance with Regulation 27 (c) of the Rules of the Federation.

F. Notices

If the Committee of Management determines misconduct under this Regulation, the National Association of the player or official concerned shall be notified in writing, specifying the details of the violation and any penalties incurred.

G. Appeals

The National Association whose player or official is charged with misconduct in connection with drug or doping misuse may request an appeal by submitting additional information for consideration by the Committee of Management and/or the ITF Medical Commission. Appeals may also be made by the individual concerned in writing.

Failure to respond to the charges within sixty (60) days of notification to the National Association concerned will be deemed as acceptance by both the National Association and the player or official concerned of the penalties imposed.

H. Drug Policy of the Men's Tennis Council, 1988

(Reproduced with permission of the Men's Tennis Council)

ARTICLE VIII. DRUG OFFENSES.

The MTC, representing the players, the International Tennis Federation ("ITF") and the MTC sanctioned tournaments and events, believes that the use of illegal drugs is inconsistent with the MTC's stated purposes.

1. *Prohibited Substances.*
   The Prohibited Substances subject to the provision of this Article are cocaine, heroin and amphetamines.

2. *Covered Persons.*
   Players, members of the MTC and its staff, members of the board and staff of the Association of Tennis Professionals, Inc. ("ATP"), MTC certified officials, the organizing committees of MTC sanctioned or recognized tournaments or events and other court officials are covered by the provisions of this Article.

3. *Prohibition.*
   Covered Persons shall not use, possess or distribute any Prohibited Substance.

4. *Penalty.*
   a. *Conviction.*
      Any Covered Person listed in Section 2 who, hereafter, pleads guilty or is convicted of a crime involving the use, possession or distribution of any Prohibited Substance shall without exception be immediately suspended and permanently disqualified from participation in or association with any MTC sanctioned or recognized tournament or event. If such person is a member of the MTC his term of office shall be terminated; if such person is a member of the staff of the MTC or ATP such employment shall be terminated. In the event of the reversal of any such conviction such suspension and disqualification shall be discontinued.
   b. *Other Procedure.*
      Any Covered Person listed in Section 2, who is found through the procedures hereinafter set forth to have used a Prohibited Substance, shall be immediately suspended and permanently disqualified from participation in or association with any MTC sanctioned or recognized tournament or event, subject to the provisions of Sections 6, 7, and 8 hereof.

5. *Independent Expert.*
   The MTC shall appoint an Independent Expert to administer on a confidential basis the provision of this Article as herein set forth. Such appointment shall be approved by the ATP Executive Director. The Independent Expert shall be a person experienced in the field of drug abuse detection and treatment. The Independent Expert shall serve until he resigns or is replaced by a successor selected in the same manner. Such Independent Expert shall be replaced at

the request of either the MTC or the ATP. The expenses and fees of the Independent Expert shall be paid by the MTC.

6. *Testing.*

The Parties agree that testing of Covered Persons may occur during each calendar year at any MTC sanctioned Grand Prix tournament as arranged by the Independent Expert.

All Main Draw Singles and Main Draw Doubles players present at such tournaments where testing is conducted shall undergo such testing procedures. All other Covered Persons present at such tournaments where testing is conducted will be subject to random testing. The time and place of the testing shall be determined by the Independent Expert with the approval of the MTC Administrator and the ATP Executive Director. All costs relating to such testing shall be paid by the MTC. The selection of the tournaments at which testing is to be conducted shall be made by the Independent Expert and shall remain confidential to all persons except those with a need to know in order to facilitate the testing procedures.

In the event that, at the completion of the testing procedures the Independent Expert determines that a positive result was produced a written report of such result shall be provided to the subject of the test promptly. Thereafter, such person shall not be subject to any penalty hereunder, provided he or she agrees to seek counseling and/or treatment from a specialist approved by the Independent Expert in the field of drug-related problems and provided he or she complies with the terms of the prescribed treatment including follow-up testing approved by the Independent Expert. All costs relating to this prescribed treatment, and any prescribed treatment hereinafter required, shall be paid by such persons.

Such person must agree that the Independent Expert shall be advised of the prescribed treatment, the progress throughout the same and the results of all tests for Prohibited Substances.

In the event that such person fails or refuses to comply with the terms of this Section, then the Independent Expert shall certify to the MTC Administrator that such Covered Person has:

(1) Refused to submit to the procedures; or
(2) Refused or failed to comply with the terms of the approved treatment.

Upon such certification the MTC Administrator shall impose the penalty set forth in Section 4b.

7. *Second Treatment.*

Notwithstanding anything to the contrary herein contained, if a person who has completed the treatment authorized above in lieu of the Penalty is again found to have used or admits to the use of a Prohibited Substance, then he or she shall not be subject to any penalty provided he or she completes a second treatment; if after a second treatment such person is again found to have used a Prohibited Substance, then he or she shall be penalized as set forth in section 4b.

Such person must agree that the Independent Expert shall be advised of the prescribed treatment, the progress throughout the same and the results of all tests for Prohibited Substances.

In the event that such person fails or refuses to comply with the terms of this Section then the Independent Expert shall certify the MTC Administrator that such Covered Person has:

(1) Refused to submit to the testing procedures; or

(2) Refused or failed to comply with the terms of the approved treatment; or
(3) Been found in violation of this Article for the third time.

Upon such certification the MTC Administrator shall impose the penalty set forth in Section 4b.

8. *Voluntary Action.*
Any Covered Person who comes forward and voluntarily notifies the Independent Expert that he or she has a problem involving the use of drugs will not be subject to any penalty hereunder, provided he or she agrees to seek treatment from a specialist approved by the Independent Expert in the field of drug related problems and provided he or she complies with the terms of such prescribed treatment as approved by the Independent Expert.

Such person must agree that the Independent Expert shall be advised of the prescribed treatment, the progress throughout the same and the results of all tests for Prohibited Substances. Notwithstanding anything to the contrary herein contained, if a person who has completed his or her first treatment under the provisions of this section produces a second positive result at any time, then he or she shall not be subject to any penalty hereunder, provided he or she completes a Second Treatment subject to the same terms and conditions as with the First Treatment.

In the event that such person fails or refused to comply with the terms of this Section then the Independent Expert shall certify to the MTC Administrator that such Covered Person has:

(1) Refused to submit to the testing procedures; or
(2) Refused or failed to comply with the terms of the approved treatment; or
(3) Been found in violation of this Article for the third time.

Upon such certification the MTC Administrator shall impose the penalty set forth in Section 4b.

9. *Limitation on Other Testing.*
Except as expressly provided in this Article, there shall be no other screening or testing for a Prohibited Substance and no Covered Person shall be required to undergo any other such screening or testing.

10. *Application for Reinstatement.*
Notwithstanding anything hereinabove set forth to the contrary, after a period of at least one (1) year from the time of permanent disqualification, any person may apply to the MTC for reinstatement. However, such person shall have no right to reinstatement under any circumstance and the reinstatement shall be granted only upon the approval of the MTC upon the affirmative vote of at least six (6) members of the MTC. The approval of the MTC shall rest in its absolute and sole discretion, and its decision thereon shall be final, binding and unappealable. With respect to Covered Persons who are not players but are members of the staff of the MTC or the ATP, such person may be reinstated at the discretion of the employer if at such time his or her prior position is vacant and available.

Among the factors which may be considered by the MTC in determining whether to grant reinstatement are the circumstances surrounding the person's permanent disqualification and whether such person has satisfactorily completed a treatment and rehabilitation program.

The granting of an application for reinstatement may be conditioned upon periodic testing of such person or such other terms as may be determined by the MTC.

11. *Confidentiality.*
a. The Independent Expert shall maintain in strict confidentiality the results

of all testing, the identities of any persons involved in proceedings under this Article, and any information disclosed to or received by the Independent Expert from any source regarding the use, possession or distribution of a prohibited substance by a Covered Person until he has certified to the MTC Administrator that the Covered Person has:

i) refused to submit to the testing procedures as authorized by this Article; or

ii) refused or failed to comply with the terms of the prescribed treatment approved by the Independent Expert; or

iii) been found in violation of this Article for the third time.

b. Upon receipt of certification, the members of the MTC, the Administrator, the ATP Executive Director and the Independent Expert shall maintain strict confidentiality until such time as the earlier of one or all of the following events occurs:

i) the Covered Person involved in proceeding under this Article VIII is suspended and permanently disqualified in accordance with the provisions of Section 4 above; or

ii) such person expressly permits in writing the disclosure of any and all information as it relates to his or her involvement in these proceedings; or

iii) disclosure of any or all of the information is compelled by order of a court of competent jurisdiction.

12. *Appointment of Independent Expert.*
The name and address of the Independent Expert duly appointed pursuant to this Article is available upon request through the offices of ATP or MTC.

13. *Testing Procedures.*
The Testing Procedures to be used as above provided shall be urinalysis, subject to such scientifically accepted techniques as specified by the Independent Expert and approved by the MTC Administrator and the Executive Director of ATP.

14. *Agreement.*
Any player, professional or amateur, who commits to enter or participate in any MTC sanctioned or recognized tournament or event, shall as a condition of such commitment, entry or participation be required to and shall be deemed to agree to the provisions of this Article and agree to release and waive any and all claims he may have against the Independent Expert, the MTC, the ITF, the ATP, the MTC Administrator, ATP Executive Director and the members, officers, directors, and employees of the MTC, ITF and ATP, arising out of or in connection with the testing procedures or the imposition of any penalties set forth in this Article.

Members of the MTC and its staff, members of the ATP staff, MTC certified officials, and representatives of MTC sanctioned or recognized tournaments or events and their staffs shall as a condition of such membership, employment, sanction, recognition or otherwise be required to and shall be deemed to agree to the provisions of this Article and that the provisions of said Article shall be deemed to be part of any existing contract of employment, whether such contract is oral, or implied by law and agrees to release and waive any and all claims they may have against the MTC, the ITF, and ATP, the MTC Administrator, ATP Executive Director and the members, officers, directors and employees of the MTC, ITF, and ATP, arising out of or in connection with the testing procedures or the imposition of any penalties set forth in this Article.

15. *Effective Date and Notice.*
    The effective date of this Article shall be January 1, 1986 and the MTC shall cause notice thereof to be publicized so as to provide satisfactory notice to all persons participating in or associated with MTC sanctioned or recognized tournaments and events.

Index

A page number in *italics* indicates a figure. A "*t*" following a page number indicates a table.